1992
YEAR BOOK OF
SPORTS MEDICINE®

The 1992 Year Book® Series

Year Book of Anesthesia and Pain Management: Drs. Miller, Abram, Kirby, Ostheimer, Roizen, and Stoelting

Year Book of Cardiology®: Drs. Schlant, Collins, Engle, Frye, Kaplan, and O'Rourke

Year Book of Critical Care Medicine®: Drs. Rogers and Parrillo

Year Book of Dentistry®: Drs. Meskin, Currier, Kennedy, Leinfelder, Matukas, and Rovin

Year Book of Dermatologic Surgery: Drs. Swanson, Salasche, and Glogau

Year Book of Dermatology®: Drs. Sober and Fitzpatrick

Year Book of Diagnostic Radiology®: Drs. Federle, Clark, Gross, Madewell, Maynard, Sackett, and Young

Year Book of Digestive Diseases®: Drs. Greenberger and Moody

Year Book of Drug Therapy®: Drs. Lasagna and Weintraub

Year Book of Emergency Medicine®: Drs. Wagner, Burdick, Davidson, Roberts, and Spivey

Year Book of Endocrinology®: Drs. Bagdade, Braverman, Horton, Kannan, Landsberg, Molitch, Morley, Odell, Rogol, Ryan, and Sherwin

Year Book of Family Practice®: Drs. Berg, Bowman, Davidson, Dietrich, and Scherger

Year Book of Geriatrics and Gerontology®: Drs. Beck, Abrass, Burton, Cummings, Makinodan, and Small

Year Book of Hand Surgery®: Drs. Amadio and Hentz

Year Book of Health Care Management: Drs. Heyssel, Brock, King, and Steinberg, Ms. Avakian, and Messrs. Berman, Kues, and Rosenberg

Year Book of Hematology®: Drs. Spivak, Bell, Ness, Quesenberry, and Wiernik

Year Book of Infectious Diseases®: Drs. Wolff, Barza, Keusch, Klempner, and Snydman

Year Book of Infertility: Drs. Mishell, Paulsen, and Lobo

Year Book of Medicine®: Drs. Rogers, Bone, Cline, Braunwald, Greenberger, Utiger, Epstein, and Malawista

Year Book of Neonatal and Perinatal Medicine®: Drs. Klaus and Fanaroff

Year Book of Nephrology: Drs. Coe, Favus, Henderson, Kashgarian, Luke, Myers, and Strom

Year Book of Neurology and Neurosurgery®: Drs. Currier and Crowell

Year Book of Neuroradiology: Drs. Osborn, Harnsberger, Halbach, and Grossman

Year Book of Nuclear Medicine®: Drs. Hoffer, Gore, Gottschalk, Sostman, Zaret, and Zubal

Year Book of Obstetrics and Gynecology®: Drs. Mishell, Kirschbaum, and Morrow

Year Book of Occupational and Environmental Medicine: Drs. Emmett, Brooks, Harris and Schenker

Year Book of Oncology®: Drs. Young, Longo, Ozols, Simone, Steele, and Weichselbaum

Year Book of Ophthalmology®: Drs. Laibson, Adams, Augsburger, Benson, Cohen, Eagle, Flanagan, Nelson, Reinecke, Sergott, and Wilson

Year Book of Orthopedics®: Drs. Sledge, Poss, Cofield, Frymoyer, Griffin, Hansen, Johnson, Simmons, and Springfield

Year Book of Otolaryngology-Head and Neck Surgery®: Drs. Bailey and Paparella

Year Book of Pathology and Clinical Pathology®: Drs. Gardner, Bennett, Cousar, Garvin, and Worsham

Year Book of Pediatrics®: Dr. Stockman

Year Book of Plastic, Reconstructive, and Aesthetic Surgery: Drs. Miller, Cohen, McKinney, Robson, Ruberg, and Whitaker

Year Book of Podiatric Medicine and Surgery®: Dr. Kominsky

Year Book of Psychiatry and Applied Mental Health®: Drs. Talbott, Frances, Freedman, Meltzer, Perry, Schowalter, and Yudofsky

Year Book of Pulmonary Disease®: Drs. Bone and Petty

Year Book of Sports Medicine®: Drs. Shephard, Eichner, Sutton, and Torg, Col. Anderson, and Mr. George

Year Book of Surgery®: Drs. Schwartz, Jonasson, Robson, Shires, Spencer, and Thompson

Year Book of Transplantation: Drs. Ascher, Hansen, and Strom

Year Book of Ultrasound: Drs. Merritt, Mittelstaedt, Carroll, and Nyberg

Year Book of Urology®: Drs. Gillenwater and Howards

Year Book of Vascular Surgery®: Dr. Bergan

Roundsmanship® '92-'93: A Student's Survival Guide to Clinical Medicine Using Current Literature: Drs. Dan, Feigin, Quilligan, Schrock, Stein, and Talbott

1992

The Year Book of SPORTS MEDICINE®

Editor-in-Chief
Roy J. Shephard, M.D., Ph.D., D.P.E.
Director, School of Physical and Health Education, and Professor of Applied Physiology, Department of Preventive Medicine and Biostatistics, University of Toronto

Editors
Col. James L. Anderson, PE.D.
Director of Physical Education, United States Military Academy, West Point
Edward R. Eichner, M.D.
Professor of Medicine, University of Oklahoma Health Sciences Center, Oklahoma City
Francis J. George, A.T.C., P.T.
Head Athletic Trainer, Brown University, Providence
John R. Sutton, M.D.
Head: Biological Sciences, Faculty of Health Sciences; Professor of Medicine and Exercise Physiology, University of Sydney
Joseph S. Torg, M.D.
Professor of Orthopedic Surgery, and Director, Sports Medicine Center, University of Pennsylvania School of Medicine, Philadelphia

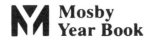

**Mosby
Year Book**

St. Louis   Baltimore   Boston   Chicago   London   Philadelphia   Sydney   Toronto

Editor-in-Chief, Year Book Publishing: Kenneth H. Killion
Sponsoring Editor: Bernadette Buchholz
Manager, Literature Services: Edith M. Podrazik
Senior Information Specialist: Terri Santo
Senior Medical Writer: David A. Cramer, M.D.
Assistant Director, Manuscript Services: Frances M. Perveiler
Associate Managing Editor, Year Book Editing Services: Connie Murray
Editorial Intern, Year Book Editing Services: David J. Lance
Senior Production/Desktop Publishing Manager: Max F. Perez
Proofroom Manager: Barbara M. Kelly

Mosby-Year Book, Inc.
11830 Westline Industrial Drive
St. Louis, MO 63146

Editorial Office:
Mosby-Year Book, Inc.
200 North LaSalle St.
Chicago, IL 60601

International Standard Serial Number: 0162-0908
International Standard Book Number: 0-8151-7702-X

Table of Contents

Journals Represented

Mosby–Year Book subscribes to and surveys nearly 900 U.S. and foreign medical and allied health journals. From these journals, the Editors select the articles to be abstracted. Journals represented in this YEAR BOOK are listed below.

Acta Orthopaedica Scandinavica
Acta Paediatrica Scandinavica
Acta Physiologica Scandinavica
American Heart Journal
American Journal of Cardiology
American Journal of Diseases of Children
American Journal of Epidemiology
American Journal of Gastroenterology
American Journal of Hypertension
American Journal of Physiology
American Journal of Public Health
American Journal of Roentgenology
American Journal of Sports Medicine
American Review of Respiratory Disease
American Surgeon
Anesthesia and Analgesia
Annals of Internal Medicine
Archives of Internal Medicine
Archives of Ophthalmology
Archives of Orthopaedic and Trauma Surgery
Archives of Physical Medicine and Rehabilitation
Arthroscopy
Athletic Training
Australian Journal of Science and Medicine in Sport
Australian and New Zealand Journal of Medicine
Australian and New Zealand Journal of Obstetrics & Gynecology
Blood
Bone and Mineral
British Heart Journal
British Journal of Dermatology
British Journal of Sports Medicine
Canadian Journal of Sport Sciences
Canadian Journal of Surgery
Canadian Medical Association Journal
Cardiology
Chest
Circulation
Clinical Orthopaedics and Related Research
Clinical Science
Clinical Sports Medicine
Complications in Orthopedics
Contemporary Orthopaedics
Critical Care Medicine
Digestive Diseases and Sciences
European Heart Journal
European Journal of Applied Physiology and Occupational Physiology
European Journal of Cancer
European Journal of Clinical Investigation
European Journal of Obstetrics, Gynecology and Reproductive Biology
Fertility and Sterility

Foot and Ankle
IEEE Transactions on Biomedical Engineering
Injury
International Journal of Nursing Studies
International Journal of Sports Medicine
Journal of Adolescent Health
Journal of Allergy and Clinical Immunology
Journal of Applied Physiology
Journal of Biomechanics
Journal of Bone and Joint Surgery (American Volume)
Journal of Bone and Joint Surgery (British Volume)
Journal of Cardiopulmonary Rehabilitation
Journal of Clinical Endocrinology and Metabolism
Journal of Computer Assisted Tomography
Journal of Foot Surgery
Journal of Gerontology
Journal of Hypertension
Journal of Long-Term Effects of Medical Implants
Journal of Musculoskeletal Medicine
Journal of Neurology, Neurosurgery and Psychiatry
Journal of Orthopaedic Research
Journal of Orthopaedic Trauma
Journal of Orthopaedic and Sports Physical Therapy
Journal of Pediatric Orthopedics
Journal of Sports Medicine and Physical Fitness
Journal of Sports Sciences
Journal of the American College of Cardiology
Journal of the American Medical Association
Journal of the National Cancer Institute
Lancet
Magnetic Resonance Imaging
Medical and Biological Engineering and Computing
Medicine
Medicine and Science in Sports and Exercise
Metabolism
Nephron
New England Journal of Medicine
Orthopaedic Review
Orthopedics
Pediatrics
Physical Therapy
Physician and Sportsmedicine
Plastic and Reconstructive Surgery
Proceedings of the National Academy of Sciences
Radiology
Research Quarterly for Exercise and Sport
S.A.M.J./S.A.M.T.—South African Medical Journal
Skeletal Radiology
Spine
Sports Medicine
Thorax
Thrombosis and Haemostatis

STANDARD ABBREVIATIONS

The following terms are abbreviated in this edition: acquired immunodeficiency syndrome (AIDS), the central nervous system (CNS), cerebrospinal fluid (CSF), computed tomography (CT), electrocardiography (ECG), human immunodeficiency virus (HIV), and magnetic resonance (MR) imaging (MRI).

Publisher's Preface

As Publishers, we feel challenged to seek ways of presenting complex information in a clear and readable manner. To this end the 1992 YEAR BOOK OF SPORTS MEDICINE now provides structured abstracts in which the various components of a study can easily be identified through headings. These headings are not the same in all abstracts, but rather are those that most accurately designate the content of each particular journal article. We are confident that our readers will find the information contained in our abstracts to be more accessible than ever before. We welcome your comments.

Introduction

The YEAR BOOK OF SPORTS MEDICINE takes a different and somewhat more standardized format this year. Each article is discussed in terms of the major headings that are being adopted by an increasing number of the leading scientific journals. It is hoped that the change will allow for a faster perusal of the articles and will allow readers to make a clearer judgment of the quality of the research described.

As usual, the 350 abstracts cover a broad and exciting range of "hot points" in sports medicine. The continued increase in participation by women in a variety of sports and active pursuits is mirrored by 31 articles covering topics that range from differences of trainability between men and women and menstrual disturbances to exercise during pregnancy and lactation, and lacerations of the vagina in water sports. In terms of environmental factors, concern is expressed about the impact of an ever-growing number of air pollutants on the urban exerciser. The problems of thermal stress that once affected the players of North American football are now surfacing in soccer as this game becomes more popular in North America. Our knowledge of methods to control obesity through appropriate combinations of exercise and dieting is becoming steadily clearer, and it is now recognized that we must take into account not only the energy expenditure added by an exercise program, but also the impact of exercise and dietary restriction upon resting metabolism.

Those interested in cardiac disease are finding that prevention is more closely associated with moderate than with intense physical activity. The extensive investigation of Shaper and colleagues illustrates what can be learned from a careful review of general practice, and it highlights the lessening of benefit that can be associated with prescribing too intensive an exercise program. Debate continues on the possible adverse myocardial effect of participation in very prolonged competitions such as ultramarathons and triathlons, and further papers on this topic are presented in this edition of the YEAR BOOK. Several papers take differing perspectives on the value of exercise in the treatment of mild hypertension, and one article makes the interesting point that whereas daytime pressures are reduced by regular physical activity, nighttime values are not. Two other articles discuss the possible diagnostic role of an excessive blood pressure response to exercise. Further articles continue to support the overall contribution of muscle strengthening exercises to rehabilitation after myocardial infarction, although one paper specifically debunks the idea that muscle training in itself is likely to improve the serum lipid profile.

Other medical diseases are well represented in the YEAR BOOK. The place of sustained moderate exercise in the prevention of colon cancer is gaining increasing acceptance, and Paffenbarger and associates contribute a valuable analysis of their prospective data on Harvard alumni supporting this hypothesis. The same authors also use the Harvard alumni database to demonstrate the value of exercise in the prevention of non–

insulin-dependent diabetes mellitus. Unfortunately, many developing societies are becoming progressively less active, with a resulting increase in the incidence of the "diseases of civilization," such as diabetes mellitus. An example of this trend is presented from the island of Mauritius. The wide potential range of benefits from an exercise program is illustrated by a paper that suggests a reduction of intraoccular pressures, and another that examines the place of exercise in the treatment of osteoarthritis.

Unfortunately, a substantial number of papers still comment on problems associated with doping. One interesting paper from Finland looks at the possible contribution of a high inherited hemoglobin level to the performance of a family of cross country skiers. Another paper, less happily, looks at the potential of masking the use of anabolic steroids by using a biologically appropriate balance of testosterone and episterone. The growing interest in exercise pharmacokinetics is represented by a paper on digoxin; exercise lowers the effective dose of this drug by increasing its binding to skeletal muscle.

In terms of injuries, sports clinics are showing a timely and growing interest in epidemiology and prevention, with reports shifting from the traditional sources of injury to some of the newer hazards such as hang gliding and snow boarding. Nevertheless, there continues to be an enormous number of reports on the treatment and rehabilitation of knee injuries, and a substantial section of the volume reviews some of the better examples of this work. It is also discouraging to read that the number of cervical spine injuries in games such as football has increased over the last few years. In ice hockey, also, the compulsory use of helmets now seems to be increasing the incidence of cervical injuries. Plainly, the sports physician must be ever vigilant to ensure that measures, theoretically sound, are in fact improving the safety of sport.

The overall quality of the research described in this volume offers vivid testimony to both the current breadth of sports medicine and the growing maturity of the discipline. It has been a stimulating task editing this collection, and I trust that you will find it equally stimulating reading.

Roy J. Shephard, M.D., Ph.D., D.P.E.

Exercise Addiction: A Dangerous Euphoria?

ROY J. SHEPHARD, M.D., PH.D., D.P.E.

School of Physical and Health Education, Department of Preventive Medicine and Biostatistics, Faculty of Medicine, University of Toronto

Introduction

A number of reports have suggested that habitual exercisers can become addicted to their physical activity program. In general, this has been regarded as a harmless medical curiosity, or a phenomenon helping compliance with an exercise prescription. In this article, the reality of the phenomenon will be discussed in relation to the intensity of physical activity that is undertaken, and the possible contribution of such an addiction to unpleasant sequelae will be examined, especially as it relates to accidents involving collisions between vehicles and joggers. Issues to be reviewed include information on the overall incidence of jogging injuries caused by collisions with motor vehicles, the potential for a prolonged bout of jogging to create a sense of invincibility where no allowance is made for the possible mistakes of other road users, and any possible lessons for the prevention of exercise-related injuries.

Exercise Euphoria and Beta-Endorphins

OPIATES AND BETA-ENDORPHINS

The pleasant sense of euphoria induced by opiates has been recognized by both physicians and addicts for many centuries. In his "Ode to the Nightingale," John Keats (a former physician at Guy's Hospital who died an early death thought to be related to opiate addiction) wrote (one presumes from personal experience):

> "My heart aches, and a drowsy numbness pains
> My sense, as though of hemlock I had drunk,
> Or emptied some dull opiate to the drains
> One minute past, and lethe-wards had sunk."

Neurophysiologists and neuropharmacologists remained puzzled about why the brain contained opiate receptors and could respond to morphine and its analogues in this fashion, until Hughes et al. (1) isolated 2 simple morphine-like compounds, the penta-peptides methionine enkephalin and leucine enkephalin, from the nerve terminals of pig brain. Hughes et al. (1) suggested that the enkephalins that they had identified were involved in the integration of sensory data, particularly information relating to pain.

One year later, Roger Guillemin (2) isolated longer-chained peptides, the endorphins, from the intermediate lobe of the pituitary gland. Equimolar concentrations of these compounds had approximately the same effectiveness as morphine in modifying sensory perceptions. When the endorphins were injected into the brain, animals became insensitive to pain for several hours; their body temperatures also dropped, and they adopted a stuporose, relaxed posture. Such effects could be reversed by adequate doses of naloxone, a morphine antagonist. It was thus suggested that the endorphins played an important role in regulating emotional responses. Exercise physiologists also speculated that such compounds might play a role in thermoregulation. In apparent confirmation of the first of these hypotheses, it was quickly noted that mental depression was associated with unusually low levels of enkephalin (3, 4).

EXERCISE AND ENDORPHIN SECRETION

It was soon discovered that exercise stimulated the secretion of endorphins by the pituitary gland (5–13), and that this response was enhanced by training (6, 14). Although enhanced secretion was first noted in response to endurance activities such as prolonged jogging or running, more recent research (reference 15 supports this; reference 16 does not) has shown that both weight-lifting and isometric exercise can also increase plasma endorphin levels. Peak exercise readings are 3–4 times baseline, and plasma endorphin concentrations may remain elevated for up to 45 minutes after endurance exercise. We may infer that such changes are transmitted across the blood-brain barrier, because morphine receptor sites in the brain show a reduced ability to bind substances such as the metenkephalins during and immediately after exercise.

The intensity of exercise needed to influence endorphin secretion is still vigorously debated. Some authors have reported a similar endorphin response in moderate and intensive activity (9), while others have claimed that the exercise intensity must reach 80%–90% of peak aerobic power for a significant increase of blood endorphin levels to occur (17–20). If the bout of physical activity is very prolonged, there may be a secondary decrease of plasma endorphin levels as exercise continues (21).

ENDORPHIN LEVELS AND MOOD STATE

Parallels were quickly noted between the "runner's high" and the euphoria that results from the ingestion or injection of opiates (22, 23). The possibility of an endorphin-mediated exercise addiction was first raised by Glasser (24). In a book entitled *Positive Addiction* he gave a graphic account of the sense of the loss of one's self, floating, euphoria, and a total integration with the act of running that occurs in the distance competitor.

ADDICTION TO ENDORPHINS

Given that morphine-like compounds are produced in the runner, and that morphine-like changes of mood-state are induced by prolonged exercise, can participants develop a biochemical addiction to running? In support of such a possibility, Baekeland (25) made the remarkable observation that some long-distance runners, like morphine addicts, pursued a relentless quest for opiates; because of this quest, they could not be persuaded to stop exercising for any amount of money.

Other authorities have supported the concept of an endorphin-related exercise addiction (26–30), drawing parallels between exercise-induced euphoria and the increased brain levels of endorphin that are found as a result of acupuncture, another procedure reducing sensitivity to pain (31, 32).

The phenomenon of endorphin addiction does not seem peculiar to human exercisers. Christie et al. (33) commented on behavioral symptoms similar to morphine withdrawal when animals that had been swimming regularly were deprived of this stimulus.

In susceptible individuals, addiction can develop over as little as 2 months of regular physical activity (34). As with direct chemical addictions, diagnosis of a physical addiction is based mainly on the presence of withdrawal symptoms, including anxiety, restlessness, guilt, irritability, tension, bloatedness, muscle twitching, and discomfort. The exercise addict may develop such symptoms if the accustomed dose of physical activity is witheld for as little as 24–36 hours (35).

The addiction may become sufficiently severe as to have negative medical and social consequences; the affected person may continue to run despite a serious injury, or they may neglect the responsibilities of work, home, and family (28). Other symptoms of addiction include "decreased ability to concentrate, lapses in judgment . . . exercise has moved to a controlling factor, eliminating other choices in life . . . the negative addict has progressed to the point where activity controls the person . . ." (34). Mandell (36) tells how "Legs and arms become light and rhythmic . . . . The fatigue goes away and feelings of power begin . . . my body, swimming, detaches from the earth . . . . A loving contentment invades the basement of my mind, and thoughts bubble up without trails . . . . After the run I can't use my mind. . . ."

Lawrence (37) cautions further that running "may create a reckless state, and the athlete should be warned not to view himself as invincible while so intoxicated." Kostrubala (38) also suggests that "endurance athletes are subject to delusions of extreme capabilities and invincibility." Whereas interactions with traffic are one danger to those who have delusions of invincibility, such a mood change would also have a potential to increase the risk of injury in almost every other type of sport.

PREVALENCE OF EXERCISE ADDICTION.

Inevitably, it is difficult to draw any clear distinction between the committed exerciser and the addict, so that the precise prevalence of exercise addiction remains uncertain. The type of individual who is particularly susceptible to a jogging addiction may be a person who is also prone to affective disorders such as depression (39), or someone with a history of other addictions such as alcohol. Such individuals may use running as a means of counteracting their depression.

WEAKNESSES IN THE ENDORPHIN HYPOTHESIS

Whereas most authors are agreed that an addiction to jogging can develop, some investigators have disputed that the endorphins are responsible. As alternative explanations, they suggest a psychological addiction to exercise, or an exercise-stimulated secretion of other chemicals in the brain, such as the monoamines involved in the transmission of nerve impulses (37, 39–44).

At the present time, there are certainly at least 2 weaknesses in the endorphin hypothesis (45). First, the technique normally used to measure β-endorphins (immunoreactivity) measures plasma levels, but it is not certain how freely the endorphins that are measured can penetrate the blood-brain barrier (32, 46, 47). Given the existence of receptors within the brain, endorphins must plainly reach the CNS to induce either a mood-altering or an addictive effect. McArthur (48) has argued for a concomitant increase of plasma and brain levels during exercise, and Barta and Yashpal (49) and Blake et al. (50) have demonstrated increased brain concentrations of endorphins when rats exercise, however, it remains unclear whether the commonly measured plasma concentrations provide a good marker of changes in brain endorphin concentrations.

A second problem is that administration of the morphine antagonist naloxone does not always inhibit the positive mood changes associated with exercise (52), as one might expect it to do if the endorphins were responsible for the euphoria. The failure to inhibit positive changes of mood could reflect no more than an inappropriate choice of naloxone dosage, because the dose used in the negative experiments was only 2 mg (52), less than in other studies where endorphin inhibition was achieved. Alternatively, it could reflect a differential distribution of endorphins within the body, so that the available naloxone reacted at sites other than the brain.

SOME POSITIVE FINDINGS

Despite significant technical problems in "proving" the endorphin hypothesis, at least one group of investigators has succeeded in demonstrating a significant correlation between plasma levels of endorphin and the lightening of mood induced by vigorous exercise (reference 53 supports this; references 9 and 13 do not).

Haier et al. (53) further noted that the exercise need not be particularly severe for a response to occur; a modest 1.6-km run at a self-selected pace was suffient to lengthen the time to the reporting of pain when a weight was placed on the fingers, and this analgesic effect of physical activity was blocked by an effective dose of the morphine antagonist naloxone (a 10-mg dose, but not the 2-mg dose that others had found ineffective). Dale et al. (54) commented further that runners who consistently stressed themselves to the point of collapse showed high levels of β-endorphins, although this observation could be related to a rise of core temperature as much as to the apparent immunity of such individuals to discomfort.

The Risks of Injury From Vehicles While Jogging

GENERAL CONSIDERATIONS

A casual review of recent issues of the YEAR BOOK OF SPORTS MEDICINE will show that there has been a steady output of research on overuse injuries in jogging and running. Many popular handbooks of aerobics and jogging (55–57), standard texts of sports medicine (58), and research studies of participants in distance-running events (59–68) provide detailed accounts of musculoskeletal injuries. It is arguable that many of these injuries are in themselves an expression of endorphin-mediated depression of warning symptoms of fatigue. Surprisingly, however, available reports make little or no mention of the potential hazard of accidents involving collision with motor vehicles.

PREVALENCE OF VEHICLE-RELATED INJURIES

A substantial proportion of the injuries sustained by joggers apparently arise from accidents involving motor vehicles (69–73).

Unfortunately, the precise risk remains poorly defined. A letter to the *American Heart Journal* claimed that in the United States, 8,300 incidents per year involved collisions between vehicles and runners or joggers (74). This item was noted by the *Medical Letter* (75), which added as a possible speculative explanation that long-distance athletes develop an "exhilarating sense of invincibility against all-comers, including vehicles."

Critics of the letter have claimed that the number of injuries cited by Burch (74) reflects the annual incidence of all pedestrian accidents in the United States (76), but as will be shown below, this is not the case. Williams et al. (76) based their criticism of Burch's letter on a survey of national newsclippings; this approach uncovered only 30 deaths and 35 injuries in joggers in the United States over a single year. However, reliance on the vigilance of the newsclipper seems likely to have underestimated the true risk incurred by the jogger. Nonfatal injuries, which typically far outnumber fatalities, are unlikely to be accorded space in major newspapers.

Koplan et al. (70) questioned participants in the 10-km Peachtree Roadrace. Their survey was unfortunately marred by uncertainty about the proportion of race participants who responded to the questionnaire, but it was estimated that at least .6% of participants had been struck by vehicles in the previous year. Assuming that 1% of the North American population are seriously involved in distance running, this would equate to 12,000 injuries per year in a population of 200 million adults. Other reports have suggested that in New Jersey alone, 20 joggers are killed each year, and that in Los Angeles, joggers account for about 1% of the 6,000 annual incidents involving pedestrians (76, 77).

ONTARIO STATISTICS

In Ontario, some 6,000 pedestrians are currently injured per year; about 180 of these incidents are fatal. Relating these figures to the overall Ontario population, the Ontario incidence of pedestrian accidents is a little lower than in Los Angeles, at 2 fatalities and some 67 accidents per 100,000 population per year. Extrapolating the Ontario figures to a total US population of about 240 million, one might well anticipate 4,800 fatalities and 160,800 accidents per year across the whole of the United States. The number of vehicle accidents that Burch ascribed to jogging, 8,300 incidents per year, would then be about 5% of this total (74). Other reports for the United States also suggest that 1%–5% of pedestrian accidents involve joggers (76).

AGE DISTRIBUTION OF INJURIES

A surprisingly high proportion of all pedestrian traffic accidents involve young adults aged 21 to 34 years. Williams et al. (76) found that 44% of injuries were in patients aged 15 to 24 years. In the 21–24-year age range, the accident rate for the 1987 Ontario sample was 43% higher than in those aged 35–44, despite the fact that sensory acuity has aged appreciably in the older age category. Some of the advantage of the older individuals probably reflects greater maturity and better judgment, but it also seems possible that at least a part of the excess of vehicle-induced injuries in the younger adults arises because a larger proportion of such individuals are engaged in running or jogging to the point of mood alterations.

LOCATION OF INCIDENT

Williams (76) estimated that 53% of jogging accidents occurred at intersections, and that the jogger was responsible for 31% of such accidents. A collision at an intersection where the pedestrian had the nominal right-of-way accounted for 8.6% of deaths and 19.7% of injuries in Ontario during 1987. Over a 5-year period, the Ontario figures showed an annual average of 1,153 accidents with right-of-way, of which 11 incidents were fatal. In a substantial proportion of accidents, particularly those with a fatal outcome, the investigating traffic officer noted as a contributing factor a disturbance of brain function from alcohol, drugs, or fatigue.

BEHAVIOR OF JOGGERS AT INTERSECTIONS

Joggers often continue to move when they reach an intersection. The more prudent continue to run on the spot, but the more foolhardy dart across the road even if there is a traffic signal opposing their movement. There are several potential medicophysiological explanations of such risk-taking behavior.

1. *Mechanical.* The more intelligent and mechanically minded jogger may be aware that a substantial amount of energy is spent in braking the body when it is moving rapidly, and that an equal amount of energy must

be expended in the opposite sense when accelerating after a stop (78). Thus, any halt to accomodate opposing traffic may be perceived as a "waste of energy."

2. *Cardiovascular.* If a person has been jogging for some minutes, there is a large blood flow to the legs, venous return being assured by the pumping action of the leg muscles (78). If the person concerned stops moving at an intersection, blood pools in the leg veins. This can cause faintness (with disturbed thinking, and even loss of consciousness). Continuing to jog (or to run on the spot) sustains venous return. Again, a person who has studied jogging carefully may realize the circulatory problems created by halting for traffic; indeed, there may be personal experience of circulatory collapse or "black-out."

3. *Muscular.* If a person jogs above a critical speed, about 70% of all-out aerobic effort, there is a progressive accumulation of lactic acid in the working muscles. This causes local muscle pain and stiffness. The rate of removal of lactate from the working muscles is greater if a jogger continues to move at least slowly (78). Thus, by study or experience, a regular exerciser may find that stopping at an intersection leads to a stiffening of the muscles.

4. *Cerebral perfusion.* As running continues, peripheral vascular pooling and an increase of skin blood flow begin to compromise the cerebral circulation, with a clouding of consciousness. One very dramatic episode of this type occurred during an international competition in London in 1908. At the end of a very warm Olympic marathon, Dorando entered the Wembley stadium and turned in the wrong direction before collapsing in a semicoma.

5. *Psychological.* Perhaps the most likely explanation of most incidents lies in the domain of exercise psychology. When asked why they jog, a large proportion of people will explain that it makes them "feel better," that it gives them a pleasant sense of exhilaration and euphoria, and that it offers an escape from the pressing realities of a harsh world (79, 80). Apter (81) speaks of physical activity as drawing the participant into "its own closed world with its own dynamic and holds his or her attention . . ." Sillitoe's *The Loneliness of the Long-Distance Runner* (82) describes a Borstal boy who finds "escape" in a jogging program sanctioned by the prison authorities. Sperryn (83) writes of the "trance-like state" induced by jogging.

A variety of factors contribute to this altered state of consciousness: the decrease of cerebral blood flow noted above, the mesmerizing effect of exactly repeated movements, increased arousal of the reticular formation of the brain by proprioceptive impulses, an increased cerebral concentration of stimulant amines, and increased secretion of β-endorphins. More information is nevertheless needed on the precise combinations of intensity and duration of effort needed to induce such effects. Do they occur in the average person who jogs gently for 2 kilometres, or are they only likely in all-out competition over a much longer distance?

6. *Psychopathic personality.* A final possibility is that the individual concerned has some psychological disturbance such as a psychopathic personality unrelated to his or her immediate exercise behaviour.

Conclusions

There seems growing evidence that regular involvement in a heavy exercise program can cause an addiction to jogging, with physical symptoms when the stimulus is withdrawn. However, it is much less certain that the moderate activity adopted by the average person will have this type of effect. It remains equally unclear whether exercise-induced alterations of mood have a major influence on the likelihood of attempting risky athletic feats, exercising beyond the point of pleasant tiredness, or ignoring otherwise obvious dangers from vehicles.

Although the exercise compliance of the exercise addict is high, it is no more desirable to produce an addiction to endogenous opioids than to externally administered drugs. A history of depression or previous addictions may increase vulnerability to exercise addiction (39), and the exercise program of such patients should be monitored with particular care. Symptoms of frustration, irritability, lack of attention, inability to concentrate, anxiety, depression, fatigue, and disturbed sleep when exercise is not possible are all clues that a person is becoming addicted to exercise (35). Failure to moderate activity in the face of pain, injury, or adverse reactions from other members of the family are other warning signs of excessive involvement.

From the viewpoint of preventing traffic injuries, it seems important to emphasize that exercise addiction is not the only hazard of the highway. Joggers bear primary responsibility for about a third of the accidents involving motor vehicles (76), and in only a small fraction of such incidents is exercise addiction a possible cause. Other factors contributing to traffic accidents, in addition to euphoria, include running in the same direction as traffic, failure to wear light-colored clothing at night, talking to a companion, and listening to taped music instead of traffic. Even where a jogger has the nominal right of way, it not always prudent to insist upon such priority. It may be much easier for the jogger to stop than for a car or a truck.

A substantial segment of vehicle-related accidents could be eliminated by ensuring that all urban roads had sidewalks, preferably with a substantial setback from the highway. However, such measures would do little to protect the addicted jogger with an endorphin-mediated sense of invincibility. Injuries related to exercise addiction may still prove to be rarities, but even a single fatality involving a healthy young adult is a tragedy. Popular handbooks for the committed roadrunner should thus give greater emphasis to the potential hazard arising from changes of mood-state.

References

1. Hughes J, et al: *Nature* 258:577, 1975.
2. Guillemin R: *N Engl J Med* 296:226, 1977.
3. Lobstein DD, Ismail AH: *Med Sci Sports Exerc* 17:209, 1985.
4. Rasmussen CL, Lobstein DD: *Med Sci Sports Exerc* 19:67S, 1987.
5. Appenzaller O, et al: *Neurology* 30:418, 1980.
6. Carr DB, et al: *N Engl J Med* 305:560, 1981.
7. Colt EWD, et al: *Life Sci* 28:1637, 1981.
8. Farrell PA: *Med Sci Sports Exerc* 17:89, 1985.
9. Farrell PA, et al: *J Appl Physiol* 52:1245, 1982.
10. Farrell PA, et al: *J Appl Physiol* 61:1051, 1986.
11. Farrell PA, et al: *Med Sci Sports Exerc* 19:347, 1987.
12. Sforzo GA, et al: *Med Sci Sports Exerc* 18:380, 1986.
13. Goldfarb AH, et al: *Med Sci Sports Exerc* 19:78, 1987.
14. Mikines KJ, et al: *Eur J Appl Physiol* 54:476, 1985.
15. Elliot DL, et al: *Life Sci* 34:515, 1984.
16. Melchionda AM, et al: *Phys Sportsmed* 12:102, 1984.
17. Langenfeld ME, et al: *Med Sci Sports Exerc* 19:83, 1987.
18. Donevan RH, Andrew GM: *Med Sci Sports Exerc* 19:229, 1987.
19. McMurray RG, et al: *Med Sci Sports Exerc* 19:570, 1987.
20. Rahkila P, et al: *Med Sci Sports Exerc* 19:451, 1987.
21. Appenzaller O, Atkinson R: Neurology of sports and exercise, in Bove AA, Lowenthal DT (eds): *Exercise Medicine: Physiological Principles and Clinical Applications.* New York: Academic Press, 1983, pp 185–227.
22. Pargman D, Baker MC: *J Drug Iss* 10:341, 1980.
23. Sachs ML: The runner's high, in Sachs ML, Buffone GW (eds): *Running as Therapy: An Integrated Approach.* Lincoln: University of Nebraska Press, 1984, pp 273–287.
24. Glasser W: *Positive Addiction.* New York: Harper and Row, 1976.
25. Baekeland F: *Arch Gen Psychiatr* 22:365, 1970.
26. Shephard RJ: *Biochemistry of Physical Activity.* Springfield, Ill: CC Thomas, 1983.
27. Little JC: *Psychiatr Ann* 9:49, 1979.
28. Morgan WP: *Phys Sportsmed* 7:56–63, 67–70, 1979.
29. Peele S: *How Much is Too Much.* Englewood Cliffs, NJ. Prentice Hall, 1981, pp 3–50.
30. Yates A, et al: *N Engl J Med* 308:251, 1983.
31. British Medical Journal (Editorial): *Br Med J* 283:746, 1981.
32. Clement-Jones V, et al: *Lancet* ii:946, 1980.
33. Christie MJ, et al: *Life Sci* 31:839, 1982.
34. Sachs ML: Compliance and addiction to exercise, in Cantu RC (ed): *The Exercising Adult.* Lexington, Mass, Collamore Press, 1982, pp 19–27.
35. Sachs ML, Pargman D: *J Sport Behavior* 2:143, 1979.
36. Mandell AJ: *Psychiatr Ann* 9:57, 61–63, 66–69, 1979.
37. Lawrence RM: Psychological aspects of exercise, in *Exercise Medicine: Physiological Principles and Clinical Applications.* New York, Academic Press, 1983.
38. Kostrubala T: Running: The grand illusion, in Sachs MH, Sachs ML (eds): *Psychology of Running.* Champaign, Ill, Human Kinetics Publ, 1981, pp 211–223.
39. Colt EW, et al: A high prevalence of affective disorders in runners, in Sachs MH, Sachs ML (eds): *Psychology of Running.* Champaign, Ill, Human Kinetics Publ, 1981, pp 234–248.
40. Ransford CP: *Med Sci Sports Exerc* 14:1, 1982.
41. Hughes JR: *Prev Med* 13:66, 1984.
42. Morgan WP: *Med Sci Sports Exerc* 17:94, 1985.
43. Brown DR: Exercise, fitness and mental health, in Bouchard C, Shephard RJ,

Stephens T, Sutton JR, McPherson B (eds): *Exercise, Fitness and Health.* Champaign, Ill, Human Kinetics Publ, 1990, pp 607–626.

44. Sime W: Discussion: Exercise, fitness and mental health, in Bouchard C, Shephard RJ, Stephens T, Sutton JR, McPherson B (eds): *Exercise, Fitness and Health.* Champaign, Ill, Human Kinetics Publ, 1990, pp 627–633.
45. Morgan WP, O'Connor PJ: Exercise and mental health, in Dishman RK (ed): *Exercise Adherence.* Champaign, Ill, Human Kinetics Publ, 1988.
46. Grossman A: *Med Sci Sports Exerc* 17:101, 1985.
47. Sutton JR: *Med Sci Sports Exerc* 17:73, 1985.
48. McArthur JW: *Med Sci Sports Exerc* 17:82, 1985.
49. Barta A, Yashpal K: *Progr Neuropsychopharmacol* 5:595, 1981.
50. Blake, MJ, et al: *Peptides* 5:953, 1984.
51. Markoff RA, et al: *Med Sci Sports Exerc* 14:11, 1982.
52. Wildmann J, et al: *Life Sci* 38:997, 1986.
53. Haier RJ, et al: *Psychiatr Res* 5:231, 1981.
54. Dale G, et al: *Br Med J* 294:1004, 1987.
55. Cooper KH: *The New Aerobics.* New York, Evans, 1970.
56. Newsholme E, Leech T. *The Runner.* Headington, Oxford, Walter L. Meacher, 1983, pp 1–152.
57. Schwartz L: *Heavyhands Walking.* Emmaus, Penn, Rodale Press, 1987.
58. Niemann DC: *Fitness and Sports Medicine: An introduction.* Palo Alto, Calif, Bull Publ, 1988, pp 1–583.
59. LaCava G: *J Sports Med Phys Fitness* 4:221, 1964.
60. Krissoff WB, Ferris WD: *Phys Sportsmed* 7:54, 1979.
61. Taunton JE, Clement DB: *Modern Med Canada* 36:476, 1981.
62. Richards R, Richards D: Providing medical care in fun runs and marathons in Australasia, in Sutton JR, Brock RM (eds): *Sports Medicine for the Mature Athlete.* Indianapolis, Benchmark Press, 1986, pp 167–180.
63. Tunstall-Pedoe D: *BMJ* 288:1358, 1984.
64. Tunstall-Pedoe D: Medical support for marathons in the United Kingdom: The London marathon, in Sutton JR, Brock RM (eds): *Sports Medicine for the Mature Athlete.* Indianapolis, Benchmark Press, 1986, pp 181–203.
65. Jacobs SJ, Berson BL: *Am J Sports Med* 14:151, 1986.
66. Lysholm J, Wiklander J: *Am J Sports Med* 15:168, 1987.
67. Holmlich P, et al: *Br J Sports Med* 22:19, 1988.
68. Robertson JW: *Sports Med* 6:261, 1988.
69. Ferstle J: *Phys Sportsmed* 6:18, 1978.
70. Koplan JP, et al: *JAMA* 248:3118, 1982.
71. Koplan JP, et al: *US Publ Health Rep* 100:189, 1985.
72. Powell KE, et al: *Phys Sportsmed* 14:100, 1986.
73. Oldridge NB: Discussion: Exercise, fitness and recovery from surgery, disease or trauma, in Bouchard C, Shephard RJ, Stephens T, Sutton JR, McPherson B (eds): *Exercise, Fitness and Health.* Champaign, Ill, Human Kinetics Publ, 1990, pp 601–606.
74. Burch GE: *Am Heart J* 97:407, 1979.
75. *Medical Letter:* New Rochelle, N.Y., 1979.
76. Williams AF: *US Publ Health Rep* 96:448, 1981.
77. Road Runners Club of America 7:10. Report cited by Williams et al: (22).
78. Shephard RJ: *Physiology and Biochemistry of Exercise.* New York: Praeger, 1982.
79. Shephard RJ: *Sports Med* 2:348, 1985.
80. Shephard RJ: *Phys Sportsmed* 13:88, 1985.
81. Apter MJ: Sport and mental health: A new psychological perspective, in Hermans GPH, Mostard WL (eds): *Sports, Medicine and Health.* Amsterdam, Excerpta Medica, 1990, pp 47–56.
82. Sillitoe A: *The Loneliness of the Long-Distance Runner.* London, W.H. Allen, 1959.
83. Sperryn P: *Sport and Medicine.* London, Butterworths, 1983.

1 Biomechanics, Muscle Training, and Overtraining

Mood State and Running Economy in Moderately Trained Male Runners
Williams TJ, Krahenbuhl GS, Morgan DW (Arizona State Univ)
Med Sci Sports Exerc 23:727–731, 1991   1–1

Introduction.—Studies have shown that running economy (RE) among trained runners can vary daily within a given subject; these variations are largely unexplained. No studies have addressed the effect of psychological factors in this relationship. The association between mood state and within-subject variation in RE was studied in 10 moderately trained male runners.

Methods.—The psychological state was measured by the Profile of Mood States (POMS) inventory. The runners had a mean age of 25.6 years, had trained for 1 year before the study, and had achieved 10-km race times of 38 to 45 minutes. Each subject performed treadmill running 5 times a week for 4 weeks at 2.68, 3.13, and 3.58 m/second. Each week before the treadmill exercise a tension, depression, anger, vigor, fatigue, confusion, and total mood disturbance (TMD) score was calculated. At each running pace oxygen consumption ($\dot{V}O_2$) was determined by the open-circuit method.

Results.—Group correlation of $\dot{V}O_2$ values, or RE and TMD scores for each week, was r = −.28, which was not significant. However, within-subject group correlation between TMD and RE was a positive r = .88 (Fig 1–1). Thus when within-subject variation was the focus of analysis, weeks with more economical values were correlated with a more positive mental health picture. The POMS subscales of tension, depression, anger, vigor, and confusion, but not fatigue, were significantly associated with average $\dot{V}O_2$.

Conclusion.—There appears to be a close association between short-term fluctuations in RE and mood state in moderately trained male runners. The POMS profile of the most economical week has the classic "iceberg" appearance, and that of the least economical week is flatter.

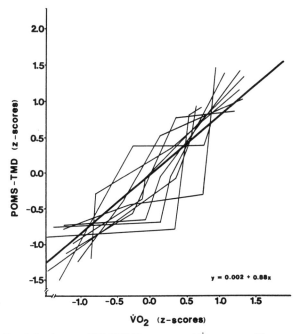

POMS-TMD (z-scores)

$\dot{V}O_2$ (z-scores)

$y = 0.002 + 0.88x$

Fig 1-1.—Correlation between POMS-TMD z-scores and $\dot{V}O_2$ z-scores. (Courtesy of Williams TJ, Krahenbuhl GS, Morgan DW: *Med Sci Sports Exerc* 23:727–731, 1991.)

The correlation could also be affected by daily variation in weight and running mechanics.

▶ Does how we feel affect how we run? Or does how we run affect how we feel? Most athletes and coaches have a firm conviction that performance and mood are related and perhaps they are causally related. In this study the profile of mood states was used as a fairly robust way of assessing "mood" while running economy (RE) was quantified as the relationship between running velocity and $\dot{V}O_2$. Here it was emphasized that this was not a training study but simply examined the within subject variability in a group of moderately trained runners whose training and "fitness" did not vary throughout the duration of the study. The observations are fascinating and suggest some interdependence although the causal relationship cannot be easily established.—J.R. Sutton, M.D.

Methods to Assess Physical Activity With Special Reference to Motion Sensors and Accelerometers

Meijer GAL, Westerterp KR, Verhoeven FMH, Koper HBM, ten Hoor F (Uni-

versity of Limburg, Maastricht, The Netherlands)
IEEE Trans Biomed Eng 38:221–229, 1991   1–2

Introduction.—Physical activity is difficult to measure. Most data on physical activity have been obtained by observational techniques that are not free of subjective observer judgment and are of no use for studying larger groups. Mechanical pedometers are motion sensors linked to a counting device that has to be calibrated for stride length. These devices do not reflect movement intensity and are not very accurate. The new generation of electronic accelerometers provides a more objective means for measuring physical activity. The present study was designed to test the reliability of the new electronic accelerometers.

Methods.—The type of accelerometer used in this study contains a 3-directional sensor connected to a data acquision unit. The unit is worn on a belt and the sensor is applied at the lower back. Four healthy individuals with a mean age of 22 years walked on a treadmill at 3, 5, and 7 km/hr for 5 minutes at each speed. Twelve different accelerometers were used for the study. Each person wore 2 of them during testing, with the sensors being placed closely together on the same waist belt. All devices were calibrated in a standardized bench test before and after each treadmill test.

Results.—Intrainstrument variation in a bench test was less than 8% during 4 measurements over a week. Intrainstrument reproducibility in a test-retest experiment was within 20%. Interinstrument variation between 2 accelerometers worn together during treadmill experiments showed a difference that was usually less than 30% and averaged 22%. This difference did not improve after adjustment for differences found in the bench test. Despite this quite large error, differences among subjects performing the same activities could be discriminated. Reproducibility of the experiment was about 76% at a treadmill speed of 3 km/hr, 85% at 5 km/hr, and 95% at 7 km/hr. Bench testing revealed that the sensitivity of a piezoelectric element is prone to shifts, probably because of mechanical, electromagnetic, or temperature shock, or all of these factors, which may be encountered in outdoor conditions.

Conclusion.—The accelerometer is accurate within 18% when used under standardized conditions in the laboratory. However, further validation studies are needed to assess its accuracy when used on individuals going through their normal daily activities.

▶ Too often researchers use equipment to make measurements and collect data without being aware of the measurement error that these instruments themselves introduce. To a certain degree, all biomechanical studies are dependent on the accuracy of the measuring instruments. In this study, the authors found that the accelerometer they used was accurate within 18% when used, under the best of conditions, in the laboratory. We can surmise that the accuracy would be further degraded if the measuring were done during normal daily activities, outside the laboratory. We need to pay more attention to the accuracy of our measuring equipment if we are to have confidence in our findings.—Col. J.L. Anderson, PE.D.

A Segment Interaction Analysis of Proximal-to-Distal Sequential Segment Motion Patterns
Putman CA (Dalhousie University, Halifax, NS)
Med Sci Sports Exerc 23:130–144, 1991   1–3

Background.—When an extremity moves freely through space, as in striking or throwing, the proximal segment typically begins forward rotation well before the more distal segments start their forward rotation. The proximal segment also reaches maximum angular velocity and begins to slow down well before the more distal segments reach maximum angular velocity. The motion-dependent interactions among the limb segments are important in determining the overall proximal-to-distal sequential pattern of both slow and fast movements.

Study Design.—Limb segment interactions were examined during kicking and in the swing phases of running and walking. The study included 4 men who were skilled in punt kicking and 2 women and 2 men who were experienced runners. High-speed film data were collected, and equations were derived to express the segmental interactions in terms of resultant joint moments at the hip and knee, as well as interactive moments that were functions of gravitational forces or kinematic variables.

Observations.—Angular motion-dependent interaction between the thigh and leg had a significant role in determining the sequential segment motion patterns seen in all activities (Fig 1–2). The interaction was comparable in all movements except when there were substantial differences in the knee angle. There was some evidence supporting summation of segment speeds, but not summation of force.

Implications.—Because of the angular velocity of the proximal segment, its effect on a distal segment is probably important in determining the pattern of most swinging motions involving human extremities. The motion patterns are not explained by general statements regarding the effect of negative thigh angular acceleration on positive leg angular acceleration.

▶ This is an excellent study which, among other things, demonstrates the complications of modeling and understanding what most of us would consider a relatively simple segmental interaction analysis. I, personally, am surprised that although support was found for the principle of summation of segment speeds, no support was found for the principle of summation of force. Similarly, no support was found for the general statements concerning the effect of negative thigh acceleration on positive leg acceleration. Many

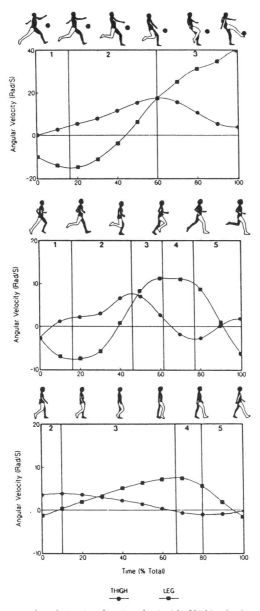

Fig 1–2.—Segment angular velocity-time functions for 1 trial of kicking (**top**), running (**middle**), and walking (**bottom**). Positive rotation is in the counterclockwise direction. The graphs have been divided into 5 sections and normalized on the basis of percent time from the beginning to the end of the movement, where these are defined as the start of forward (positive) thigh rotation and ball contact in kicking and as toe-off and foot strike in running and walking. Note that the ordinate scale for kicking is twice that of running and walking. (Courtesy of Putman CA: *Med Sci Sports Exerc* 23:130–144, 1991.)

of us learned from Dyson about the summation of segment speeds as well as the summation of forces (1). However, this investigation found that there was no evidence that the forward swing motion of the lower extremity in kicking, running, or walking was initiated by the larger muscle groups of the proximal segment and continued by the smaller muscles of the distal segment. Whether this finding will hold true in replication or with studies of other motion patterns, such as the overhand throwing pattern, awaits further research. This study points out that the interaction between segments is complex and it is difficult to quantify the roles played by different muscle groups to produce proximal-to-distal sequential patterns of segment motions.—Col. J.L. Anderson, PE.D.

Reference

1. Dyson G: *The Mechanics of Athletics,* ed 6. London, University of London Press, 1973, pp 38–39, 189.

Three-Dimensional Measurement System for Functional Arm Motion Study
Safaee-Rad R, Shwedyk E, Quanbury AO (University of Manitoba; Rehab Centre for Children, Winnipeg, Manitoba)
Med Biol Eng Comput 28:569–573, 1990   1–4

Introduction.—A three-dimensional system was created for measuring functional arm motion, based on a photographic method using televi-

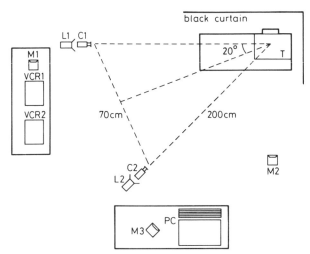

Fig 1–3.—Diagram of system set-up. *Abbreviations: T,* area of table that is used to perform different tasks (table area of activity); M1 and M2, black-and-white monitors; VCR1 and VCR2, video cassette recorders; C1 and C2, video cameras; L1 and L2, video lights; M3, image-processing system monitor; PC, personal computer with video digitizer board. (Courtesy of Safaee-Rad R, Shwedyk E, Quanbury AO: *Med Biol Eng Comput* 28:569–573, 1990.)

sion cameras. It is an accurate and inexpensive way of acquiring a permanent visual record of movements — clinically a very important attribute.

Methods.—The hardware includes spherical reflective markers, 2 charge-coupled devices monochrome video cameras, and 2 black-and-white video monitors. One of the video cassette recorders is used for image digitization; it has freeze, frame-by-frame replay, and frame-counting capabilities. A frame of ping pong balls serves to calibrate the system. The angle between the optical axes of the cameras is 40 degrees (Fig 1–3). Software is available for system calibration, image acquisition and processing and kinematic analysis of movement.

Application.—Typically, kinematic data are acquired in 1 hour. Dynamic error was less than 3% when studying functional arm motion during feeding. The system proved easy to use for this purpose. It is important that this system can be readily assembled using standard commercial products. Hopefully, this will encourage physicians and researchers to use video imaging in analyzing movements.

▶ This 3-dimensional measurement system presents some interesting alternatives for acquiring kinematic data in a rather short period of time. However, it appears to me that there are also some clear limitations when it comes to analyzing fast or extremely fast movements such as we find in the sports setting. Coaches may be able to use this technique as a method of improving the knowledge they gain from visual observations.—Col. J.L. Anderson, PE.D.

Development of a Three-Dimensional Finite Element Model of a Human Tibia Using Experimental Modal Analysis
Hobatho MC, Darmana R, Pastor P, Barrau JJ, Laroze S, Morucci JP (Hôtel Dieu; INSA; ENSAE, Toulouse, France)
J Biomech 24:371–383, 1991   1–5

Objective.—An accurate 3-dimensional finite element analysis of a human tibia was attempted with the goals of interpreting vibrational measurements of resonant frequencies in vivo and quantifying the effects of elastic properties on these frequencies. The modal analysis included estimates of the tibia's natural frequency, damping ratio, and mode shapes.

Methods.—Experimental modal analysis was carried out to measure the frequency response function of a grossly normal male human tibia. A finite element model, or structural model, was constructed by condensing 3 substructures (the proximal epiphysis, diaphysis, and distal epiphysis). Values for mechanical properties were taken from the literature. The experimental model served to optimize the structural model.

Analysis.—After optimization, differences between the experimental and structural models were caused only by mechanical properties and mass distribution. The finite element model eliminated effects of boundary conditions and geometric properties (e.g., length). Relative error between the 2 methods was about 3%, corresponding to the standard deviation of the measured frequencies. Modal shapes included bending in the lateromedial and sagittal planes of vibration and a slight torsional effect stemming from the twisted geometry of the bone.

▶ This study is excellent in that it helps us to realize some of the complexities of the human body. In this case, one bone, the tibia. The human tibia possesses a complex structure. It has no axial symmetry, its crest twists along the length, and its material properties are inhomogeneous. There are many other variables that we do not understand about this one bone. Just think about the many more complications that must be studied and understood before we can really perform biomechanical studies of complex movements and still be confident in the accuracy of our findings. Yet, every study such as this that is well done becomes a building block for our eventual understanding of complex movements.—Col. J.L. Anderson, PE.D.

Three-Dimensional Kinematics of Glenohumeral Elevation
An K-N, Browne AO, Korinek S, Tanaka S, Morrey BF (Mayo Clinic and Found, Rochester, Minn)
J Orthop Res 9:143–149, 1991   1–6

Objective.—The shoulder exhibits more motion than any other joint. A protocol was developed to measure the 3-dimensional orientation of the humerus with reference to the scapula and to define the kinematics of the glenohumeral joint.

Methods.—A magnetic tracking system was used to monitor humeral orientation with respect to the scapula. Two sets of coordinate systems were defined to describe joint motion: a reference system fixed on the glenoid and a moving system attached on the humerus (Fig 1–4). Humeral motion was described by the Eulerian angle system based on a 1–3'–1" rotation sequence. The kinematics of the humerus and scapula were monitored by the 3Space Isotrak System.

Findings.—The maximal humeral elevation in the 9 specimens studied ranged from 95 degrees to 120 degrees. Maximal elevation differed by as much as 30 degrees at different planes of elevation, with peak elevation occurring anterior to the plane of the scapula at about 23 degrees. Anterior to the scapular plane, external humeral rotation allowed greater elevation. Further posterior to the plane, internal rotation was required for maximal humeral elevation.

Conclusion.—These findings confirm the value of describing glenohumeral motion by maximum arm elevation rather than by maximum flexion or abduction.

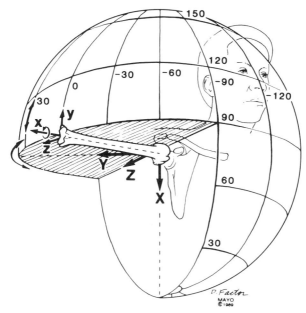

Fig 1–4.—Definition of the reference coordinate system. The X, Y, Z represents the reference fixed coordinate system affixed on the scapula. The *x, y, z* represents the moving coordinate system affixed on the humerus. The latitude on the globe represents the amount of humeral elevation, and the longitude on the globe represents the plane of elevation. The humeral axial rotation takes place about the *x* axis along the humeral shaft. (Courtesy of An K-N, Browne AO, Korinek S, et al: *J Orthop Res* 9:143–149, 1991.)

▶ Anyone who is interested in sports medicine should be pleased to see this study on the kinematics of the glenohumeral joints. Here at West Point injuries to the shoulder during physical activity have replaced knee injuries as the most costly. It is my belief that there is a real increase in the number of shoulder injuries. Why this is so is not definitively known; however, I feel that it is connected with the fact that our youth are not as physically active between the ages of 3 and 16 years. All of our fitness studies support the fact that our youth are less fit today than in the past.—Col. J.L. Anderson, PE.D.

Force-Velocity Relationship of Human Elbow Flexors in Voluntary Isotonic Contraction Under Heavy Loads
Kojima T (University of Tokyo)
Int J Sports Med 12:208–213, 1991   1–7

Objective.—Because the force-velocity (F-V) relationship of human muscles is an important property relating to sports activities, the F-V relationship of the elbow flexors was examined in 7 men, aged 19–38 years, who were moderately active in various recreational activities.

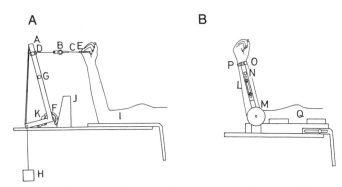

Fig 1–5.—Schematic illustration of experimental arrangements. *Abbreviations*: A and L, lever and bar; B, force transducer; C, stainless wire; D, handle clamp; E, handle; F and M, potentiometers; G and N, accelerometers; H, external load; I and Q, blocks; J, stopper; K, ratchet; O, aluminum plate; and P, rubber belt. (Courtesy of Kojima T: *Int J Sports Med* 12:208–213, 1991.)

Methods.—The elbow flexors were studied as a single muscle in maximum voluntary contraction using isotonic lever systems. Measurements were made at an elbow angle of 90 degrees (Fig 1-5) using external loads of up to 90% of maximum voluntary isometric force. The effect of muscle fatigue was minimized by adjusting the initial elbow angle at the onset of flexion to the size of the load and reducing the duration of flexion with heavy loads.

Findings.—The Hill equation fitted fairly well with F-V data obtained with loads up to 90% of maximum voluntary isometric force. Predicted maximum isometric force was larger than that observed experimentally by a mean of 6%. The overall coefficient of correlation was .97.

Conclusion.—In moderately active males, observed F-V relationships of the elbow flexors in maximal voluntary contraction, subjected to isotonic loading, obey the Hill equation fairly well. Deviation at low velocity and high force output may reflect the contractile properties of the muscles rather than CNS inhibition.

▶ For those who may have forgotten, here is the Hill equation:
$$(F + a)(V + b) = b(F_o + a)$$
where: "F" is the muscular force, "V" is the shortening velocity of the contractile component of the muscle, "F_o" is the maximum isometric force, and "a" and "b" are constants.—Col. J.L. Anderson, PE.D.

Biomechanical Changes at the Ankle Joint After Stroke

Thilmann AF, Fellows SJ, Ross HF (Alfried Krupp Krankenhaus, Essen, Germany; The Medical School, Birmingham, England)
J Neurol Neurosurg Psychiatry 54:134–139, 1991   1–8

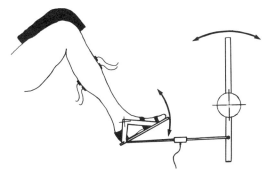

Fig 1–6.—Experimental set-up. (Courtesy of Thilmann AF, Fellows SJ, Ross HF: *J Neurol Neurosurg Psychiatry* 54:134–139, 1991.)

Background.—Muscular hypertonia is a major disability in persons with spasticity, impeding and even preventing voluntary movements. Those having spasticity for some time reportedly exhibit increased stiffness at the ankle in the absence of reflex activity.

Study Plan.—The resistance of the relaxed ankle to slow displacement over the range of joint motion was measured in 15 hemiparetic subjects who had had unilateral cerebral ischemia in the middle cerebral artery area at least 1 year earlier. None had clinical signs of contracture. Ten normal subjects and 5 orthopedic patients with abnormal feet but no functional problems also were studied using the arrangement shown in Figure 1-6.

Findings.—Normal subjects had increased stiffness only when the foot was dorsiflexed beyond 70 degrees, and a lesser increase occurred on plantar flexion. Hemiparetic patients were significantly stiffer in dorsiflexion on the involved side. Curves on the "healthy" side were identical to those in normal subjects.

Interpretation.—Hemiparetic patients exhibit altered passive biomechanics at the affected ankle, presumably reflecting loss of compliance in the Achilles tendon. Increased stiffness of the triceps surae may play a role.

▶ All of the patients in this study were screened to exclude clinically defined contracture from the results, and all cases of activation of the ankle musculature were excluded. The authors have determined that the observed increase in stiffness must arise as the result of passive biomechanical changes. Because no differences from the normal condition were found in plantar-flexion, the increased stiffness must be a property of the ankle extensor musculature or of its tendons and connective tissue. The authors therefore feel justified to conclude that, although some change in the passive mechanical properties of the muscle fibers of the triceps surae may have occurred, the major factor behind the increased resistance to dorsiflexion at the paretic ankle is an increase in the passive stiffness of the Achilles tendon.—Col. J.L. Anderson, PE.D.

Simultaneous Measurement of Changes in Length of the Cruciate Ligaments During Knee Motion
Kurosawa H, Yamakoshi K-I, Yasuda K, Sasaki T (Hokkaido University, Sapporo, Japan)
Clin Orthop 265:233–240, 1991   1–9

Background.—Several methods have been described for measuring changes in length of the anterior cruciate ligament (ACL) and posterior cruciate ligament (PCL) to evelute their biomechanical function. A technique of simultaneously measuring changes in length of various parts of the fiber bundles of the ligaments during motion in the cadaver knee was examined.

Methods.—A strain gauge-type elongation transducer was modified to be implanted along the length of the ligament fiber. Four of these transducers were gathered into a bundle at the proximal part for the ACL and 3 were made into a bundle for the PCL (Fig 1–7). A strain amplifier was used to measure changes in elongation. Knee specimens from 3 adults (2 men and 1 woman, ranging in age from 50 to 65 years) were tested.

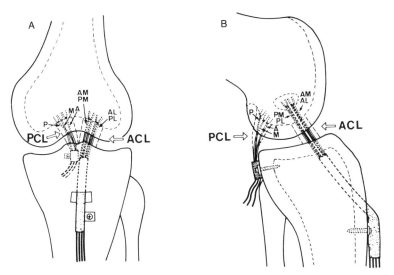

Fig 1–7.—Installation of the strain-gauge transducers in the anterior cruciate ligaments (ACL) and posterior cruciate ligaments (PCL) in the anteromedial (AM), anterolateral (AL), posteromedial (PM), posterolateral (PL), anterior (A), middle (M), and posterior (P) bundles. **A,** anteroposterior and (**B**) lateral views. (Courtesy of Kurosawa H, Yamakoshi K-I, Yasuda K, et al: *Clin Orthop* 265:233–240, 1991.)

Results.—During unconstrained joint flexion and extension, the ACL transducers indicated that the maximum shortening peak was at about 30 degrees of flexion. Beyond this point, the transducers in the anterior bundle increased in length, whereas those in the posterior bundle remained shortened. In the PCL, transducers in the anterior bundle had their maximum lengthening peak at about 50 degrees of flexion and those in the posterior bundle had their maximum lengthening peak at about 0 degrees. A lesser change occurred in the middle bundle. On simulated application of quadriceps forces, the ACL transducers lengthened and the PCL transducers shortened; these changes decreased at more than 90 degrees. Quadriceps force caused increased shortening of the PCL after the ACL was cut.

Conclusion.—A strain gauge technique for simultaneous measurement of elongation of various parts of the ligament fibers of the ACL and PCL, which minimizes disturbance of the ligaments, was studied. Results of such testing suggest that the 2 ligaments may be considered functionally specialized aggregates of parallel fibers rather than as distinctly separate bundles. Quadriceps force appears to strongly affect changes in ligament fiber length, with those of the ACL lengthening to nearly the same degree as those of the PCL shorten.

▶ These authors feel that their results strongly suggest that the ACL should be regarded functionally as the aggregate of 2 fiber bundles and that, to some degree, those bundles work mutually as a restraint for hyperextension and as a stabilizer for knee motion. To a considerable degree, they feel that these findings agree with the anatomical findings reported by Girgis (1). Furthermore, these authors report that their findings have proved that the ACL plays an important role as a static stabilizer that is antagonistic to the quadriceps force from 10 degrees to about 60 degrees of knee flexion. They suggest that these findings confirm the consensus of clinical practitioners that the ACL is one of the most important structures contributing to the function of the knee joint and that a patient sustaining a severe injury to the ACL should be considered for surgical treatment.—Col. J.L. Anderson, PE.D.

Reference

1. Girgis FG, et al: *Clin Orthop* 106:216, 1975.

Short Crank Cycle Ergometry
Schwartz RE, Asnis PD, Cavanaugh JT, Asnis SE, Simmons JE, Lasinski PJ (Sports Medicine/Rehabilitation of Manhasset; North Shore Univ Hosp, Manhasset, NY)
J Orthop Sports Phys Ther 13:95–100, 1991   1–10

Background.—Ergometric cycling is an excellent rehabilitation technique, but its early use is limited by the requirement for at least 90 de-

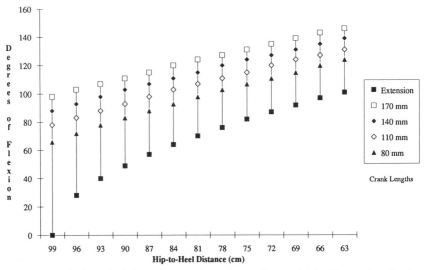

Fig 1–8.—The hip-to-heel distance can be obtained by setting seat height. The arc of motion for that seat height can be read on the vertical axis. The shorter the crank length, the smaller the arc of knee motion required to bring the pedal through its complete cycle, extension being the lowest point and flexion being the highest. The longer the crank length, the larger is the arc of motion required to bring the knee around a complete cycle rotation. (Courtesy of Schwartz RE, Asnis PD, Cavanaugh JT, et al: *J Orthop Sports Phys Ther* 13:95–100, 1991.)

grees of knee motion. A new cycle ergometer was designed as an alternative to continuous passive motion machines to expedite rehabilitation in patients who have had knee surgery.

Methods.—The change in knee angle during cycling was analyzed. Shortening of the crank length of the cycle ergometer could reduce the arc of knee motion needed to perform the cycling exercise (Fig 1–8). A computer program was written representing this model and using a patient's leg lengths to create an individualized range-of-motion profile. A standard cycle ergometer was used, a spindle was installed to allow for exchangeable crank arms of 80, 110, 140, and 170 mm. This allowed adjustment to achieve a specific range of motion for an individual patient.

Discussion.—A modified cycle ergometer was described as an alternative to continuous passive motion machines for patients after knee surgery. This equipment can be used for patients who lack knee motion as well as those who need a limited arc of motion in their therapeutic protocol. Clinical protocols are given for patients who may start full extension and those who must avoid it.

▶ This study presents a clever way to use cycle ergometry to expedite knee rehabilitation. I have often wondered if there could be a way found for patients to begin using the cycle ergometer before they can attain nearly full extension or flexion of the affected knee. These authors seem to have answered the question.—Col. J.L. Anderson, PE.D.

Spondylogenic Disorders in Gymnasts

Weber MD, Woodall WR (Univ of Mississippi, Jackson)
J Orthop Sports Phys Ther 14:6–13, 1991   1–11

Background.—Participation in gymnastics is increasing in the United States, and many of these athletes will sustain spondylogenic injuries. The evaluation and treatment of these injuries, including the mechanism of stress reaction in bone, were studied.

Etiology and Diagnosis.—Most pars fractures in gymnasts are stress fractures. The mechanism of these injuries is unknown. The first pain usually occurs during hyperextension, leading some clinicians to hypothesize that the injury results from hyperextension. It has also been suggested that the hypolordotic lumbar spine is at risk for flexion overload pars fracture because of the decreased angle of the posterior ligamentous system. Signs and symptoms are fairly consistent, almost always beginning with increasing low back pain, which is often noticed during a back walkover or flip. It is exaggerated by hyperextension or twisting. Single-leg standing with extension of the lumbar spine usually caused increased unilateral pain. Muscle strength and flexibility testing should be done, and simple radiographs can be diagnostic. If radiographs are negative, a technetium bone scan may show the stress reaction.

Treatment and Prevention.—Many treatments have been evaluated including restricted activity, bracing, casting, and surgical fusion. All of these are more successful in relieving symptoms than in achieving bony union. Rest and rehabilitation exercises are universally accepted; such a program should be started as soon as possible. The athlete must not return before completing adequate rehabilitation, or the stress fracture cy-

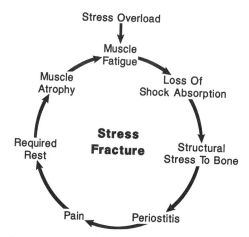

Fig 1–9.—Schematic representation of Clement's theory of the stress fracture cycle. (From Weber MD, Woodall WR: *J Orthop Sports Phys Ther* 14:6–13, 1991. Adapted from Clement DB: *Am J Sports Med* 2:81–85, 1974.)

cle will recur (Fig 1-9). Most reported programs have been vague, including pelvic tilts, knees to chest, and hamstring stretching. Lumbar spine stabilization exercises enhance neutral positioning of the lumbar spine and pelvis. Stabilization must be maintained through education when the athlete returns to limited practice. Advanced exercises must only be done when abdominal and paraspinal control of the spine is complete. Prevention is hard to discuss because the causative factors are not completely understood; however, most of the predisposing factors are modifiable, including hours of practice per week; muscular and skeletal imbalances; and repeated hyperextension, flexion, and rotation.

Conclusions.—Health-care professionals are likely to see more gymnasts with spondylogenic disorders. These conditions, including exercises for a spinal stabilization program, are examined.

▶ At West Point we have found that people with low back pain that is the result of muscular imbalance can be treated with an exercise protocol that brings both some immediate relief from pain and long-term rehabilitation that appears to ultimately eliminate the problem. This exercise procedure results in fully stretching the hamstring and lower back muscles and properly strengthening the buttocks and lumbar muscles. The exercises are performed while lying on your back, with a belt allowing optimum isolation of the lumbar muscles. This procedure has proved to be amazingly effective in hundreds of cases for the treatment of low back pain, with very little if any risk.—Col. J.L. Anderson, PE.D.

A Comparison of Three Muscle Pennation Assumptions and Their Effect on Isometric and Isotonic Force
Scott SH, Winter DA (University of Waterloo, Ontario)
J Biomechanics 24:163–167, 1991   1–12

Introduction.—Mathematical models that predict muscle forces have been used to clarify normal and abnormal movement patterns. Elaborate models that consider the complex architecture and spatial features of muscle and provide information on the internal structure of muscle have been developed, but these models are too complex to be of use in a generalized musculoskeletal model. Simpler models that provide computational ease have also been developed, but these contain assumptions and simplifications of the actual situation. The suitability of 3 representations of muscle pennation was analyzed.

Methods.—The pennation of a muscle is defined as the angle between muscle fibers and the line of action of the muscle. The effect of muscle pennation on muscle force output was modeled by using 3 different assumptions, and the error associated with each muscle pennation assumption was calculated. The first model assumed that pennation has little effect on force output and thus can be neglected. The second model assumed that the pennation angle remains constant. The third model assumed that pennation is variable and dependent on fiber length. To examine these 3 assumptions, a single unit length fiber located within a unipennate muscle was modeled with unity isometric maximal force. For each assumption fiber force/length and force/velocity characteristics were transformed to muscle properties.

Results.—The fixed pennation model provided the worst estimate of muscle force output for all conditions except for resting length isometric contractions. Neglecting muscle pennation entirely actually gave a better estimate of muscle force output. The assumption that the pennation angle changes with fiber length gave the smallest error and provided the best estimate of muscle force output. However, this variable pennation model slightly underestimated the true pennation change resulting from fiber length and did not perfectly mimic actual physiologic phenomena.

Conclusion.—A variable pennation model that assumes a constant muscle thickness and volume while attempting to correct for change in pennation angle most accurately predicts muscle force output for skeletal muscles.

▶ These authors, Scott and Winter, have reported that the models used in this study calculated the error associated with different muscle pennation assumptions. They found it surprising that the fixed pennation model provides the worst estimate of muscle force output for all situations except resting length isometric contractions. In fact, a better estimate of force output would be provided by neglecting muscle pennation entirely. The model that assumes a constant volume and thickness and attempts to correct for change in pennation angle provided the best fit to the regression curve results. However, they determined that the variable pennation model slightly underestimates the true pennation change caused by fiber length and thus does not perfectly follow the physiologic phenomena.—Col. J.L. Anderson, PE.D.

The Relationship Between Muscle Kinetic Parameters and Kinematic Variables in a Complex Movement
Jarić S, Ristanović D, Corcos DM (Institute for Medical Research, Belgrade, Yugoslavia; School of Medicine, Belgrade; Univ of Illinois, Chicago)
Eur J Appl Physiol 59:370–376, 1989   1–13

Introduction.—In the field of sports medicine, a number of analytical methods have been used to determine the relative contribution of a muscle group to the performance of a complex human movement. The relative contribution of active muscle groups to the complex movement mechanics should be separable into the effects of their particular kinetic parameters. Kinematic variables of the vertical jump were measured in a group of trained subjects.

Patients and Methods.—Participants included 39 young men (aged 20–22 years) who were physical education students. All had considerable experience in the vertical jump exercise and in an additional isometric force exertion task. In the first part of the experiment, kinematic variables from a maximal voluntary vertical jump in the standing erect position with the preparatory counter-movement (the counter movement jump) were measured. Then, in isometric conditions, kinetic parameters of the hip and knee extensors and the plantar flexors were recorded for the same subjects.

Results.—There were significant positive correlations between kinetic parameters of the active muscle groups and jumping height. Knee extensors were responsible for the dominant effect on these correlations. The correlations between these parameters and the duration of the jump phases were much weaker. Fast force production in 1 muscle group was related to a significant decrease in the joint angles of distant body segments. Kinetic parameters appear to explain more than 25% of the variability in the jump.

Conclusions.—Future investigations of complex human movements could show how certain parameters, derived from the musculoskeletal system, determine the performance of these movements. Such results would be of value to coaches, rehabilitation therapists, and designers of exercise programs.

▶ The authors of this study understand that because they found significant coefficients of correlation between these kinetic and kinematic parameters does not necessarily mean there exists a causal relationship. They understand that only through further research of complex human movements, using other variables such as force-velocity relationships, angle-torque measurements, and anthropometric measurements, can we more accurately understand human movement.—Col. J.L. Anderson, PE.D.

A Correlation Between Muscular Strength and Hydroxyproline Concentration in Human Patellar Tendon
Lemley PV, Welch MJ (U.S. Military Academy, West Point, NY)
J Sports Med Phys Fitness 31:104–107, 1991   1–14

Introduction.—Athletes, particularly those involved in contact sports, often injure the connective tissue of the knee. It would be important in the prevention of injury and in the strategy of physical fitness training to know whether the connective tissue is modified in response to athletic stress or training. Preliminary studies in immobilized rabbits suggested that changes in the connective tissue of the knee do occur. The present study was designed to investigate whether collagen in the connective tissue of the knee changes in response to athletic stress or training. Specifically, a correlation was sought between a variability in the concentration of hydroxyproline and leg strength parameters.

Methods.—Four men and 1 woman with a mean age of 21 years underwent anterior cruciate ligament (ACL) reconstruction during which the patella tendon was removed from the knee. All patients were actively participating in a vigorous physical fitness program and playing a sport before their knee injury. Leg strength data from the nonoperated legs were obtained an average of $4\frac{1}{2}$ months after operation. The samples of patella tendon tissue were used to determine the concentration of hydroxyproline, a posttranslationally modified amino acid found mainly in collagen protein.

Results.—No correlation was found between concentrations of hydroxyproline in the samples of patellar tendon and any of the leg strength parameters measured. These findings suggest that the concentration of hydroxyproline in connective tissue is not modified in response to athletic stress or training, but rather it appears to be relatively constant across a range of leg strengths.

Conclusion.—Further studies are needed to determine what type of biochemical modification does occur if there is modification in the connective tissue of the knee in response to athletic stress or training.

▶ Although the investigators lacked enough subjects to allow them to draw strong conclusions, this study is included here because it presents an interesting protocol that might be adopted or adapted by other researchers who are interested in studying injuries to the connective tissue. Understanding what type of biochemical modification occurs, if any, may be important in injury risk assessment, enzyme therapy, and injury prevention, and in tailoring strategies of physical fitness strategies.—Col. J.L. Anderson, PE.D.

Effect of Propelling Surface Size on the Mechanics and Energetics of Front Crawl Swimming
Toussaint HM, Janssen T, Kluft M (Vrije Universiteit, Amsterdam, The Netherlands)
J Biomech 24:205–211, 1991   1–15

Background.—Swimmers create propulsive force by giving a velocity change to masses of water. However, in so doing, they transfer energy to the water that is not used for propulsion. In theory, increasing the size of the propelling surface should reduce this loss of energy (Fig 1–10). The effect of enlarging the propelling surface artificially with paddles was evaluated.

Methods.—The subjects were 6 male and 4 female nationally and internationally competitive swimmers, all of whom trained at least 6 hours per week. Subjects performed several 400-meter swims at varying velocities, swimming each velocity once with and once without paddles. The stroke used was the front crawl with arms alone, the legs being floated with a small buoy. In each swim, the rate of energy expenditure, or

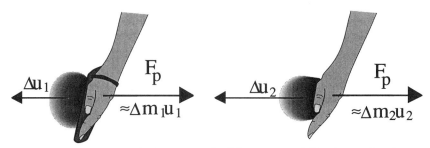

Fig 1–10.—In swimming, a fixed point to push off from is not available. The propulsive force is generated by pushing off against masses of water and will equal the impluse (mΔu) of the pushed away water. During the push-off, energy ($\frac{1}{2}m\Delta u^2$) is transferred from the swimmer to the water. A propulsive force generated by giving a big mass of water a small velocity change will cost less energy compared with the same force generated by giving a small mass of water a large velocity change. This may be accomplished by artificially enlarging the hands with paddles. (Courtesy of Toussaint HM, Janssen T, Kluft M: *J Biomech* 24:205–211, 1991.)

power input; power output; work per stroke cycle; distance per stroke cycle; work per unit distance; and propelling efficiency were measured.

Results.—Use of paddles decreased power input by 6%, power output by 7.6%, and work per unit distance by 7.5% at the same average velocity. It increased propelling efficiency by 7.8% and work per stroke cycle by 7%. Power transferred to the water decreased from 27.1 to 21.7 W, and propelling efficiency increased from 63.7% to 69%. The actual increase in distance per stroke cycle and the decrease in stroke cycle frequency precisely matched the predicted values.

Conclusions.—Swimming with paddles can maintain velocity with a 6% decrease in energy expenditure. Paddle swimming may be a useful and rather specific form of strength training for competitive swimmers.

▶ Swim paddles such as these have been used by a number of American swimming coaches to help swimmers strengthen their arms and shoulders. However, I doubt that many have had the opportunity to see the scientific explanation that is presented by these authors.—Col. J.L. Anderson, PE.D.

The Effect of Pre-Performance Massage on Stride Frequency in Sprinters
Harmer PA (Willamette Univ, Salem, Oreg)
Athlet Train, JNATA 26:55–59, 1991   1–16

Background.—Precompetition massage is often done on the assumption that it will improve the athlete's performance or decrease the likelihood of injury. Studies of the efficacy of massage have had conflicting results. The effects of preperformance massage on stride frequency in male sprinters were assessed.

Methods.—Subjects were 14 trained sprinters, mean age 21.6 years. Two 10-second trials of maximal running in place were performed on 2 successive days. On the first day, 1 group performed both trials without massage and the other group received a massage by a licensed massage technician before the trials. The groups were reversed on the second day. Exercise was performed on a force platform, and stride frequency was determined by counting the vertical component of the ground reaction force.

Results.—Stride frequency scores tended to decrease from the first to the second trial in all testing periods. There was no difference between scores after and without massage. All subjects had a positive response to massage, however, and felt that it allowed them to cope better with physical exertion. Some stated that massage could improve their performance for several days afterward.

Conclusions.—Stride frequency is not significantly increased by preperformance massage. Use of massage as an ergogenic aid should be the responsibility of the coach or the athletes, rather than the athletic trainer. However, trainers may wish to consider the affective benefits of massage.

▶ In this study massage did not improve the stride frequency of sprinters. I agree with the author's statement that massage as a performance ergogenic aid should not be the responsibility of the athletic trainer. We do use massage in many forms to treat our injured athletes. Please read Abstract 1–17 and my comments on the physiologic effects of massage.—F.J. George, A.T.C., P.T.

A Physiologic Evaluation of the Sports Massage
Boone T, Cooper R, Thompson WR (Univ of Southern Mississippi, Hattiesburg)
Athlet Train, JNATA 26:51–54, 1991   1–17

Background.—Massage is widely agreed to be an important part of coaching and athletic conditioning, but its physiologic benefits remain unproved. A study was done to determine whether massage has positive physiologic responses during submaximal exercise and whether these responses are central or peripheral in origin.

Methods.—Subjects were 10 healthy male volunteers, mean age 28 years. All subjects performed submaximal treadmill exercise designed to elicit 80% of their maximal heart rates, both with and without prior 30-minute massage. Steady-state responses were determined by the Beckman Metabolic Measurement Chart; cardiac output was assessed by indirect cardon dioxide Fick Method; and mixed venous carbon dioxide pressure (tension) was calculated by the equilibrium carbon dioxide rebreathing method.

Results.—Exercise performance did not improve with massage. Heart rate, stroke volume, cardiac output, and arteriovenous oxygen responses were not significantly different between the 2 exercise sessions, suggesting that exercise oxygen consumption was derived from similar central and peripheral adjustments. There were no significant differences in lactic acid or blood pressure responses.

Conclusions.—Massage performed immediately before submaximal exercise appears to have no cardiovascular effects. Claims made for the physiologic benefits of massage thus appear to be questionable.

▶ Please read Abstract 1–16 for related information on the use of massage as an ergogenic aid. The present study is another one that rejects any theory that preperformance massage has any beneficial cardiovascular effects on submaximal exercise. Many athletes do state that massage helps them perform better; however, the benefits may be more psychological than physiologic.—F.J. George, A.T.C., P.T.

The Intensity of Exercise in Deep-Water Running
Ritchie SE, Hopkins WG (University of Otago, Dunedin, New Zealand)
Int J Sports Med 12:27–29, 1991   1–18

Background.—Deep-water running (DWR) has gained in popularity as a training exercise for runners because it appears to cause less musculoskeletal stress than normal running. However, its effectiveness, particularly as an endurance training activity, is unclear. The maximum achievable intensity of DWR was compared to that of running.

Methods.—The subjects were 8 male runners, 2 of whom were experienced and 6 of whom were inexperienced in DWR. The inexperienced runners received 1 training session in the technique of DWR. Buoyancy vests were not used. Over 2 weeks, the subjects performed DWR 3 times, 20 minutes at the first session and 30 minutes for the latter 2 sessions. Oxygen consumption ($\dot{V}O_2$), respiratory quotient (RQ), heart rate, perceived effort, and aches and pains in the legs were monitored to assess intensity. The findings were compared to those of 30-minute runs on a treadmill at difficult and normal paces and a 30-minute outdoor run at normal pace.

Results.—At the last session of DWR, $\dot{V}O_2$ reached 73% of maximum. This was not significantly different from the 78% $\dot{V}O_2$ of the difficult treadmill run but was significantly higher than the 62% $\dot{V}O_2$ of the normal treadmill run. Comparisons of RQ, perceived effort, and aches and pains gave similar results. Heart rate, however, was similar in DWR and normal training and significantly lower in DWR than in the difficult treadmill run.

Conclusions.—Performed hard enough and long enough, DWR can achieve a level of exercise intensity sufficient to maintain or improve aerobic power. The observed disparity in $\dot{V}O_2$ and heart rate may result from cooling or increased venous return. Deep-water running may not be specific for training of competitive runners. Use of a buoyancy vest may result in a lower exercise intensity.

▶ Many of our runners have been using DWR in their regular training schedule to prevent injuries and as an alternative workout when they are injured. We have been using buoyancy vests for this training. After reading this study, I will discuss the removal of the vests with our track coach in an attempt to increase the intensity of the workout. We are well aware of the authors' "slight reservations about the specificity of DWR for the training of competitive runners." However, we feel the benefits of DWR for preventing injury, or for continuance of training when injured, outweigh the reservations.—F.J. George, A.T.C., P.T.

Torque Development in Insokinetic Training
Esselman PC, de Lateur BJ, Alquist AD, Questad KA, Giaconi RM, Lehmann JF (Univ of Washington, Seattle)
Arch Phys Med Rehabil 72:723–728, 1991   1–19

Background.—In skeletal muscle, torque decreases as concentric velocity increases. There are varying reports about the velocity at which torque is gained in response to isokinetic training. Torque gains and

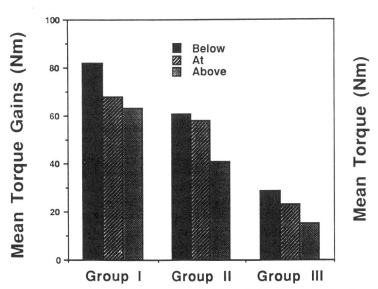

Fig 1–11.—Pretraining to posttraining mean torque gains at velocities faster than (*above*), equal to (*at*), and slower than (*below*) the training velocity, calculated for each group. (Courtesy of Esselman PC, de Lateur BJ, Alquist AD, et al: *Arch Phys Med Rehabil* 72:723-728, 1991.)

muscle adaptations in men performing an isokinetic training program were studied, including the effects of training velocity.

Methods.—Twenty healthy men (mean age, 27 years) were randomized into 4 groups; 3 groups performed maximal isokinetic knee extensions 5 days a week for 12 weeks, and the fourth group served as a non-exercise control. For each subject, the protocol was different for the opposite lower extremity: group I trained at 36 degrees per second with 20 or 60 repetitions; group II trained at 36 degrees per second with 20 repetitions with 1 limb, and at 108 degrees per second with 60 repetitions with the other limb; and group III trained at 108 degrees per second with 20 or 60 repetitions. Biopsies of the vastus lateralis muscle were performed before and after training, and the specimens were examined for muscle fiber area and enzyme activity. Every 2 weeks during the study, maximal torque velocity tests were done from 0 to 234 degrees per second at intervals of 18 degrees per second.

Results.—On analysis of the torque-velocity curves, the men who trained at 36 degrees per second made significant gains in torque overall and in comparison with those who trained at 108 degrees per second (Fig 1–11). Those gains occurred mainly during the first 4–8 weeks of training. Muscle fiber area did not increase significantly, but glycolytic and mitochondrial enzyme activity did.

Conclusion.—At least in isokinetic training, the amount of torque developed during training appears to be the most important variable for developing strength. If eccentric contractions are the stimulus for muscle hypertrophy, this stimulus would not be provided. Neural factors also play an important role. The contralateral effect seems more important in strength gain than any direct effect of performing more repetitions; however, this does not confound the main findings of the present study.

▶ The authors of this abstract have reinforced the concept that torque is more important than velocity when attempting to develop strength with an isokinetic training program. They go on to state that "if isokinetic training is being used as part of a general training program, even for a sport or activity that requires rapid muscular movements, isokinetic training at low velocity would probably contribute to optimal performance as long as specific skill training in that sport was a significant portion of the training."—F.J. George, A.T.C., P.T.

The Relationships Among Isometric, Isotonic, and Isokinetic Concentric and Eccentric Quadriceps and Hamstring Force and Three Components of Athletic Performance
Anderson MA, Gieck JH, Perrin D, Weltman A, Rutt R, Denegar C (Univ of Oklahoma Health Science Ctr, Oklahoma City; Univ of Virginia, Charlottes-

ville; Texas Woman's Univ, Dallas; and Slippery Rock Univ, Penn)
J Orthop Sports Phys Ther 14:114–120, 1991   1–20

Introduction.—Quadriceps and hamstring force variables were assessed for predictability of athletic performance. Three components of athletic performance were examined.

Methods.—Thirty-nine college-aged male athletes were evaluated for bilateral quadriceps and hamstring muscle torque for concentric, eccentric, isotonic, and isometric contractions. Vertical jump performance, 40-yard dash time, and agility run time were used to assess athletic performance.

Results.—Quadriceps and hamstring force and vertical jump were not significantly correlated. The 40-yard dash time significantly correlated with right peak isokinetic concentric hamstring force at 60 degrees/second, and agility run time correlated with left mean isokinetic eccentric hamstring force at 90 degrees/second.

Conclusions.—Little functional relationship was discovered between the ability to generate quadriceps or hamstring force and athletic performance in 3 specific events.

▶ When I read the title of this abstract, I did expect to find a higher relationship between quadriceps force and athletic performance. It was interesting to note that, for different legs and different speeds, hamstring force was correlated with the 40-yard dash time and the agility run, and quadriceps force was not. However, in the authors conclusions, they state, "there is little, if any, functional relationship between the ability to generate quadriceps or hamstring force and the 40-yard dash, vertical jump, or the agility run."—F.J. George, A.T.C., P.T.

The Effect of Eccentric Strength Training at Various Speeds on Concentric Strength of the Quadriceps and Hamstring Muscles
Bishop KN, Durrant E, Allsen PE, Merrill G (Cleveland State Univ; Brigham Young Univ, Provo, Utah)
J Orthop Sports Phys Ther 13:226–230, 1991   1–21

Background.—Controversy has arisen as to the benefits of the increased use of eccentric contractions in strength training. Whether an isokinetic eccentric strength training program could improve concentric strength of the quadriceps and hamstring muscles and whether there was a differential effect at the speeds of 60 and 180 degrees/second was investigated in 43 male college students enrolled in a physical fitness class.

Methods.—Pretesting of the concentric strength of the subjects' dominant legs was done using a Kinetic Communicator dynamometer at speeds of 60 and 180 degrees/second. Subjects were then divided into 3 groups: the 2 treatment groups trained the dominant leg 3 times/week for 8 weeks at either 60 or 180 degrees/second and the control group did not train. Subjects evaluated their muscle soreness before each training session, and treatment effects were assessed by a concentric posttest.

Results.—The subjects' ability to participate in the eccentric training program was not affected by delayed muscle soreness. Both training groups showed no significant improvement in quadriceps strength. Concentric hamstring strength, however, was significantly increased in both groups. Most muscle soreness was reported during the first week of training.

Conclusions.—Concentric hamstring strength can be developed by eccentric training; the effectiveness of this training is unaffected by training speed. Eccentric training should be an ideal method for rehabilitation of the injured hamstring. Allowing a day of rest between training sessions can avoid extensive muscle pain.

▶ The authors recommend that eccentric training be used for rehabilitating hamstring injuries. They also recommend a day of rest between eccentric training sessions to avoid delayed onset muscle soreness. We have made a change in the positioning of our patients with hamstring injuries when exercising. To work the muscles in a more functional position, we have the athletes do their exercises standing or prone. We rarely use the sitting position for strengthening hamstring muscles.—F.J. George, A.T.C., P.T.

Comparison of Isokinetic Strength and Flexibility Measures Between Hamstring Injured and Noninjured Athletes
Worrell TW, Perrin DH, Gansneder BM, Gieck HJ (Univ of Virginia, Charlottesville)
J Orthop Sports Phys Ther 13:118–125, 1991   1–22

Background.—Hamstring injuries are common in sports that require maximal running, and they appear to be associated with a high rate of reinjury. Isokinetic strength and flexibility were compared in athletes with and without a history of hamstring injury.

Methods.—Thirty-two highly skilled male athletes, mean age 20.7 years, were studied. Sixteen of the athletes who had a history of hamstring injury were matched for motor dominance, sport, and position played to 16 athletes who had no history of hamstring injury. Both groups were tested on a Kinetic Communicator dynamometer for concentric and eccentric quadriceps and hamstring peak torque and reciprocal muscle groups ratios. Testing speeds were 60 degrees/second and 180 degrees/second. Each athlete's knee was also passively extended with the hip in 90 degrees of flexion to determine hamstring flexibility.

Results.—On hamstring strength analysis, greater strength values were obtained during eccentric than concentric testing. On analysis of variance, the injured extremity was significantly less flexible than the uninjured extremity within the hamstring injured group. This group also had significantly less flexibility than the noninjured group. The 2 groups showed no significant differences in strength on any isokinetic measure. The hamstring-injured group was symptomatic and had a high rate of reinjury.

Conclusions.—In athletes with a history of hamstring injury, hamstring flexibility is less than in athletes with no history of hamstring injury, and the injured extremity is less flexible than the noninjured extremity. Clinically, accurate and periodic assessment of hamstring flexibility and a supervised hamstring stretching program are recommended. More research is needed on the role of hamstring strength and flexibility, and hamstring stretching techniques should be reevaluated.

▶ This study supports the concept that the lack of hamstring flexibility is the most important cause of hamstring injuries. It also indicates that hamstring stretching and flexibility programs now being used are either not appropriate or are not being done properly. Athletes with prior hamstring injuries must be supervised and instructed in proper hamstring flexibility programs. We have found that using a contract-relax type of proprioceptive neuromuscular facilitation program can be beneficial for these athletes. Many of these athletes tend to return to participation too soon, before they are completely rehabilitated, and are often reinjured. The best advice to give a hamstring-injured athlete is to *avoid reinjury.*—F.J. George, A.T.C., P.T.

Dynamic Joint Forces During Knee Isokinetic Exercise

Kaufman KR, An K-N, Litchy WJ, Morrey BF, Chao EYS (Mayo Clinic and Found, Rochester, Minn; Children's Hosp and Health Ctr, San Diego)
Am J Sports Med 19:305–315, 1991   1–23

Introduction.—Rehabilitation is an important aspect of treating knee injuries and isokinetic exercise has been widely used in rehabilitation as well as in conditioning and research. An analytical biomechanical model was used to analyze forces in the tibiofemoral and patellofemoral joints during isokinetic exercise in 5 men (mean age, 27 years) who took part in the study. None of the men had previously undergone surgery or had a history of knee disorders.

Methods.—A triaxial electrogoniometer, mounted on the individual's knee, was used to measure angular displacement of the knee and 3-dimensional motion of the lower limb. A load was provided by a Cybex II isokinetic dynamometer, and a load cell placed on the Cybex arm measured the 3 orthogonal force components acting on the shank.

Results.—A biomechanical model predicted the dynamic forces generated during isokinetic exercise. This exericse was shown to produce large loads on the tibiofemoral and patellofemoral joints, especially during extension exercises. The tibiofemoral compressive force (4 body weight) during isokinetic exercise approximates that obtained during walking, but occurs at 55% of knee flexion. Anterior shear forces exist during extension and load the anterior cruciate ligament between 40 degrees of knee flexion and full extension. The maximum posterior shear force, 1.7 body weight, occurred at a knee position of 75 degrees during the flexion portion of isokinetic exercise.

Conclusion.—The joint forces occurring during knee isokinetic exercise are not high compared with those experienced during athletic events. Nevertheless, these results suggest that this form of exercise should be used with care in patients with knee injuries or abnormalities. Forces in the patellofemoral joint, for example, reached a level of 5.1 body weight at 70–75 degrees of knee flexion, about 10 times the force generated by level walking or straight leg raises.

▶ This is a superb study and was the recipient of the 1989 American Orthopaedic Society for Sports Medicine award for excellence in research. The original paper is recommended reading for all those involved in knee surgery and rehabilitation.—J.S. Torg, M.D.

Mechanisms Underlying the Training Effects Associated With Neuromuscular Electrical Stimulation

Trimble MH, Enoka RM (Indiana Univ, Bloomington; Univ of Arizona, Tucson)
Phys Ther 71:273–282, 1991   1–24

Introduction.—Neuromuscular electrical stimulation (NMES) can increase muscle strength in appropriate conditions, but the mechanism is uncertain. Activation of muscle occurs by a different means in NMES and voluntary control. The recruitment order of motor units elicited by over-the-muscle electrical stimulation was studied to ascertain whether it is different from that in voluntary activation.

Methods.—Muscle twitch response elicited by Hoffman reflexes (H-reflexes) and direct motor responses (M-responses) was compared in 22 volunteers, 15 men and 7 women, ranging in age from 19–53 years. In addition, the effect of submotor NMES on twitch force associated with H-reflexes was examined. Variation in the time to peak twitch force indicated changes in the population of motor units contributing to the response, because H-reflexes represent the summed activity of many motor units in a way consistent with volitional action.

Results.—Peak force and time to peak force were similar in H-reflex-elicited twitches in both the quadriceps femoris and triceps surae. Both parameters changed with stimulus strength, and time to peak force decreased as peak force increased. In M-responses, however, time to peak twitch force increased with stimulus strength, with significant variation in time to peak force and peak force across stimulus intensity. Percutaneous application of NMES thus activated a faster-contracting set of motor units during H-reflex.

Conclusion.—Neuromuscular electrical stimulation appears to preferentially activate faster-contracting motor units, possibly those that are normally active at high intensities of voluntary exercise. The mechanisms of these alterations involve direct activation of large efferent axons and the feedback effects of cutaneous afferents. High-threshold motor units may be trained more effectively with NMES, in conjunction or alternation with voluntary exercise.

▶ In response to a commentary on their study, the authors state in their conclusion "that submaximal electrical stimulation of nerve results in the activation of a faster contracting population of motor units than that associated with a submaximal voluntary activation has profound clinical applications." They explain that "NMES may provide a therapeutic means to activate high threshold motor units that are normally only activated under voluntary conditions at high exercise intensities." Please read Abstract 1–25 for related information.—F.J. George, A.T.C., P.T.

The Effect of Electrical Stimulation on Isometric and Isokinetic Knee Extension Torque: Interaction of the Kinestim Electrical Stimulator and the Cybex II+
Locicero RD (Crowl Physical Therapy Ctr, Inc, Sacramento, Calif)
J Orthop Sports Phys Ther 13:143–148, 1991   1–25

Background.—Kots et al. reported that electrical stimulation increased muscle strength 30% to 40% more than conventional training methods. While electrical stimulation strengthens muscles, isometric or isokinetic strength changes with electrical stimulation are no greater than with conventional training. The Kinestim electrical stimulator's ability to induce an isometric contraction torque of the quadriceps was evaluated. The differences in torque production during maximal volitional contraction (MVC) and electrical stimulation with MVC during isometric and isokinetic knee extension were compared.

Methods.—Thirty healthy volunteers participated in a practice session and a testing session. The Kinestim electrical stimulator delivered a 2,500-Hz, sinusoidal waveform current modulated to 50 bursts per second to the quadriceps femoris musculature.

Results.—During the superimposed contraction (SC) conditions, torque output ranged from 93% to 104% MVC. At 0 degrees per second and 240 degrees per second, there was no difference in torque production between the SC and the MVC; but at 60 degrees per second, it was significantly less for SC than MVC.

Conclusions.—Isometric and isokinetic SCs produced a high percentage of a subject's MVC torque but did not produce a torque higher than volitional contraction. Isometric SC torque production was similar to isometric MVC torque production. Isokinetic torque production was significantly less for SC than MVC at 60 degrees per second but not at 240 degrees per second.

▶ The authors of this abstract comment on a study done by Williams et al., which states that isokinetic strength gains after ES training appear to be speed specific because the ES group showed gains at faster speeds (240 and 300 degrees/second) and the control group did not (1). Please read Abstract 1–24 and the conclusion that NMES activates high-threshold motor units and the clinical implications.—F.J. George, A.T.C., P.T.

Reference

1. Williams RA, et al: *J Orthop Sports Phys Ther* 8:143.

Exercise-Induced Muscle Soreness After Concentric and Eccentric Isokinetic Contractions
Fitzgerald GK, Rothstein JM, Mayhew TP, Lamb RL (Virginia Commonwealth Univ, Richmond; Univ of Illinois at Chicago)
Phys Ther 71:505–513, 1991   1–26

Background.—Some reports have indicated that exercises involving eccentric muscle contractions result in greater muscle soreness than those that involve mainly concentric contractions. The effect of isokinetic exercises has not been evaluated. Two experiments were done to determine whether there are any differences in muscle soreness between subjects who perform concentric and eccentric isokinetic quadriceps femoris exercises.

Methods.—Experiment 1 involved 20 nondisabled volunteers who were randomly assigned to perform either eccentric or concentric exercises at a power level of 90% of the maximum power produced during concentric quadriceps contractions. Experiment 2 involved 20 different subjects who were randomly assigned to perform either concentric or eccentric muscle contractions at maximum effort, with no specific power level. Muscle soreness was rated on a visual analogue scale immediately before exercise and 24 and 48 hours afterward. One-way analysis of variance was used to compare changes in muscle soreness ratings between exercise groups in both experiments.

Results.—In groups exercising at equal power levels, there was no difference in the change in muscle soreness before and after exercise. However, greater increases in muscle soreness were noted in subjects who performed eccentric contractions at maximal effort compared with those who performed concentric contractions.

Conclusions.—The dependent factor in producing exercise-induced muscle soreness appears to be the intensity rather than the type of the muscle contraction. Subjects who perform eccentric isokinetic contractions appear to have greater changes in muscle soreness at 24 hours than those who perform concentric isokinetic contractions at maximal effort. This is probably because greater torque is produced during eccentric isokinetic contractions than during concentric isokinetic contractions at maximal effort.

▶ This study indicates that the degree of exercise-induced muscle soreness is determined by the intensity of the isokinetic exercise performed rather than by the type of exercise (i.e., eccentric or concentric). The authors recommend that either concentric or eccentric exercises can be done without experiencing delayed-onset muscle soreness if the exercise is controlled and submaximal.—F.J. George, A.T.C., P.T.

Effects of Ultrasound and Trolamine Salicylate Phonophoresis on Delayed-Onset Muscle Soreness
Ciccone CD, Leggin BG, Callamaro JJ (Ithaca College NY)
Phys Ther 71:666–678, 1991   1–27

Background.—In phonophoresis, ultrasound is used to drive a drug through the skin and into underlying tissue. It has the potential advantage, therefore, of delivering a drug in a relatively safe, pain-free, easy fashion to structures lying deep within the body. The effects of ultrasound and phonophoresis on delayed-onset muscle soreness (DOMS) were tested using an anti-inflammatory/analgesic cream.

Methods.—Delayed-onset muscle soreness was induced in the elbow flexors of 40 college-aged women through repeated eccentric contractions. The women were randomly assigned in equal numbers to 1 of 4 groups. Group 1 received sham ultrasound and placebo cream; group 2, sham ultrasound and trolamine salicylate cream; group 3, ultrasound and placebo cream; and group 4, ultrasound plus trolamine salicylate cream. Treatment was applied on 3 consecutive days. Before each treatment, muscle soreness and active elbow range of motion was assessed.

Results.—Delayed-onset muscle soreness was increased in group 3 but not in group 4. The ultrasound enhancement of DOMS therefore appeared to be offset by the anti-inflammatory/analgesic action of salicylate phonophoresis. Soreness was not reduced in the arms of women receiving daily treatments of only ultrasound or only salicylate cream (Fig 1–12).

Conclusions.—Used alone, ultrasound increases the symptoms associated with DOMS. The ability of ultrasound to enhance the mechanisms underlying DOMS, however, seemed to be offset by the pharmacologic activity of trolamine salicylate. The technique of salicylate phonophoresis

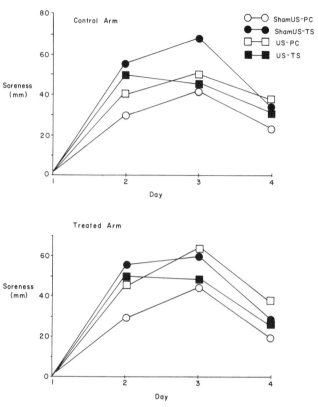

Fig 1–12.—Ratings of elbow flexor soreness in control (untreated) and treated arms of 4 subject groups on days 2-4 of the study. (Courtesy of Ciccone CD, Leggin BG, Callamaro JJ: *Phys Ther* 71:666-678, 1991.)

may be indicated when a clinician wishes to administer ultrasound without promoting cellular changes that mimic an inflammatory response.

▶ Susan Michlovitz, M.S., P.T., has written a commentary to this study that questioned the use of DOMS as a model for studying the effects of ultrasound and trolamine salicylate (1). She did agree with the authors that, because of the addition of heat from ultrasound, the symptoms of DOMS may be exacerbated. Because of this she recommends that ultrasound be used for its nonthermal effects during the acute stages of an injury. She did commend the authors for including a sham ultrasound-salicylate group in their study. She recommends that we plan ultrasound treatments carefully and that we scrutinize the use of phonophoresis.—F.J. George, A.T.C., P.T.

Reference

1. Michlovitz S: *Phys Ther* 71:675, 1991.

Does the Pressor Response to Ischemic Exercise Improve Blood Flow to Contracting Muscles in Humans?
Joyner MJ (Mayo Clinic and Found, Rochester, Minn)
J Appl Physiol 71:1496–1501, 1991   1–28

Background.—Inadequate blood flow and oxygen delivery to rhythmically contracting skeletal muscles can elicit reflex increases in arterial blood pressure. The gain in reflex pressor response that occurs when perfusion pressure to rhythmically contracting muscles is reduced was determined. Also, whether the pressor response improves blood flow to the contracting muscles was investigated.

Methods.—Six normal subjects performed light, moderate, and heavy rhythmic forearm contractions at a rate of 30/minute with the forearm enclosed in a Plexiglas box. Pressure in the box was increased by 10 mm Hg each minute up to 50 mm Hg to reduce transmural pressure in the arterial system of the forearm. The mean arterial pressure (MAP) was measured continuously.

Findings.—During light exercise there was no reflex increase in MAP until box pressure reached 50 mm HG, but MAP increased with box pressure increases on only 10–20 mm Hg during moderate or heavy exercise. The gain in reflex pressor responses observed during moderate and heavy exercise was less than that observed in experiments on dogs. Oxygen saturation was measured to assess how a 50 mm Hg increase in box pressure and subsequent reflex increase in MAP altered the blood flow to the contracting muscles during heavy rhythmic exercise. Although the increased box pressure evoked a pressor response, the increase in arterial pressure failed to improve the delivery of oxygen to the contracting muscles.

Conclusions.—The gain of reflex increases in arterial pressure in response to reductions in muscle perfusion pressure was less in human beings than in previous dog studies. During exercise with reduced muscle blood flow the increased sympathetic outflow evoked by chemosensitive afferent activation can constrict resistance vessels in contracting muscles sufficiently to prevent the increases in MAP from improving blood flow to the working muscles.

▶ The compressing force that is developed by a contracting muscle begins to occlude local blood flow when effort exceeds 15%–25% of maximal voluntary force, and occlusion becomes complete at about 70% of maximal voluntary force. The local accumulation of metabolites stimulates a reflex increase of blood pressure and heart rate, and it has been held that this counters the local compressing force of the muscles, restoring muscle blood flow. Some evidence in support of this hypothesis was obtained by Kay and Shephard (1). During moderate aerobic exercise (around 70% of maximal oxygen intake), lactate at first accumulated, but later plateaued and gradually declined as systemic blood pressures rose. However, given that the phenomenon was only observed at a relatively low intensity of aerobic exercise, the increase of pressure was plainly only effective in countering a moderate compressing force. Moreover, because the exercise was aerobic in type, the subjects were able to sustain it for an extended period, giving full scope to the local vasodilator action of accumulating metabolites.

The present paper shows that the response of the systemic blood pressure to external compression of the muscle vascular supply is not fixed, the intensity of the response being enhanced by moderate or vigorous exercise. This reflects our current understanding of the circulation during vigorous exercise: there is a general peripheral vascular constriction that is reversed locally in the active muscles as metabolites accumulate. The evidence that blood flow was not increased by the rise of systemic pressure was derived from a drop in the oxygen saturation of blood collected from a deep vein (30%–33% falling to 15%–16%, and interpreted as a 20%–25% reduction of flow). However, the increment of pressure under discussion (< 20 mm Hg) was much less than might be expected during very vigorous bouts of exercise. It would be interesting to know whether blood flow was better compensated in situations where large increases of blood pressure developed and the venous effluent had already dropped to a minimum value.—R.J. Shephard, M.D., Ph.D., D.P.E.

Reference

1. Kay C, Shephard RJ: *Int Z Angew Physiol* 27:311, 1969.

2 Growth, Aging, Female Athletes

Survey of Health Care Available to Child Athletes
Bennett JT, Urmson L, Binder AJ, Brunet ME, Thomas KA (Tulane Univ, New Orleans)
Orthopaed Rev 20:983–988, 1991   2–1

Background.—Children and adolescents commonly participate in sports activities in the United States, but they often are coached by volunteers who lack expertise in treating athletic injuries. A questionnaire was drafted to determine the number and characteristics of sports medicine clinics throughout the United States designed to treat the child athlete.

Methods.—The survey defined a child athlete as being between the ages of 4 and 12 years. The questionnaire was sent to the directors and administrators of 84 children's hospitals and 397 sports medicine clinics that cared for 4- to 12-year-old athletes. The hospitals and clinics were free-standing, part of a university, or a section of a general hospital.

Results.—Of the 481 facilities identified, 209 responded (43%) to the survey. Sixty of the 209 stated they did provide care for the child athlete. Fourteen offered separate clinic services for the child athlete, representing 25% of their outpatient visits. Of these 14 institutions, 3 were part of a children's hospital, 4 were associated with a university medical center, 2 were located in a general hospital, and 5 were free-standing sports medicine clinics. The patients actually treated in these 14 facilities were older, with most falling into the 11- to 20-year-old categories. The most common presenting symptoms were musculoskeletal injuries, particularly sprains and strains. In the 14 specialized clinics, the young patient had easier access to orthopedists, pediatricians, and cardiologists than at the 46 affiliated facilities that stated they treated children's sports injuries. Most of the centers (85%) were established to fill a community need, and most (74%) were funded by private insurance. About 35% of the injuries could have been treated by a primary care physician, but 77% of respondents believed that the children benefited from the specialized care in terms of eduction, injury prevention, proper use and fitting of sports equipment, and on-field management of injuries.

Implications.—Most of the sports medicine clinics surveyed had provided services for 5 years, were need-based, and were located in cities with more than 100,000 inhabitants. Most institutions without specific sports medicine programs for young children indicated that no such clinic existed in the community.

▶ It appears that the lack of health care available to a child athlete is of significantly lesser import when compared to the availability of acute medical care for the pediatric population in general. As pointed out in a recent cover story by *U.S. News and World Report* (Jan. 27, 1992), "most hospitals and rescue squads aren't really prepared to deal with childrens' medical crises." The article further points out that "every day, some of America's children die, or almost die, because they are taken to the wrong hospital, treated with improper equipment, given wrong doses of medicine, or not diagnosed properly." This article in a lay publication clearly defines the scope of the greater problem, putting the question of availability of health care for the child athlete into perspective.—J.S. Torg, M.D.

Aerobic Responses to Walking Training in Sedentary Adolescents
Rowland TW, Varzeas MR, Walsh CA (Baystate Med Ctr, Springfield, Mass)
J Adolesc Health 12:30–34, 1991   2–2

Background.—Adolescence appears to be a crucial period in the development of regular exercise habits. The effects of a structured school-based walking program on the aerobic activity of previously sedentary adolescents are reported.

Methods.—Fifteen high school students, mean age 15.7 years, volunteered for the program as an alternative to a regular physical education class. Fourteen of the subjects were girls; most were obese. The subjects walked 3 days per week for 11 weeks. Average distance per session was 1.8 miles and average heart rate was 151 beats/min, representing 79.6% of maximum. Maximal treadmill testing was done to measure physiologic responses to exercise before and after training and during a 3-month control period preceding the program.

Results.—Average precontrol skinfold sum was 52 mm; this did not change significantly during training. Mean maximum oxygen uptake improved from 3.7 to 33.3 mL/kg/min, and treadmill endurance time increased from 9.16 to 1.85 min.

Conclusions.—A program of walking training can have small but significant aerobic effects in previously sedentary adolescents. The results in weight-relative maximal oxygen uptake are comparable to those observed in adults.

▶ This study shows that walking training in sedentary, obese adolescents can be effectively conducted, even in an inner city school setting. Potential benefits are manifold. Aerobic fitness here improved 10% and, likely, mood and self-esteem improved in tandem. One can also hope to help shape a lifelong habit of physical activity. How fast to walk? The subjects here walked at a speed of nearly 4 miles per hour. A recent randomized study among 102 sedentary Dallas women aged 20 to 40 years looked at an aerobic program of 3 different walking speeds, 3, 4, and 5 miles per hour, in comparison to remaining sedentary. After 24 weeks, the gain in physical fitness correlated with walking speed, but all 3 groups of walkers had equivalent beneficial increases in serum levels of high-density lipopotein cholesterol (1). It appears, then, that even slow, regular walking, although it may improve fitness little, can improve the cardiovascular risk profile. When it comes to kids and fitness, how can we help? A recent study found familial aggregation in physical activity (i.e., children of active and less active parents had physical activity patterns similar to those of their parents) (2). Another recent study showed that when physicians refer obese kids to a YMCA lifestyle modification program, the kids show long-term benefits (3).—E.R. Eichner, M.D.

References

1. Duncan JJ, et al: *JAMA* 266:3295, 1991.
2. Freedson PS, Evenson S: *Res Quart Exerc Sport* 62:384, 1991.
3. Cohen CJ, et al: *J Sports Med Phys Fit* 31:183, 1991.

An Unusual Stress Fracture in a Multiple Sport Athlete
Sterling JC, Calvo RD, Holden SC (Fort Bend Orthopaedics and Sports Medicine Associates, Sugar Land, Tex)
Med Sci Sports Exerc 23:298–303, 1991   2–3

Background.—Cross-training is becoming widely accepted in training and competition, and overuse injuries have become a major problem in athletes who cross-train. An unusual case of a stress fracture of the upper extremity in a multiple-sport athlete is reported.

Case Report.—Male, 14, who competed as a swimmer and a baseball third baseman felt and heard a pop in his arm on throwing the baseball. He had experienced aching and tenderness in the midhumeral area but continued to participate in sports. He was in constant discomfort, had severe pain when he moved his arm, and had pain that radiated to his shoulder. The arm was swollen, ecchymotic, and extremely tender on passive motion. A closed, comminuted spiral fracture of the humerus was seen on radiograph. Bone scans done to rule out benign or malignant humeral lesions showed increased uptake at the fracture site and no cold spots or other bone pathology. A cuff and collar was then placed. One week later, a humeral fracture brace was applied and the fracture was well aligned. At 3 weeks, the patient had no complaints. Rehabilitation was instituted, along with instruction on overuse injuries and appropriate training techniques. He had no problems or complaints at 3 years of follow-up.

Conclusion.—Humeral stress factors may be precipitated by repetitive stresses, low-grade external forces, rapid application of muscular force, or underlying disease or bone weakness. In dealing with cross-training athletes, the physician, coach, and trainer need to listen to the athlete with an open mind and be aware of the problems that can result from participation in multiple sports.

▶ A poignant plea for coach, trainer, team physician—somebody!—to ask about and heed warning signs in cross-training athletes. This boy was working out in swimming and baseball for 3–4 hours a day, plus taking part in weekly swim meets. Part of his regimen was weight lifting 3 times a week, instituted by his junior high school condition coach (too many coaches here?). This boy had deep aching arm pain and tenderness in the mid-humerus—hallmarks of a stress fracture—prior to his final injury, but continued to practice and compete. Finally, during the deceleration phase of throwing, his "occult" stress fracture progressed to a spiral fracture.—E.R. Eichner, M.D.

Conversion Reactions in Pediatric Athletes

Dvonch VM, Bunch WH, Siegler AH (Univ of South Florida, Tampa; Univ of Chicago)
J Pediatr Orthop 11:770–772, 1991
2–4

Background.—Sports for teenagers can provide an outlet for energy and an opportunity to socialize, but participation may also be stressful because of the pressure to perform well and meet parents' expectations. Five patients aged 9–19 years displayed a conversion reaction in response to stresses induced by athletic competition. The conversion reaction is a maladaptive attempt to deal with stress or anxiety in one's life.

Patients.—In 1 case, an 11-year-old boy was placed on the senior football team at his father's request. During preseason practice he was tackled and became "paraplegic." His behavior was notable in that in physical therapy, he dragged himself to the pool but swam freely with both arms and legs moving. When the physician recommended that he not play football competitively, he started to walk within 12 hours, and his paraplegia resolved completely within 3 days.

Discussion.—Patients with conversion reactions are frequently younger than their peers in the sport and are characterized as high achievers. Although the parents may contribute to the stress the child feels, it is often the perfectionist child who generates internal stress associated with an inability to deal with failure or poor performance. When allowed a hearing separate from his or her parents, one-on-one supportive conversation with the child identified the conflict in 4 of 5 children described. Physical therapy can help resolve symptoms of an acute episode. Psychotherapy is recommended only for patients with persistent maladaptive behavior or for children unable to identify the source of conflict.

Conclusion.—Diagnosis of conversion reaction may be difficult if practitioners ignore the obvious inconsistencies. The physician should be aware of atypical physical examination findings and an extreme emotional response of the patient. In making treatment decisions, confrontation should be avoided and one-on-one supportive conversation should be initiated without the parents' presence.

▶ Besides the "paraplegic" reaction described above, reported here are a 9-year-old female ice skater who developed performance-limiting "foot pain" and a 13-year-old female swimmer who developed a strange, performance-limiting "shoulder injury." Two other athletes with conversion reactions, a 16-year-old swimmer and a 19-year-old soccer player, are mentioned. Reasons for these reactions include performance anxiety, fear of losing, fear of disappointing parents, coaches, or teammates, fear of injury, fear of losing a scholarship, and/or perfectionistic personality. In most cases, a perceptive physician who talks supportively in private with the young athlete can discern the problem and begin to bring the solution, including the chance to "escape with honor," which often enables the child to recover fast.—E.R. Eichner, M.D.

Bilateral Chronic Exertional Compartment Syndromes of Forearm in an Adolescent Athlete: Case Report and Review of Literature
Wasilewski SA, Asdourian PL (Lahey Clinic Med Ctr, Burlington, Mass)
Am J Sports Med 19:665–667, 1991   2–5

Introduction.—Chronic exertional compartment syndrome develops most often in athletes and usually involves the anterior or deep posterior compartments of the lower extremities. Exertional compartment syndromes of the upper extremities are rare. Chronic exertional compartment syndrome of both forearms and, eventually, in all 4 extremities, was evaluated in 1 patient.

Case Report.—Girl, 14 years, reported a 6-month history of activity-related pain and swelling in the forearms associated with weakness in the hands and wrists during vigorous athletic activities, (e.g., gymnastics or field hockey). She had no history of severe trauma to either upper extremity. The symptoms resolved quickly on stopping the activity, but they recurred with its resumption. Neurologic, vascular, and radiographic examinations of the upper extremities were normal. After 3 months of conservative treatment, the symptoms persisted and a chronic exertional compartment syndrome was suspected. The diagnosis was confirmed with compartment pressure measurements. Bilateral superficial forearm flexor compartment fasciotomy was performed and the symptoms resolved. About 10 months after she was first seen, bilateral anterior tibial compartment syndromes were diagnosed and treated by percutaneous bilateral anterior and lateral tibial compartment fasciotomy. She remained symptom-free for 3 months; but 7 months after leg fasciotomy, the patient required bilateral open fasciotomy to all 4 compartments in the lower extremities through 2 extensive skin incisions. The patient has since become an All-State field hockey player and continues playing field hockey at the college level. At her last follow-up visit, 3½ years after the last operation, she had no complaints of pain in the arms or legs.

Conclusion.—Chronic exertional compartment syndrome should be suspected whenever a patient complains of activity-related pain in the forearm associated with weakness in the fingers and wrist.

▶ A dramatic and unique case report of exertional compartment syndromes of all 4 extremities, along with a concise review of the literature. When exercised, a muscle can expand in volume by as much as 20% as a result of capillary dilatation and increased permeability. Exertional compartment syndrome, then, begins with an increase in compartmental contents and causes pain as the intracompartmental pressure rises abnormally high and compresses arterioles, with anoxic injury to tissues. Presumably, this patient's symptoms were the result of her intensive athletic training during early adolescence, which may have caused rapid muscle hypertrophy in an intrinsically tight fascial compartment. The diagnosis was suspected clinically, confirmed by measuring compartmental pressures, and cured surgically.—E.R. Eichner, M.D.

Low-Back Pain in Adolescent Athletes: Detection of Stress Injury to the Pars Interarticularis With SPECT
Bellah RD, Summerville DA, Treves ST, Micheli LJ (Children's Hosp, Boston)
Radiology 180:509–512, 1991   2–6

Background.—Early detection of stress injury of the pars interarticularis is vital. The ability of bone scintigraphy to localize the diagnosis is improved by single photon emission computed tomography (SPECT). Results of planar and SPECT scintigraphy in young patients referred for low-back pain were reviewed to determine whether SPECT increases detection of the pars interarticularis injury.

Methods.—One hundred sixty-two patients were referred during 1 year. One hundred were female and 62 male; mean age was 16.4 years. About 130 patients were athletes, and 72% had symptoms referable to the posterior elements. All patients underwent both planar and SPECT bone scintigraphy.

Results.—Scintigraphic studies showed no abnormality in 56% of patients. The abnormalities demonstrated on planar imaging were also detectable on SPECT. An abnormal focus of radiotracer uptake was found with SPECT in 71 patients. In 32, the abnormality was also seen on planar scintigraphy. The abnormality was demonstrated with SPECT alone in 39 patients (Fig 2–1). Of 56 patients with normal radiographic results, 16 had scintigraphic abnormalities that could be revealed only by SPECT.

Conclusions.—Single photon emission CT is capable of detecting stress injuries that are not demonstrated by planar bone imaging or radi-

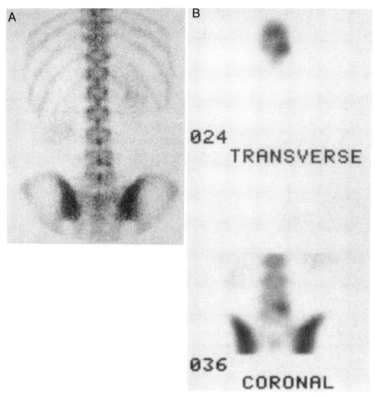

Fig 2–1.—A, plantar skeletal scintigram in a patient with low-back pain is normal; **B,** use of SPECT shows focal area of increased radiotracer uptake in L-4, on the left, representing stress injury to the pars interarticularis. (Courtesy of Bellah RD, Summerville DA, Treves ST, et al: *Radiology* 180:509–512, 1991.)

ography. With the use of SPECT, soft-tissue mechanical causes can be separated from osseous causes of low-back pain in young athletes; this differentiation is vital for selecting the proper mode of therapy.

▶ This report of a 1-year clinical experience in evaluating 162 young athletes referred for skeletal scintigraphy because of suspected stress injury to the pars interarticularis, or spondylolysis, proposes a diagnostic advance. SPECT seems more sensitive than most other methods for demonstrating stress injury to the pars interarticularis, and can often be positive even when the plantar bone scan is entirely normal. This group goes on to suggest that SPECT may even be "better than computed tomography (CT)" for demonstrating a pars defect. Although more research with SPECT is needed, this group recommends that skeletal SPECT be performed on any young patient with symptoms suggesting injury to the pars interarticularis, even if routine x-rays and bone scan are normal. For a timely, comprehensive, practical review on low back pain in young athletes, see reference (1).—E.R. Eichner, M.D.

Reference

1. Harvey J, Tanner S: *Sports Med* 12:394, 1991.

Flow Limitation and Regulation of Functional Residual Capacity During Exercise in a Physically Active Aging Population
Johnson BD, Reddan WG, Pegelow DF, Seow KC, Dempsey JA (Univ of Wisconsin, Madison)
Am Rev Respir Dis 143:960–967, 1991   2–7

Background.—The decline in airflow generation with age may affect ventilation and breathing patterns during exercise even if they are not affected under normal eupneic states. The effects of age-related loss of elastic recoil on exercise hyperpnea were studied in a group of elderly physically trained individuals capable of achieving high-intensity exercise with substantial ventilatory requirement.

Study Design.—Whether a mechanical limitation to expiratory flow rates is achieved during exercise, and whether this limitation influences maximal ventilation, breathing pattern, and/or the regulation of end expiratory lung volume (EELV) throughout progressive exercise, were investigated. Twenty-nine individuals aged 68–70 years participated in 2 sessions of laboratory pulmonary function testing and progressive exercise tests.

Subject Characteristics, Lung Volumes, and Flow Rates in Subjects Divided
Into the Most Fit and the Least Fit

	Most Fit (n = 14)			Least Fit (n = 15)		
	(mean)	(SEM)	(% pred)	(mean)	(SEM)	(% pred)
Age, yr	69	1		70	1	
Height, cm	174	2		174	2	
Weight, kg	66.6	2.4		70.0	2.3	
TLC, L	6.798*	0.212	102	7.179	0.257	108
VC, L	4.201	0.150	111	4.257	0.216	111
FRC, L	3.916*	0.131	95	4.240	0.167	105
RV, L	2.487	0.095	80	2.546	0.134	83
$\dot{V}max_{50}$, L/s	3.405*	0.181	93	2.748	0.254	75
FEV_1, L	3.245*	0.099	116	2.987	0.132	108

*Significant difference between most fit and least fit groups at $P < .05$.
(Courtesy of Johnson BD, Reddan WG, Pegelow DF, et al: *Am Rev Respir Dis* 143:960–967, 1991.)

Findings.—With mild-to-moderate exercise (50%–75% of maximum oxygen uptake), the mean EELV was reduced, expiratory airflow limitation was present over more than 25% of the tidal volume, and the EELV was within closing capacity in 11 subjects. As exercise intensity progressed, the tidal volume plateaued at 58% of the vital capacity, and increased airflow rates were achieved by significantly increasing the EELV back to near resting levels. A portion of the expiratory tidal flow-volume envelope moved away from the constraints of the effort-independent portion of the maximal flow-volume curve. At maximal exercise, the EELV remained similar to the previous intensity of exercise and a significantly greater portion of the tidal expiratory flow-volume envelope became flow limited. The least fit subjects had a reduced capacity for expiratory flow generation relative to the fittest subjects, were more hyperinflated during exercise, and incurred greater expiratory flow limitation for a given respiratory minute volume (table).

Conclusion.—With loss of elastic recoil with age, subjects may simply use all of the airflow and volume reserve they have to achieve an appropriate respiratory minute volume (and ventilatory response), sufficient for their maximal carbon dioxide output and maximum oxygen uptake. The loss of elastic recoil with aging appears to parallel the loss of maximum oxygen uptake with age.

▶ The present group of subjects illustrate well how regular physical activity can conserve aerobic function. Despite ages in the range 61–79 years, maximal oxygen intakes averaged 44 mL/kg/min, with 1 subject scoring as high as 62 mL/kg/min. Ventilation was correspondingly large (an average of 114 L/min during maximal exercise, corresponding to a surprising 91% of the 15-second maximal voluntary ventilation). Nevertheless, loss of elastic tissue from the lungs, almost an inevitable consequence of aging, led to some limitation of expiratory flow. Airway collapse occurred even with moderate effort, and in a move to compensate for this problem during more vigorous activity, subjects exploited the inspiratory part of their flow/volume curves. The cost was a substantial increase of respiratory workrate. Ventilatory problems would have been more severe if maximal exercise had not induced a substantial bronchodilation, as previously observed in our laboratories (1). Although ventilatory function was quite closely correlated with maximal oxygen intake in the present study, Johnson and associates wisely do not infer that there is necessarily a causal relationship; they suggest rather that high values for both variables are serving as indicators of a low biological age.—R.J. Shephard, M.D., Ph.D., D.P.E.

Reference

1. Shephard RJ: *Clin Sci* 32:167, 1967.

Effects of Gender, Age, and Fitness Level on Response of $\dot{V}O_{2\ max}$ to Training in 60–71 Yr Olds

Kohrt WM, Malley MT, Coggan AR, Spina RJ, Ogawa T, Ehsani AA, Bourey RE, Martin WH III, Holloszy JO (Washington Univ, St Louis)
J Appl Physiol 71:2004–2011, 1991   2–8

Introduction.—Several studies have assessed the degree to which endurance exercise training can affect the maximal aerobic power ($\dot{V}O_{2max}$) in elderly individuals, but direct comparisons of the training response in older men and older women are not available. This study examined the gender-related differences in the cardiac response to vigorous endurance exercise performed by men and women 60 years and older. The role of age and initial fitness level in the cardiac response to exercise was also examined.

Study Design.—The study was carried out with 181 nonsmoking, healthy volunteers, aged 60–71 years, who had been sedentary for at least 2 years. Another 48 elderly persons were enrolled as non-exercise controls. Of the 229 people entered into the study, 100 exercisers and 35 controls completed it. The 9- to 12-month supervised exercise program consisted primarily of walking on a treadmill and running on an indoor track. Some also used an exercise cycle or a rowing machine. Individual exercise prescriptions were updated weekly from activity logs. A

TABLE 1.—Physiologic Responses to 9 or 12 Months of Endurance Exercise Training in Older Men

			Month of Training Program		
	Baseline	3	6	9	12
		12 mo of training (n = 24)			
$\dot{V}O_{2\ max}$					
$ml \cdot min^{-1} \cdot kg^{-1}$	27.6±4.6	31.7±5.5*	33.7±6.0*	33.8±5.2	35.2±6.0†
l/min	2.22±0.29	2.51±0.39*	2.62±0.40*	2.63±0.40	2.71±0.49†
RER_{max}	1.23±0.09	1.16±0.08*	1.18±0.05	1.17±0.06	1.18±0.07
$\dot{V}E_{max}$, l/min	78.4±15.8	84.6±14.6*	87.6±12.7	88.0±14.5	90.8±15.7
HR_{max}, beats/min	169±11	168±10	167±10	165±9	166±9
HR_{rest}, beats/min	83±11	77±15†	75±13	73±14	73±10
Weight, kg	81.5±11.9	80.0±11.0*	78.7±10.5*	78.4±9.9	77.6±9.8†
		9 mo of training (n = 29)			
$\dot{V}O_{2\ max}$					
$ml \cdot min^{-1} \cdot kg^{-1}$	28.1±3.8	31.5±4.9*	32.8±4.7†	34.2±4.9*	
l/min	2.37±0.39	2.58±0.39*	2.66±0.39†	2.72±0.39	
RER_{max}	1.25±0.09	1.18±0.07*	1.17±0.07	1.18±0.06	
$\dot{V}E_{max}$, l/min	81.2±14.6	87.0±14.4*	89.0±13.6	90.8±13.1	
HR_{max}, beats/min	170±11	167±12	169±8	168±8	
HR_{rest}, beats/min	79±13	73±11†	75±11	73±12	
Weight, kg	84.9±13.5	82.9±12.8*	81.9±11.9†	80.6±11.0	

Note: Values are means ± SD.
Abbreviations: RER, respiratory exchange ratio; $\dot{V}E$, expired ventilation.
*$P < .01$; significantly different from preceding value.
†$P < .05$; significantly different from preceding value.
(Courtesy of Kohrt WM, Malley MT, Coggan AR, et al: *J Appl Physiol* 71:2004–2011, 1991.)

TABLE 2.—Physiologic Responses to 9 or 12 Months of Endurance Exercise Training in Older Women

	Baseline	3	Month of Training Program 6	9	12
12 mo of training (n = 19)					
$\dot{V}O_{2\,max}$					
ml·min⁻¹·kg⁻¹	22.1±3.0	24.1±3.4*	24.9±3.2†	25.6±3.1	26.7±3.8†
l/min	1.40±0.22	1.49±0.21*	1.54±0.20†	1.58±0.21	1.61±0.22
RER_{max}	1.20±0.12	1.16±0.09	1.20±0.09	1.19±0.08	1.20±0.07
$\dot{V}E_{max}$, l/min	48.4±8.6	49.6±7.7	53.0±8.8†	54.2±6.6	57.0±7.2†
HR_{max}, beats/min	166±11	163±15	165±13	166±13	167±11
HR_{rest}, beats/min	88±14	80±13†	76±15	81±15	82±13
Weight, kg	63.9±11.6	62.7±11.0†	62.5±10.4	62.2±9.4	61.1±9.9*
9 mo of training (n = 38)					
$\dot{V}O_{2\,max}$					
ml·min⁻¹·kg⁻¹	21.3±2.8	23.8±3.1*	25.2±3.6*	26.0±3.8*	
l/min	1.49±0.21	1.62±0.19*	1.69±0.21*	1.74±0.23*	
RER_{max}	1.20±0.12	1.14±0.07*	1.16±0.07†	1.16±0.07	
$\dot{V}E_{max}$, l/min	50.8±10.1	53.7±8.7†	57.0±9.5*	58.4±10.4†	
HR_{max}, beats/min	166±11	163±13	163±12	165±10	
HR_{rest}, beats/min	86±13	82±13	78±12	78±12	
Weight, kg	70.7±12.0	69.1±11.6*	66.6±15.5	67.8±12.2	

Note: Values are means ± SD.
*P < .01; significantly different from preceding value.
†P < .05; significantly different from preceding value.
(Courtesy of Kohrt WM, Malley MT, Coggan AR, et al: *J Appl Physiol* 71:2004–2011, 1991.)

group of 46 young sedentary controls were studied for comparison on 1 occasion.

Results.—After walking and running for 9–12 months for an average of 3.9 days per week, 45 minutes a day, at 80% of maximal heart rate, the average improvement in $\dot{V}O_{2max}$ was 24%. The average improvement in $\dot{V}O_{2max}$ was 26% for men (Table 1) and 23% for women (Table 2). The difference was statistically not significant. When exercisers were divided into 3 groups according to age, there were no significant differences in the relative increase in $\dot{V}O_{2max}$ between the different age groups. Pretraining $\dot{V}O_{2max}$ correlated with absolute improvement in $\dot{V}O_{2max}$.

Conclusion.—In healthy individuals between the ages of 60 and 71 years, the $\dot{V}O_{2max}$ adapts to endurance exercise training to the same relative extent as it does in young persons. This adaptation is independent of gender, age, and initial fitness level.

► It is sometimes quite remarkable how reputable U.S. journals can publish papers that fail to acknowledge earlier work! The present authors claim novelty for a report on subjects 60–71 years of age that found a 26% training response in men and a 23% response in women. However, in summarizing the studies of Sidney and Shephard (published in 1978), I wrote 5 years ago "At one year, the final gain averaged 24 per cent, much as anticipated in younger subjects. As in some other comparisons (Roskamm, 1967; Kilbom,

1971; Getchell & Moore, 1975), increases were shown equally by women and men!" (1). To judge from their reference list, the present authors remain blissfully ignorant of all 4 of the papers that have previously demonstrated much the same thing!

It is encouraging that such substantial gains of maximal oxygen intake can be attained at the age of retirement, and the data reinforce the value of conditioning even for those who have not previously been active.—R.J. Shephard, M.D., Ph.D., D.P.E.

Reference

1. Shephard RJ: *Physical Activity and Aging*, ed 2. Rockwood, Md, Aspen Publications, 1987.

Effects of a Three-Year Exercise Program on Motor Function and Cognitive Processing Speed in Older Women
Rikli RE, Edwards DJ (California State Univ, Fullerton; Saddleback College Emeritus Inst, Mission Viejo, Calif)
Res Q Exerc Sport 62:61–67, 1991   2–9

Background.—Many motor functions have been found to decline with age. These include reaction time, balance, flexibility, and grip strength. The effects were studied of a 3-year exercise program on motor performance and cognitive processing speed of formerly sedentary elderly women.

Methods.—The participants were 31 women, aged 57–85 years, who were first-time enrollees in exercise classes taught at a retirement complex. Simple and choice reaction time (CRT), balance, sit and reach flexibility, shoulder flexibility, and grip strength were tested. The exercise classes, which met 3 times a week, were designed to meet American College of Sports Medicine guidelines.

Results.—Performance was improved significantly on all measures throughout the study, except for the sit and reach test. When the exercise group was compared with a comparable group of sedentary control subjects, significant interactions were noted between treatment and time on all variables except CRT and grip strength. The exercise group's pretest to posttest scores tended to improve over the 3-year period, whereas those of the control group declined (table).

Conclusions.—Physical activity appears to be an effective intervention for reversing or at least slowing certain age-related declines in cognitive and motor functions. These findings also suggest that it is never too late for sedentary persons to enjoy the benefits of exercise.

▶ A variety of problems lead to the eventual institutionalization of the elderly. Sometimes there is an acute medical crisis such as a stroke, and sometimes the loss of key support, for example when a child moves to another

Pretest and Posttest Means, Standard Deviations (in Parentheses),
and Univariate ANOVA F Values for Significant Interaction Effects
of Exercise Vs. Control Subjects

		Pretest	Posttest	F	p
Simple reaction time (ms)	Exercise	287.05 (29.12)	274.43 (29.86)	6.69	.014
	Control	285.46 (36.72)	291.23 (34.31)		
Choice reaction time (ms)	Exercise	352.00 (45.45)	317.95 (43.59)	4.89	.034[*]
	Control	380.20 (78.60)	392.20 (62.71)		
Balance (s)	Exercise	37.90 (19.94)	42.80 (20.18)	7.29	.011
	Control	26.62 (11.89)	20.85 (9.92)		
Sit & reach flexibility (cm)	Exercise	-1.69 (3.01)	-.02 (2.98)	7.35	.011
	Control	-5.0 (7.92)	-5.46 (6.22)		
Shoulder flexibility (cm)	Exercise	-1.10 (2.48)	.88 (2.94)	15.04	.001
	Control	-5.00 (6.09)	-6.46 (4.22)		

[*]Approached, but did not reach significance at the .01 level.
(Courtesy of Rikli RE, Edwards DJ: *Res Q Exerc Sport* 62:61-67, 1991.)

city. But often, the problem is a progressive deterioration of function, so that residual abilities are no longer adequate to deal with the demands of daily living. Sometimes the functional loss is physical, but often the primary problem is a deterioration of cognitive skills. There has thus been considerable interest in reports such as the 4-month study of Dustman et al., which suggested that regular exercise can reverse age-related deteriorations of motor performance and cognitive processing (1). The present report confirms these findings, although the underlying mechanism of benefit remains uncertain. Some investigators have suggested that exercise improves cerebral blood flow (2), but any effect from an increase of systemic blood pressure is very short-lived. A second possibility is an increase of cerebral arousal, whether through the liberation of neurotransmitters, or an increased input of proprioceptive impulses to the reticular formation of the brain. It is also important to remember that exercise cannot be administered in a double-blind fashion, and part of the apparent response may be a reaction to greater attention or to a new focus of interest in what had become a rather uninteresting life.—R.J. Shephard, M.D., Ph.D., D.P.E.

References

1. Dustman RE, et al: *Neurobiol Aging* 5:35, 1984.
2. MacRae PG: Physical activity and central nervous system integrity, in Spirduso WW, Eckert HM (eds): *Physical Activity and Aging.* Champaign, Ill: Human Kinetics Publ, 1989, pp 69–77.

The Impact of Daily Exercise on the Mobility, Balance and Urine Control of Cognitively Impaired Nursing Home Residents
Jirovec MM (Wayne State Univ, Detroit)
Int J Nurs Stud 28:145–151, 1991   2–10

Background.—Nursing home residents have limited opportunities to exercise, especially those residents who need any type of assistance with ambulation. The impact of a daily exercise program on mobility, balance, and urine control was studied in 15 cognitively impaired elderly nursing home residents.

Methods and Results.—The director of nurses in 2 suburban nursing homes identified those residents who had episodes of urinary incontinence. Fourteen participants were women; ages ranged from 70 to 97 years. Seven participants were restrained for all or part of the day. Data on walking distance, speed of walking, balance ability, ability to rise from a chair unassisted, ability to walk unassisted, and incidence of urinary incontinence were obtained before and after a month of daily assisted walking. After the program, the participants were able to walk significantly greater distances before tiring. There was also a significant reduction in the incidence of urinary incontinence (table).

Mobility, Balance, and Urine Control Before and After 4 Weeks of Daily Exercise

	Before	After
Walking distance (feet)*	50	73
Balance (seconds)	24	26
Speed (inches per second)	5.5	7.7
Incidence of incontinence (7 a.m.–3 p.m.)	2.3	1.0
Incidence of incontinence (7 a.m.–10 p.m.)	2.8	2.5

*$P < .05$.
(Courtesy of Jirovec MM: *Int J Nurs Stud* 28:145–151, 1991.)

Conclusions.—Daily exercise appears to improve the mobility and urine control of cognitively impaired nursing home residents. Thus urinary incontinence frequency in this population may be more amenable than commonly believed to nursing interventions designed to enhance rather than inhibit mobility.

▶ There are some weaknesses in the design of this experiment. The sample size was quite small, there was no independent control group, and the hourly recording of continence may have reminded some disturbed patients of the need to use the toilet. Some of the observed gains could reflect a greater sense of self-efficacy, or even a strengthening of pelvic muscles. Nevertheless, anyone who has heard the frantic calls of "bottle, nurse" from a bedbound elderly patient can appreciate that measures to increase mobility and thus the ability to reach the toilet unaided would be the most likely explanation of the decreased incidence of incontinence reported in this paper.

Given that patients were capable of achieving a higher level of mobility, it is disturbing to note that they had previously been restrained by physicians and nursing staff—one more unfortunate example of iatrogenic disease.—R.J. Shephard, M.D., Ph.D., D.P.E.

Muscle Cross-Sectional Area, Force Production and Relaxation Characteristics in Women at Different Ages
Häkkinen K, Häkkinen A (University of Jyväskylä; Central Hospital of Central Finland, Jyväskylä, Finland)
Eur J Appl Physiol 62:410–414, 1991   2–11

Introduction.—Under normal conditions, human muscle strength peaks at ages 20–30 years and remains relatively unchanged for 20 years thereafter. However, a steep decline in maximal muscle strength sets in after age 50 years. This decline has been attributed to a reduction in the size of individual muscle fibers and a loss of muscle fibers. However, it is not known whether aging also affects maximal strength per cross-sectional area (CSA) of the muscle. In addition, explosive force production and relaxation capacity of the activated muscle may have a role in the loss of muscle strength.

Methods.—To assess muscle CSA, force production, and relaxation characteristics in women of different ages, 10 young women (YW) with a mean age of 30 years, 10 middle-aged women (MW) with a mean age of 50 years, and 10 elderly women (EW) with a mean age of 70 years were studied. All of the women were healthy and habitually active, but they had no experience in strength training or competitive sports. Bilateral isometric leg extension force-time curves, maximal force, maximal rates of force development, and relaxation-time curves were measured on an electromechanical dynamometer. The CSA of the quadriceps femoris (QF) muscle of the right thigh was measured with an ultrasonic apparatus. Percentage body fat was estimated from skinfold thickness measurements.

Results.—The CSA of the QF muscle in YW was slightly larger than that in MW and much larger than that in EW whose values were markedly smaller than those in MW. Maximal force in YW was slightly greater than that in MW and much greater than that in EW whose values were markedly smaller than those in MW. Individual CSA values correlated with maximal force for all 3 age groups. Isometric force-time curves differed among the 3 age groups, but relaxation times did not.

Conclusion.—The decline in maximal strength with aging could well be related to the decline in muscle CSA. However, the time it takes to produce explosive force may worsen even more with aging than does maximal strength, especially at older ages. The atrophying effects of aging may be greater on fast twitch muscle fibers than on slow twitch fibers, suggesting that in addition to the decline in maximal strength, the rate of neural muscle activation may also be affected by aging.

▶ These investigators present an excellent paper telling us how things are for active subjects who regularly participate in aerobic physical activities such as walking, jogging, swimming and biking. However, the next 2 papers by Charette et al. (Abstract 2–12) and by Smidt et al. (Abstract 2–13) appear to show that the loss of strength through the reduction in size of muscle fibers and loss of muscle fibers can be slowed by participating in a well-designed strength maintenance/development program. I still feel that we make a mistake when we extol the virtues of aerobic exercise to the exclusion of muscular strength and endurance activities. As we get older, we need both if we are to maintain a healthy lifestyle.—Col. J.L. Anderson, PE.D.

Muscle Hypertrophy Response to Resistance Training in Older Women
Charette SL, McEvoy L, Pyka G, Snow-Harter C, Guido D, Wiswell RA, Marcus R (Stanford Univ, Stanford, Calif; VA Med Ctr, Palo Alto, Calif)
J Appl Physiol 70:1912–1916, 1991   2–12

Introduction.—The age-related decreases in muscle strength may be partly reversible by resistance training. Studies in young and elderly men and young women have examined hypertrophy of muscle fibers as a result of resistance training. In elderly women, an increase in muscle hypertrophy could lead to increased bone strength and a reduction in the risk of falls. The results of an experiment with resistance training in elderly women were reviewed.

Methods.—The 27 healthy women, aged 64–86 years, were randomly assigned to a nonexercising control group or a 12-week resistance-training group. After initial testing of baseline maximal strength, the exercisers began a regimen of 7 exercisers that stressed primary muscle groups of the lower extremities. Biopsy material was obtained from the midlateral thigh of 6 controls and 13 exercisers at the end of the training period.

Results.—The exercisers had increases of 28% to 115% in muscle strength compared with baseline values in all muscle groups. The cross-sectional area of type II muscle fibers significantly increased in the exercisers, but type I fibers showed no change in either group. The control group showed no significant strength changes or changes in type II muscle fibers.

Conclusion.—The gains in muscle strength in the elderly women who underwent resistance training were partly the result of increased type II muscle fiber hypertrophy. Resistance training can be safely performed by elderly women and may provide a useful model to examine the effects of exercise on posture, gait, and bone mass in older women.

▶ This study reminds us again that physical exercise can and should be used by our aging population to help them to maintain their quality of life. There are many groups around the world that are working to promote this idea, but we still aren't getting the message out fast enough. I am convinced that getting our aging population involved in exercise programs will save more in health care costs than the programs themselves will cost.—Col. J.L. Anderson, PE.D.

The Effect of Trunk Resistive Exercise on Muscle Strength in Postmenopausal Women

Smidt GL, O'Dwyer KD, Lin S-Y, Blanpied PR (Univ of Iowa, Iowa City; Hand and Orthopaedic Rehabilitation Associates, Raleigh NC; Hfieu-Chang Lin, Taipei, Taiwan; Univ of Rhode Island, Kingston)
J Orthop Sports Phys Ther 13:300–309, 1991   2–13

Background.—Trunk muscle strength is important in maintaining optimal function and preventing musculoskeletal injury. There have been few reports of trunk muscle strengthening programs; most have been short-term programs in young subjects with chronic low back pain. The effects of a quantitatively based resistive exercise program on the trunk muscle strength of older women were studied.

Methods.—The study sample was comprised of 55 women, average age 56 years, who volunteered for the study. Subjects were randomized to maintain their current lifestyle or participate in the exercise program. The program involved progressive resistance exercise of the trunk muscles, performed 3–4 times per week for 10 months. Trunk strength was tested in the same positions used in the exercise program; the external forces generated were measured with the trunk attachment of the Muscle Evaluation and Exercise Dosimeter (MEED) 3000 System. The program used body segments and cuff weights to achieve desired resistance

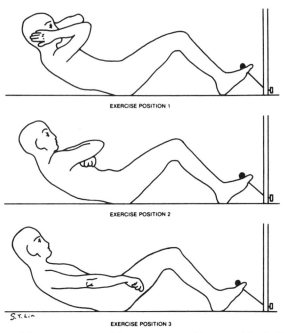

Fig 2–2.—Three different positions used for sit-up exercise. (Courtesy of Smidt GL, O'Dwyer KD, Lin S-Y, et al: *J Orthop Sports Phys Ther* 13:300–309, 1991.)

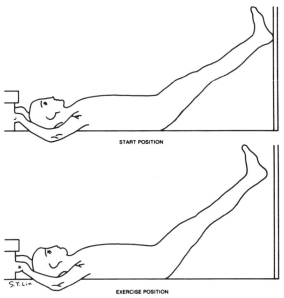

Fig 2–3.—Two different positions used for double-leg flexion exercise. (Courtesy of Smidt GL, O'Dwyer KD, Lin S-Y, et al: *J Orthop Sports Phys Ther* 13:300–309, 1991.)

levels for sit-up (Fig 2–2), prone trunk extension, and double-leg flexion exercises (Fig 2–3).

Results.—In each exercise task, the women who participated in the exercise program showed significant gains in strength of 25% to 30%. At 12 months, their performance was superior to that of the control group in every activity. The strength tests were reliable according to interday trials using the MEED 3000, with all correlations reaching at least r = .93.

Conclusions.—Long-term controlled, progressive resistive exercise is feasible and effective in increasing trunk muscle strength in older women. The MEED 3000 is a reliable system for assessing trunk muscle strength. The exercise program evaluated may be useful in the treatment of patients with low back dysfunction.

▶ This is an excellent study for several reasons. The subjects are women with an average age of 56 years. The length of the training program was sufficient that it should be expected to produce a training effect. The controls, to include an adequate control group, were sufficient. It involved concerns for trunk strength and endurance that are normally neglected even though low back pain is one of our most prevalent concerns for our aging population. It would be interesting to see a follow-up on the exercise subjects to determine how many have continued with the exercise routine.—Col. J.L. Anderson, PE.D.

Strength and Skeletal Muscle Adaptations in Heavy-Resistance-Trained Women After Detraining and Retraining
Staron RS, Leonardi MJ, Karapondo DL, Malicky ES, Falkel JE, Hagerman FC, Hikida RS (Ohio Univ, Athens)
J Appl Physiol 70:631–640, 1991   2–14

Background.—There have been several studies of neuromuscular adaptations to resistance training in men, but few comparable investigations in women. Current evidence suggests that women, like men, can increase muscle fiber strength and size at a sufficient training intensity and duration. There have been few studies of strength training-detraining. The effects of long-term detraining in strength-trained women, the effects of retraining, and the effects of short-term weight training on detrained and untrained women were studied in 15 college-age women.

Methods.—Eight of the women were previously trained and 7 were untrained. The strength-trained women had participated in a 20-week study of strength training for the lower limb. Those subjects then detrained for 30 to 32 weeks, after which they and the previously untrained women participated in a 6-week "retraining" phase. Four subjects in each group continued this training for an additional 7 weeks.

Results.—Maximal dynamic strength increased, hypertrophy of all 3 major muscle fiber types occurred, and percentage of type IIb fibers decreased in response to the initital 20-week training program. Fiber cross-sectional area was little affected by detraining, but percentage of type IIb fibers increased and IIa fibers decreased. Although maximal dynamic strength decreased, it did not decline to pretraining levels. After retraining, cross-sectional areas of both fast fiber types increased compared with detraining values, and percentage of type IIb fibers decreased. In the 8 subjects who had an additional 7 weeks of training, cross-sectional areas continued to decrease and IIb fibers were absent. The previously untrained women showed similar changes.

Conclusions.—In previously trained women and those who have never trained, strength training appears to cause rapid muscular adaptations. Some adaptations, such as fiber area and maximal dynamic strength, may not be lost during long periods of detraining, thus contributing to a rapid return to form.

▶ More and more we seem to be learning that the muscle adaptation of women to strength training is very similar to the muscle adaptation of men to the same type of training. However, I don't think anyone is saying that the hypertrophy of muscle tissue is the same in women as in men.—Col. J.L. Anderson, PE.D.

A Physiological Comparison of Female Body Builders and Power Lifters
Johnson GO, Housh TJ, Powell DR, Ansorge CJ (Univ of Nebraska-Lincoln)
J Sports Med Phys Fitness 30:361–364, 1991   2–15

Introduction.—Although there have been several studies of the physiologic characteristics of male body builders and power lifters, there are few of females. Muscular strength, body composition and build, and anaerobic power and capacity were compared in 10 female body builders (FBB), with a mean age of 30.4 years, and 10 female power lifters (FPL), with a mean age of 25.2 years. The minimum duration of training in both groups was 2 years. All of the women had competed, 12 on the national level.

Methods.—Measures of body build and composition were obtained through hydrostatic weighting, 7 skinfold measurements, 13 circumference measurements, and 9 diameter measurements. A Cybex II dynamometer at 60 degrees per second was used to measure flexion and extension strength of the dominant forearm and leg. The Wingate Anaerobic Test was used to assess anaerobic power and capacity.

Results.—Mean body weight was 68.60 kg for FPL compared with 56.47 kg for FBB, and relative fat was 21.47% for FPL and 13.51% for FBB. Both of these measures, as well as sum of skinfolds, sum of diameters, and sum of circumferences, were significantly greater in FPL than in FBB. The groups did not differ significantly in fat-free weight, muscular strength, or anaerobic power and capacity.

Conclusion.—These differences are related to the leaner physique and smaller skeletal structure of FBB, as dictated by the definition and symmetry sought by body builders. The basic training techniques of the 2 groups were similar, as reflected by the lack of differences in the strength and anaerobic characteristics.

▶ Probably the most significant difference in the way women power lifters and women body builders prepare for competition has more to do with their nutritional intake than with their strength training techniques. Of course, power lifters must train specifically for the 3 lifts they are going to have to attempt, and the body builders are looking more for body symmetry. However, it is much more important for the body builders to be concerned with reduction of body fat than it is for power lifters.—Col. J.L. Anderson, PE.D.

Comparison of Hemodynamic and Left Ventricular Responses to Increased After-Load in Healthy Males and Females
Sagiv M, Metrany R, Fisher N, Fisman EZ, Kellermann JJ (Tel-Aviv University, Tel-Hashomer, Israel)
Int J Sports Med 12:41–45, 1991   2–16

Background.—In men, sustained isometric exercise increases mean arterial blood pressure in relationship with the size of the muscle mass and the intensity and duration of contraction. No such data have been gathered in women, however. Hemodynamic and left ventricular response to large muscle mass isometric exercise in healthy, nonathletic men and women were compared.

Methods.—The subjects were 20 men, mean age 31.5 years, and 20 women, mean age 30.4 years. All were sedentary and in good health, and none was participating in any sports or fitness program. At a single session, subjects performed isometric deadlift exercise, during which their maximal voluntary contraction was measured. Subjects then performed the same exercise for 3 minutes at 30% of maximal voluntary contraction (Fig 2–4). Echocardiography was performed during both rest and exercise to measure hemodynamic and left ventricular responses.

Results.—Women exerted a maximal tension of 87.4 kg vs. 127.3 kg for the men. Both sexes showed significant increase in heart rate and contractility index during exercise, but the men had significantly higher mean arterial pressure both at rest and during exercise. In men, exercise increased ejection fraction from 62% to 65% and increased fractional shortening from 32% to 35%; these parameters were unchanged in the women. Neither group had significant changes in end-diastolic dimen-

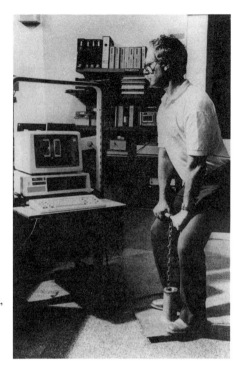

Fig 2–4.—Deadlift isometric exercise maneuver. (Courtesy of Sagiv M, Metrany R, Fisher N, et al: *Int J Sports Med* 12:41–45, 1991.)

sion or stroke volume. Both sexes had significantly lower end-systolic dimension during exercise.

Conclusions.—Submaximal isometric exercise appears to result in augmented hemodynamic and left ventricular function in normal, healthy men and women. Women, however, have a relatively lower afterload because they use less active muscle mass in performing the exercise.

▶ This study demonstrates again that sex differences in body size and composition account for a significant fraction of the intergender variance in maximal force exerted. Most of us realize that maximal force exerted is highly correlated with the mass of skeletal muscle tissue that is active during exercise. Because body weight and lean body mass is generally lower in women, none of us should be surprised with the findings that the men were capable of exerting greater isometric forces than were the women. A study of men and women of equal weight might produce some interesting results.—Col. J.L. Anderson, PE.D.

Responses to Eccentric and Concentric Resistance Training in Females and Males

Colliander EB, Tesch PA (Karolinska Institutet, Stockholm)
Acta Physiol Scand 141:149–156, 1990   2–17

Background.—Short-term resistance training benefits both males and females by similar relative increases in lower limb strength. The sexes have similar eccentric peak torque, normalized for body weight, but males have higher concentric peak torque than females. The effects of a program of short-term accommodated resistance training, which consisted of coupled concentric and eccentric maximum voluntary quadriceps muscle actions in men and women, were assessed.

Methods.—The subjects were 11 women, mean age 27 years, and 11 men, mean age 26 years, with asymptomatic knee function. All were physically active, but none had ever participated in a regular strength training program. Each volunteer performed 4–5 sets of 6 maximum bilateral coupled concentric and eccentric quadriceps muscle actions 3 times per week. Angular velocity was constant at 1.05 rad s^{-1}. Before and after this training program, each subject had measurement of unilateral and bilateral concentric and eccentric peak torque at angular velocities of .52, 1.57, and 2.62 rad s^{-1}; 3 repetition maximum half-squat; and vertical jump height.

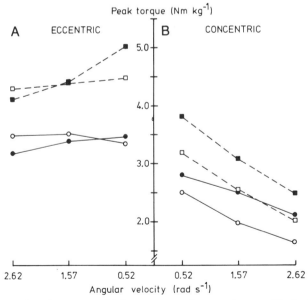

Fig 2–5.—**A** Unilateral eccentric and (**B**) concentric quadriceps peak torque (Nm kg^{-1}) in females (*open symbols*) and males (*filled symbols*) before (*open circle, filled circle*) and after (*filled square, open square*) training. Values are mean. (Courtesy of Colliander EB, Tesch PA: *Acta Physiol Scand* 141:149–156, 1990.)

Results.—Concentric and eccentric peak torque increased significantly in both sexes at all angular velocities. They had similar relative increases in unilateral concentric—26% for both sexes—and eccentric peak torque—28% in women vs. 36% in men—across speeds (Fig 2–5). Corresponding increases were seen in bilateral concentric—20% vs. 28 %—and eccentric peak torque—24% vs. 39% in females and males. The sexes showed equal increases in 3-repetition maximum half-squat and vertical jump height.

Conclusions.—Short-term accommodated resistance training appears to increase concentric and eccentric peak torque and functional strength at a rate that is independent of sex. However, the relationship between torque and velocity appears to change in men, indicating that they experience relatively greater enhancement of maximum voluntary force in the slow-speed, high-force region.

▶ This study again shows that eccentric peak torque, normalized for body weight, is similar between men and women. However, concentric peak torque is greater in men than in women. Because eccentric but not concentric peak torque relative to body weight was similar in the 2 groups, the increase in the eccentric to concentric peak torque ratio as a function of increased angular velocity was greater in women than in men. Other investigators have suggested that the muscle force generated during the performance of slow speed, maximum voluntary, concentric or eccentric muscle actions is impaired, probably through neural inhibitive mechanisms. The findings of this study do show that the largest changes in response to training occurred in this part of the torque-velocity curve.—Col. J.L. Anderson, PE.D.

The Effect of Exercise Duration on Serum Cholesterol and Triglycerides in Women
Hughes RA, Housh TJ, Hughes RJ, Johnson GO (Cameron Univ, Lawton, Okla; Univ of Nebraska-Lincoln)
Res Q Exerc Sport 62:98–104, 1991   2–18

Introduction.—Most studies on the effects of exercise training on lipoprotein profiles in women have used exercise training periods lasting 30 minutes or less. The lack of training-induced changes in lipoprotein profiles in women may be the result of the duration of exercise. A study was conducted to determine whether the duration of a single period of submaximal exercise affects the serum concentrations of triglycerides, cholesterol, and cholesterol subfractions in women.

Methods.—Body composition, maximal oxygen uptake ($\dot{V}O_{2max}$), and ventilatory threshold (VT) were evaluated in 32 normolipidemic women, aged 19–32 years. Submaximal treadmill evaluations were conducted after cessation of each woman's last menstrual bleeding. Blood lipid parameters were measured before and after exercise.

Results.—Hematocrit levels were unchanged by exercise and all changes in lipid and lipoprotein concentrations were greater than any estimated changes in plasma volume. The $\dot{V}O_{2max}$, Vt, and body composition characteristics were not related to lipid and lipoprotein concentrations. There were no among-group differences in any of the lipid or lipoprotein levels, suggesting that exercise duration does not influence lipid or lipoprotein concentrations in women after a single period of submaximal exercise of 45 minutes or less.

Conclusion.—Training or acute bouts of exercise have been shown to positively affect the serum lipoprotein levels of men. However, in this study, a single bout of submaximal exercise had little effect on the serum lipoprotein levels of women. Previous studies had similar results, suggesting that neither short periods of exercise nor a single exercise period affected lipoprotein concentrations in women. Women may have to exercise for longer sessions or undertake extended training programs to produce the positive changes in lipoprotein levels seen in exercising men.

▶ There is a concern around the United States that not enough research has been done using women subjects to gain knowledge on the prevention of coronary heart disease. Most studies have been done on men. This study helps to demonstrate the need for more research on this topic using women subjects. We used to consider coronary heart disease to be a man's disease. Today we know better.—Col. J.L. Anderson, PE.D.

Exercise Intensity: Effect on Postexercise O_2 Uptake in Trained and Untrained Women
Chad KE, Quigley BM (University of Queensland, Brisbane, Australia)
J Appl Physiol 70:1713–1719, 1991   2–19

Background.—It is well known that metabolism remains elevated for long periods after exercise; however, there have been few studies of how this phenomenon is affected by the intensity and duration of exercise. The effect of constant exercise duration and varying exercise intensities on postexercise metabolic rate was examined in 10 female volunteers, 5 trained cyclists (mean age, 25.2 years), and 5 untrained women (mean age, 27.2 years).

Methods.—The athletes trained an average of 300 km/week, whereas the untrained women participated in no formal exercise. Physical characteristics and maximal oxygen consumption ($\dot{V}O_{2max}$) were measured. The subjects performed 30 minutes of cycle ergometer exercise at intensity levels of 50% and 70% of $\dot{V}O_{2max}$. The effects on 3-hour recovery of $\dot{V}O_2$ and respiratory exchange ratios were measured by open-circuit spirometry.

Results.—After exercise at 50% $\dot{V}O_{2max}$ postexercise $\dot{V}O_2$ was greater in both trained and untrained subjects than after exercise at 70% $\dot{V}O_{2max}$. Respiratory exchange ratios were also lower in both groups after 50% $\dot{V}O_{2max}$ exercise than after 70% $\dot{V}O_{2max}$ exercise. This finding suggested that increased fat metabolism may play a role in the elevation of metabolism. In support of this, fatty acid oxidation was greater after 50% $\dot{V}O_{2max}$ exercise than after exercise at 70% $\dot{V}O_{2max}$.

Conclusions.—Moderate exercise, performed for 30 minutes, appears to produce an increase in metabolism. This may have important implications for weight loss, especially in older people who are at increased cardiac risk with high-intensity exercise. It remains unclear what effect high-intensity, short duration exercise may have on long-term elevation of metabolism.

▶ This study presents some interesting points. Not many of us would suspect that exercising at 50% $\dot{V}O_{2max}$ for 30 minutes would be more effective in producing an extended excess postexercise O_2 consumption (EPOC) than exercising at 70% $\dot{V}O_{2max}$ for the same length of time. We would probably guess that the EPOC for trained individuals might be greater that for the untrained. We still need to gain a better understanding of the precise mechanisms for increased fat metabolism in recovery from exercise.—Col. J.L. Anderson, PE.D.

Health Effects of Recreational Running in Women: Some Epidemiological and Preventive Aspects
Marti B (University of Zurich)
Sports Med 11:20–51, 1991   2–20

Introduction.—Women who run but not at an elite level have a peak oxygen uptake 40% to 100% higher than the general female population. Part of the difference—but not all of it—can be ascribed to low body weight, endurance training, and not smoking. Sedentary women are able to improve their cardiorespiratory fitness by undertaking aerobic exercise.

General Health Effects.—Women who exercise regularly have a significantly lower risk of both fatal and nonfatal coronary events. Changes in the blood lipids consequent to exercise training remain unclear, although increased high-density-lipoprotein cholesterol levels have been found in distance runners. Better fitness relates to a lower risk of hypertension developing, and moderately intense aerobic exercise can lower the blood pressure in patients with hypertension. In addition, an athletic life-style may correlate with a reduced risk of adult-onset diabetes.

Endocrine Function.—The prevalence of secondary amenorrhea in runners varies widely. Factors contributing to the risk include low body fat, the mileage run, and nutritional status. Athletes with amenorrhea tend to have lower vertebral bone density that improves when the menses resume. Ongoing exercise itself correlates with increased spinal bone density in both pre-menopausal and postmenopausal women.

Injuries.—As many as half of recreational runners report activity-related injuries, depending on how injury is defined. Female gender by itself is not a major risk factor in those who are habitually active, but it may be more significant when sedentary persons begin to jog. Exercise at reasonable levels is not likely to cause significant joint injury.

Mental Factors.—Those who exercise regularly tend to be less anxious and depressed than others, and have increased self-esteem. Anorexia is not more prevalent in competitive distance runners, although it is the best runners who are the most likely to be anorectic. Relatively few runners smoke.

Recommendation.—There is a broad consensus that jogging 2½–6 km/day—entailing energy expenditure of 150–400 kcal/day assuming moderately intense exercise—is a reasonable goal for health-oriented running.

▶ This is an excellent review of the literature on the health effects for women who run for recreation. There are no real surprises to be found here. It points out the overwhelming benefits of aerobic training for women and mentions the concerns, including exercise-induced amenorrhea, injuries, and anorexia. I like the fact that it reports a broad consensus in the literature that jogging from 2½–6 km/day, which causes an energy expenditure of 150–400 kcal/day, is a reasonable goal for health-oriented running. Hopefully, we can eventually get this same kind of information for people who walk or perform other types of aerobic exercise. We also need to remind people that aerobic exercise alone may not be enough to maintain good health. Proper muscular balance and muscle tone should not be forgotten.—Col. J.L. Anderson, PE.D.

Maximal Exercise Performance and Lean Leg Volume in Men and Women
Winter EM, Brookes FBC, Hamley EJ (Bedford College of Higher Education, Bedford, England; Loughborough University of Technology, England)
J Sports Sci 9:3–13, 1991   2–21

Background.—There have been many reports comparing the maximal exercise capabilities of men and women, and interest has intensified with the advent of all-out cycle ergometry protocols using friction-braked ergometers. The effects of mechanical, physiologic, and cultural factors have also come to be of interest. Cycle ergometric exercise testing was used to compare maximal exercise performance of men and women.

Methods.—The subjects were 47 female and 34 male physical education students. Mean age was 21.2 years for the women and 22.1 years for

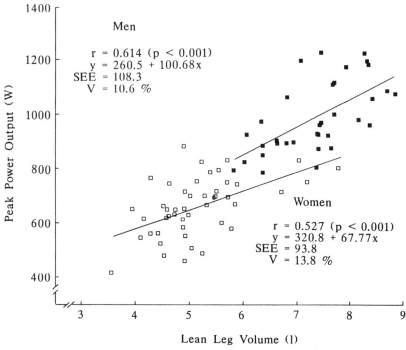

Fig 2–6.—The relationship between optimized peak power output and lean leg volume in men (*filled square*) and women (*open square*). V% = coefficient of variation of points about the regression line. (Courtesy of Winter EM, Brookes FBC, Hamley EJ: *J Sports Sci* 9:3–13, 1991.)

the men. A friction-braked cycle ergometer optimization procedure was used to evaluate external peak power output (OPP) and optimized pedal rate in each subject. The anthropometric technique of Jones and Pearson was used to calculate lean leg volume (LLV) and lean upper leg volume (LULV).

Results.—Mean OPP was 1,007 W in men vs. 673 W in women, and mean optimized pedal rate was 119.5 rev min^{-1} in men vs. 104.5 rev min^{-1} in women. Lean leg volume was 7.41 in men vs. 5.19 in women, and LULV was 4.96 in men vs. 3.35 in women. There was no significant difference in the ratio standards OPP/LLV and OPP/LULV between the sexes; and in both OPP was related to both of the anthropometric parameters (Figs 2–6 and 2–7). On analysis of covariance, there were no differences between the sexes in variance about regression and the regression coefficients, but the elevation of the regression lines was different.

Conclusions.—The differences between maximal exercise performance in men and women appear to be unrelated to estimated LLV. Men have a greater power output for a given volume of lean leg, but the rate of increase in performance with increasing volume is the same for

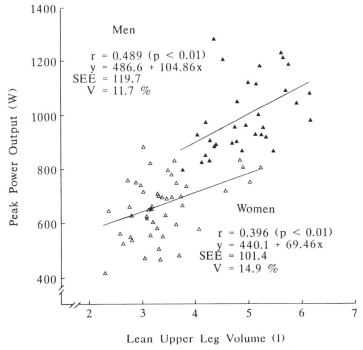

Fig 2–7.—The relationship between optimized peak power output and lean upper leg volume in men *(filled triangle)* and women *(open triangle)*. V% = coefficient of variation of points about the regression line. (Courtesy of Winter EM, Brookes FBC, Hamley EJ: *J Sports Sci* 9:3-13, 1991.)

both sexes. Comparisons of this type using ratio standards are misleading; it is more appropriate to consider regression standards.

▶ These authors make an excellent point by showing the problems associated with using ratio standards for the purpose of statistical analysis. They point out that 40 years ago, Tanner suggested that the use of ratio standards may produce misleading results by misrepresenting the variables under scrutiny, resulting in incorrect conclusion. They point out that within their study, using ratio standards produced a type II error on 2 occasions. They felt that the differences in performance between the men and women in this study clearly were not explained simply by the intergroup differences in the anthropometric indices of the lower limb, but rather are independent of size. The analysis of covariance, they demonstrate, adjusts for the differences, but the use of ratio standards does not provide the sensitivity. By the use of ratio standards to express performance, it may suggest that there are no intergroup differences—an incorrect interpretation that is pointed out in this study by use of regression standards.—Col. J.L. Anderson, PE.D.

Response of Plasma Immunoreactive β-Endorphin and Corticotropin to Isometric Exercise in Uncomplicated Pregnancy and in Pregnancy-Induced Hypertension

Räisänen I, Salminen K, Laatikainen T (Helsinki University Central Hospital)
Eur J Obstet Gynecol Reprod Biol 35:119–124, 1990   2–22

Introduction.—The increased response of plasma adrenaline to an isometric exercise has been reported in pregnancy-induced hypertension (PIH). These findings suggest that the catecholamine response to stress is changed in PIH. Increased plasma concentrations of corticotropin-releasing hormone have also been reported in women with PIH.

Methods.—The basal levels of immunoreactive β-endorphin (ir-βE) and corticotropin were compred and the effects of isometric exercise on these hormones were investigated in 9 women with uncomplicated pregnancies and 10 women with pregnancy-induced hypertension in the third trimester of pregnancy. Gestational age and maternal age were matched in the 2 groups. The response of plasma ir-βE and corticotropin to isometric exercise was tested with a handgrip test.

Results.—The mean basal concentration of corticotropin was 3 times higher in the PIH group compared with the control goup; there was no significant difference in basal ir-βE levels. The corticotropin and ir-βE concentrations uncreased significantly in all the pregnant women in response to the handgrip test.

Conclusion.—There was no abnormality in the corticotropin and endorphin responses to isometric exercise related to PIH. Isometric exercise was sufficient to increase the secretion of these hormones in both the pregnant subjects with PIH and the normal controls. The increased basal concentrations of corticotropin in women with PIH may be explained by significantly increased circulating corticotropin-releasing hormone.

▶ This study shows again how remarkable the human body really is. It demonstrates that a stress such as a physiologic isometric exercise, the handgrip, is sufficient to increase corticotropin and β-endorphin secretion in pregnant women. Yet other studies have shown that the same isometric exercise did not produce the same response in nonpregnant women. This suggests that adaptation to a stress response occurs during pregnancy, possibly to help the mother withstand the stress of labor.—Col. J.L. Anderson, PE.D.

Pregnancy-Induced Changes in the Maximal Physiological Responses During Swimming

McMurray RG, Hackney AC, Katz VL, Gall M, Watson WJ (Univ of North Carolina, Chapel Hill)
J Appl Physiol 71:1454–1459, 1991   2–23

Background.—Because swimming is a non-weight bearing exercise, it may be ideal for pregnant women. Water improves exercise heat dissipation, and its buoyancy reduces the adverse effect of the additional mass of pregnancy. There are few data on the maximal oxygen uptake ($\dot{V}O_{2max}$) of gravid women and none on their response during swimming. The effect of pregnancy on $\dot{V}O_{2max}$, maximal ventilation ($\dot{V}_{max}$), and hemodynamics was examined during tethered swimming. The results were compared with the results of cycle ergometry.

Methods.—Ten women were tested during the 25th and 35th weeks of pregnancy and between 9 and 11 weeks post partum by an incremental exercise test to volitional maximum ($\dot{V}O_{2peak}$) on land with a cycle ergometer and in the water with a tethered swim ergometer. Maternal heart rate, blood pressure, and blood samples were obtained after an initial rest period and after exercise.

Results.—Resting heart rates were significantly increased during pregnancy, but maximal heart rates were not significantly altered by pregnancy or exercise. Respiratory exchange ratios during the last minute of exercise were significantly lower during pregnancy and were lower during swimming than during cycling. The cycling $\dot{V}O_{2peak}$ was not affected by pregnancy. The postpartum swim $\dot{V}O_{2peak}$ was similar to the cycle results, but during pregnancy it was significantly lower than the cycling $\dot{V}O_{2peak}$. Hemoglobin, hematocrit, and total plasma concentrations of protein were reduced significantly while resting during pregnancy and were increased during exercise. All the hematologic variables were significantly lower during pregnancy than post partum.

Conclusions.—Unlike the findings during cycling, the $\dot{V}O_{2peak}$ of pregnant women during swimming was reduced. The reduction in $\dot{V}O_{2peak}$ during swimming was associated with a decreased peak ventilation, but it was not correlated with exercise-induced hemoconcentration. The exercise-induced increases in hemoconcentration during pregnancy may be related to pregnancy-induced changes in capillary dynamics.

▶ There is increasing evidence that moderate exercise is beneficial to the pregnant woman, not only in helping to avoid a loss in her general physical condition, but also by contributing to a favorable pregnancy outcome. The main hazard is a substantial rise of core temperature, which can have adverse effects upon the development of the fetus, particularly during the first trimester. Because of the lower core temperature and buoyancy support, swimming is a popular type of exercise for those who are pregnant. The difference of peak oxygen intake between swimming and cycling apparently increases as pregnancy develops, and given the close relationship of this discrepancy to a parallel difference of peak ventilation, mechanical problems in synchronizing breathing with the swimming stroke seem to be responsible. The discrepancy of aerobic power between the 2 modes of exercise at 35 weeks of gestation (about 25%) is large enough that it should be noted when developing a swim prescription for the pregnant woman.—R.J. Shephard, M.D., Ph.D., D.P.E.

Maximal Aerobic Exercise in Pregnant Women: Heart Rate, O_2 Consumption, CO_2 Production, and Ventilation

Lotgering FK, Van Doorn MB, Struijk PC, Pool J, Wallenburg HCS (Erasmus University, Rotterdam, The Netherlands

J Appl Physiol 70:1016–1023, 1991   2-24

Introduction.—The question of whether pregnancy affects the ability to perform physical exercise has been studied but not definitively answered. A study was done to see whether pregnancy influences maximal aerobic power.

Methods.—Heart rate, oxygen (O_2) uptake ($\dot{V}O_2$), carbon dioxide production ($\dot{V}CO_2$), and ventilation at rest and during bicycle and treadmill exercise tests were measured. Rapidly increasing exercise intensities were studied at 16, 25, and 35 weeks of gestation and at 7 weeks after delivery.

Observations.—Compared with nonpregnant states, maximal heart rate was slightly lower throughout pregnancy during bicycle and treadmill exercises. Pregnancy did not affect maximal $\dot{V}O_2$ during these exercises. Because of increased $\dot{V}O_2$ at rest, the amount of O_2 available for exercise tended to drop with increasing gestation, becoming statistically significant only during treadmill exercise at 35 weeks' gestation. Power was positively correlated with O_2 availability during bicycle as well as treadmill exercise. The relationship was not affected by pregnancy. Carbon dioxide production at maximal exercise was lower during pregnancy than at 7 weeks after the birth. Maximal ventilation was increased during gestation. The relationship between ventilation and $\dot{V}CO_2$ was not influenced by gestation, except for the hyperventilation of pregnancy, which was maintained at maximal aerobic exercise.

Conclusions.—Pregnancy does not markedly influence either maximal heart rate or maximal O_2 uptake. The increased O_2 uptake at rest tends to reduce the amount of O_2 available for exercise at very high levels of treadmill exercise in late gestation. Pregnancy does not affect the relationship between power and O_2 uptake.

▶ This study is well done and complements other studies looking at the same or similar questions. The authors do note 2 points where they feel their study can be criticized. They did not perform the bicycle and treadmill tests in random order, and the control measurements were taken 7 weeks postpartum and may not represent the true nonpregnant state. However, they were aware of these design flaws before they did the study and made conscious decisions to accept these flaws for the greater good of being able to conduct the study.—Col. J.L. Anderson, PE.D.

Exercise and Breast-Feeding Mothers
Shelkun PH (Chicago)
Phys Sportsmed 19:109–116, 1991   2–25

Background.—Most mothers continue to breast-feed their baby in the first weeks, but many express concern about returning to exercise during lactation. Current thinking on exercise for lactating mothers is reviewed.

Discussion.—Research into this area has begun only recently, but moderate aerobic exercise appears to have no effect on the mother's milk or the infant's growth. In underdeveloped countries, lactation is remarkably consistent: where nutrition is inadequate, energy is mobilized from tissue reserves. In Western cultures, however, diet does not appear to be an important consideration. Exercise may induce hormonal and metabolic changes that counter balance the increased demands on energy; therefore, milk volume and energy output in milk may even be higher in lactating women. Exercise causes a temporary increase in serum prolactin, which may or may not affect lactation, and accumulation of lactic acid is unlikely to affect lactation.

Although some physicians recommend that a woman wait 2 weeks after delivering a baby to resume exercise, others suggest that she can begin exercising as soon as she feels ready. A slow return to exercise is generally recommended. It is up to the mother's individual preference when to feed in relation to exercise. The patient must have an adequate caloric intake to meet her increased energy demands if she is exercising to reduce weight, although recent research suggests that the Recommended Daily Allowance of 2,700 calories may be too high for the postpartum level of activity.

The breasts must be well supported during exercise. Nipple soreness may result from improper breast support. Breast pain may also be a sign of infection.

Conclusions.—For nursing mothers, exercise may increase energy levels and reduce fatigue. Exercise may also help to prevent postpartum depression. Moderation in such exercise is widely recommended.

▶ This article presents reasonable advice to nursing mothers, or for that matter, for most people, men and women. That is, under almost all circumstances, moderate exercise will be beneficial to you if you will listen to your body.—Col. J.L. Anderson, PE.D.

The Menstrual Cycle: Does it Affect Athletic Performance?
Quadagno D, Faquin L, Lim G-N, Kuminka W, Moffat R (Florida State Univ, Tallahassee)
Phys Sportsmed 19:121–124, 1991   2–26

Background.—There have been few studies of the association between athletic performance and phases of the menstrual cycle, and the reported results have been conflicting. Nonetheless, coaches and athletes commonly believe that performance is impaired during certain menstrual phases. The effect of the menstrual cycle on performance was investigated in swimmers and weight lifters.

Methods.—The weight-lifting group included 12 recreational weight lifters, mean age 24.3 years, who trained at least 30 minutes per day, 3 days a week. Those athletes were tested by bench and leg presses in the premenstrual, menstrual, and postmenstrual phases of 3 menstrual cycles. The swimmers were 15 competitive swimmers who trained 2 to 3 hours per day, 6 days a week. Those athletes were tested on the 100-m and 200-m freestyle events, during the same 3 phases of 3 menstrual cycles.

Results.—Neither group showed any significant differences in performance in any of the 3 trials, according to 2-way analysis of variance. On the bench press, values ranged from 12.5 to 13.8 repetitions of 70% of maximum weight. In the 100-m freestyle event, times ranged from 68.4 seconds to 70.7 seconds.

Conclusions.—In female weight lifters and swimmers performing events of short duration, there appears to be no effect of menstrual cycle on athletic performance. Further research should include events of both long and short duration. Ideally, the subjects would be unaware of the nature of the research.

▶ Results of studies of women's athletic performance in relation to their menstrual cycles have varied greatly. This one is no different. Possibly this is a case where the psychological effects are greater than the physiologic effects. Another weakness we find when attempting to compare results of various studies is the lack of control and so many important variables.—Col. J.L. Anderson, PE.D.

Exercise and "The Pill": Putting a Rumor to Rest
Schelkun PH (Chicago)
Phys Sportsmed 19:143–152, 1991   2–27

Background.—There is a persistent rumor that oral contraceptives reduce peak athletic performance, but none of the few studies assessing the question have confirmed this idea.

Performance Effects and Advantages.—The newer biphasic and triphasic oral contraceptives have minimized side effects. Some studies have suggested that oral contraceptives reduce functional aerobic and endurance capability, but these have been small and inconclusive. Some female athletes continue to have fears about using these drugs, however. Generally, the advantages of the contraceptives outweigh their disadvantages, notably in the beneficial effects on the symptoms of dysmenorrhea. The athlete, with medical guidance, can also manipulate her menstrual cycle around the date of an important competition; this is only recommended for world-class athletes, however. Oral contraceptives also protect against endometrial hyperplasia and bone loss.

Menstrual Dysfunction.—The mechanism of "athletic amenorrhea" remains unclear, but oral contraceptives may be the solution to this problem. Many women fail to seek medical attention for various reasons. The problem appears to progress in severity from luteal phase deficiency to hypoestrogenic amenorrhea. Anovulatory amenorrhea may increase the risk of endometrial hyperplasia, adenocarcinoma, and breast cancer; this may also be treated with oral contraceptives. Amenorrheic athletes should have other causes of menstrual dysfunction ruled out, and should undergo progesterone challenge. Oral contraceptives are probably the most convenient of several therapeutic options. Some physicians recommend oral contraceptives to help minimize calcium loss in younger women who are at risk of amenorrhea and are unaware of its dangers.

Discussion.—The use of oral contraceptives is convenient and may be protective for women at risk of menstrual dysfunction. There appear to be few, if any, effects on athletic performance.

▶ I recall when the YEAR BOOK OF SPORTS MEDICINE was first published. Any discussion such as the effects of oral contraceptives on physical performance and concerns about the causes and effects of "athletic amenorrhea" would have been quite unsophisticated by today's standards. We are making some progress in our understanding, but we all must know that we still have a long way to go.—Col. J.L. Anderson, PE.D.

Spinal Bone Loss and Ovulatory Disturbances
Prior JC, Vigna YM, Schechter MT, Burgess AE (University of British Columbia, Vancouver)
N Engl J Med 323:1221–1227, 1990   2–28

Introduction.—Bone loss accelerates with the cessation of menstruation and in women with menstrual disorders such as exercise-related amenorrhea. A prospective 1-year trial was undertaken to determine whether spinal bone loss occurs in ovulatory premenopausal women who exercise intensively.

Methods.—The density of cancellous bone from T12 to L3 was estimated by quantitative CT at a 1-year interval in 66 women aged 21–42 years, all of whom had 2 consecutive ovulatory cycles at the outset. Twenty-one women were training for a marathon and 22 others ran regularly but less intensively.

Results.—Overall spinal bone density decreased by 3 mg/ml/year, or 2% per year. No woman became amenorrheic, but 29% of the subjects had ovulatory disturbances, and these correlated closely with bone loss. Thirteen women with anovulatory cycles lost bone mineral at a rate of 4.2% per year. Menstrual cycle patterns in the women who trained for a marathon run did not differ significantly from those in the other groups.

Discussion.—This study failed to confirm more marked bone mineral loss in women who train intensively. It appears that inadequate progesterone production is associated with accelerated bone loss, even if the cycle interval remains normal. This association could be confirmed by a controlled trial in which anovulatory but menstruating women receive progesterone for 10 days per cycle in a dose equivalent to the amount produced in the normal luteal phase.

▶ The seminal study of Drinkwater et al. in 1984 (1) showed significant bone mineral content loss in amenorrheic compared with eumenorrheic athletes. In that paper we were presented with the picture of an amenorrheic runner in her mid-20s with a lumbar bone mass equivalent to a postmenopausal female. Since then our consciousness has been alerted to the significant morbidity associated with athletic amenorrhea. It was, in addition then, implicit that these changes were primarily estrogen-dependent. The present study by Prior and colleagues is of interest for 2 reasons. FIrst, the 66 premenopausal women came from a larger pool of subjects who were going to train, but none of whom developed amenorrhea, although many developed ovulatory distrubances. The principal findings were that the decreases in bone mineral density over this 1-year period were much more closely related to the disturbance of ovulation (without amenorrhea) but not with the intensity of the physical activity. Perhaps the second conclusion is even more interesting in that the authors suggest that it is the decrease in progesterone production that is the primary culprit in this bone demineralization. If this hypothesis turns out to be true, it will also be very important. There may well be a much larger group of athletes previously not suspected of being at risk of developing osteoporosis who we may need to consider; that is, women with short luteal phases or anovulatory cycles who may appear to be cycling in a relatively normal manner and therefore are assumed to be relatively normal hormonally. However, if the prior hypothesis is true, then such an assumption is not warranted.—J.R. Sutton, M.D.

Reference.

1. Drinkwater BL, et al: *N Engl J Med* 311:277, 1984.

The Application of Historical Data for Evaluation of Osteopenia in Female Runners: The Menstrual Index

Grimston SK, Sanborn CF, Miller PD, Huffer WE (University of Calgary, Can-

ada; Texas Women's Univ, Denton; Univ of Colorado, Denver)
Clin Sports Med 2:108–118, 1990   2–29

Introduction.—The female long-distance runner with athletic amenorrhea may be predicted to have low bone mass, or osteopenia, and low bone mineral density (BMD) of the lumbar spine. It has been postulated that the reduced level of estrogen as reflected in amenorrhea is the mechanism underlying the low bone mass. A study was designed to develop a simple, objective menstrual index (MI) that would define menstrual history numerically and would determine the association between MI, prior calcium intake, and bone mass in female distance runners.

Subjects.—Twelve white female runners and 5 sedentary women had bone mass measured at the distal radius, lumbar vertebrae (L2-L4), and femoral neck using photon absorptiometry. Nine of the runners were currently menstruating regularly and 3 were currently amenorrheic. A menstrual index derived from a questionnaire about current and previous menstrual status reflected menstrual patterns since menarche. A dietary calcium history through childhood, adolescence, and early adulthood was determined.

Findings.—There was a significant relationship between MI and BMD at L2-L4 and also between calcium intake from 12 to 18 years of age and BMD. A history of menstrual irregularity and perhaps a marked decrease in calcium intake between ages 12-18 years may be associated with osteopenia in female runners. Current calcium intake was not related to current BMD.

Conclusions.—Bone mineral density in this group of female runners was associated with a history of menstrual irregularity and a decrease in calcium intake in adolescence but not with current calcium intake. The menstrual index, derived from menstrual history since menarche, may be an effective method for numerically defining menstrual history.

▶ These authors call into question the automatic assumption that below normal BMD of the lumbar spine is the result of secondary amenorrhea brought on by exercise. Their findings indicate that low calcium intake between the ages of 12–18 years may play some significant role. It has been reported that children in that age range should consume 1,200 mg of calcium per day. These are interesting findings. Coaches and parents of adolescent female athletes should pay more attention to the nutritional need of these athletes.—Col. J.L. Anderson, PE.D.

Relationships Among Strength, Endurance, Weight and Body Fat During Three Phases of the Menstrual Cycle
Dibrezzo R, Fort IL, Brown B (Univ of Arkansas, Fayetteville)
J Sports Med Phys Fitness 31:89–94, 1991   2–30

Background.—Women were prevented from competing in running events longer than 1,500 meters in the Olympics until 1984. This lack of knowledge of the effect of the menstrual cycle on the athletic performance of women coupled with societal myths about the influence of the menstrual cycle are slowly changing. The relationships among body weight, body fat, and dynamic strength and muscular endurance were studied during different phases of the menstrual cycle.

Subjects.—Twenty-one healthy women, aged 18–36, with normal menstrual cycles were assessed for body weight and percent body fat. The women were tested for strength and endurance of the knee flexors and extensors on a Cybex II isokinetic dynamometer. Testing was perfomed at 3 speeds of the dynamometer during the mensus phase (within 24 hours of onset), ovulation phase (13–14 days from onset), and luteal phase (10 days from ovulation) of the menstrual cycle in all the women.

Findings.—The phases of the menstrual cycle had little or no effect on the relationships among body weight, percent body fat, knee extension flexion strength or endurance. The correlations of peak torque variables between the cycle phases indicated a consistency of performance.

Conclusions.—In this study, performance of strength and endurance testing was consistent during all phases of the menstrual cycle in 21 women tested. The phases of the menstrual cycle had little or no effect on the relationships among body weight, percent body fat, knee extension and flexion strength or endurance.

▶ This study joins a list of works that tend to show that the different phases of the menstrual cycle have little or no effect on physiologic performance variables. Of course, it is possible that the gross motor skills that generally have been used in these studies may not be affected, but fine motor skills might be. However, most investigators tend to support the conclusion that physical performance is not adversely affected during the different phases of the menstrual cycle. Also, younger women who are less experienced in dealing with their menses may be more affected.—Col. J.L. Anderson, PE.D.

The Association Between Weight, Physical Activity, and Stress and Variation in the Length of the Menstrual Cycle
Harlow SD, Matanoski GM (Univ of North Carolina, Chapel Hill; Johns Hopkins Univ, Baltimore)
Am J Epidemiol 133:38–49, 1991   2–31

Introduction.—Previous studies have associated variation in the length of the menstrual cycle with age, body weight, exercise, and life stress, but few studies have quantified the magnitude of risk associated with specific exposure levels. The present study was designed to prospectively quantify the association between menstrual cycle length and weight, physical activity, and stress in population of college women.

Study Design.—In 1985, a total of 563 eligible college freshman women were invited to enroll in a 12-month menstrual diary study. No incentives were offered. Participants maintained a daily record of their menstrual bleeding and completed a self-administered questionnaire on weight, dieting, physical activity, recent major life events, use of contraceptives, smoking, and use of alcohol at enrollment. Information was updated monthly by mailed questionnaire. Height and weight were measured at enrollment, in the middle, and at the end of the 12-month study.

Results.—Of the 179 women who enrolled in the study, 162 contributed sufficient data for at least 1 segment. The women ranged in age from 17 to 19 years. The unadjusted probability of a menstrual cycle being longer than 43 days was 5%. Women with a history of long cycles were more likely to have a long cycle during the study. Situations that created a demand for performance or required adjustment to new demands also increased the risk of a long cycle. Starting college increased the risk of long cycles, regardless of whether the student had left home. Moderate exercise minimally increased the probability of a long cycle. Weight changes and being overweight were independently associated with the probability of long cycles. When 17- to 43-day cycles were evaluated, a history of long cycles increased the expected cycle length by a mean of 1.42 days, whereas dieting tended to shorten the expected cycle length by a mean of 1.38 days, living on campus shortened it by .90 day, and starting college shortened it by .64 days.

Conclusion.—Expectations of performance while coping with a new set of circumstances or with an increased burden increases the probability of long menstrual cycles. Moderate activity has a small but consistent positive effect on the probability of having a cycle longer than 43 days. Menstrual history and stress are more important than either body weight or physical activities in explaining variations in length of menstrual cycles.

▶ This study agrees with the major findings of the study we conducted here at West Point in 1976 and 1977. At that time, we reported that the increased cycle lengths to include secondary amenorrhea probably were caused by something other than physical activity, dieting, or low body fat. We suggested that psychological stress should also be considered. This study, although more complete and more sophisticated than ours, seems to confirm our findings.—Col. J.L. Anderson, PE.D.

The Role of Endogenous Opiates in Athletic Amenorrhea
Samuels MH, Sanborn CF, Hofeldt F, Robbins R (Univ of Colorado, Denver)
Fertil Steril 55:507–512, 1991   2–32

Introduction.—Menstrual cycle abnormalities in female athletes are associated with decreased luteinizing hormone (LH), follicle-stimulating hormone (FSH), and resting prolactin levels (PRL) and may contribute to decreased bone density and increased fracture rates. In some studies, elevated endogenous opioids suppressed LH secretion, but data on female athletes are sparse and conflicting. It was hypothesized that menstrual disturbances in female athletes arise from opioid-induced abnormalities in gonadotropin and/or prolactin secretion. The effects of menstrual status, acute exercise, releasing hormone stimulation, and opiate blockade on gonadotropin and PRL secretion, were investigated.

Methods.—Luteinizing hormone, FSH, and PRL levels were measured in 6 eumenorrheic and 6 amenorrheic athletes. Levels of LH, FSH, and PRL were measured during thyrotropin-releasing hormone and gonadotropin-releasing hormone tests at baseline, after naloxone infusions, after exercise to exhaustion, and after similar exercise during naloxone infusions.

Results.—Contrary to the original hypothesis, amenorrheic runners did not have significant alterations in basal, postexercise, or stimulated hormone levels compared with eumenorrheic runners. Opioid blockade by naloxone had little effect on gonadotropin release in amenorrheic athletes. Resting prolactin level was slightly augmented, not inhibited, by naloxone.

Conclusions.—Elevated opioid levels did not suppress gonadotropin or elevate PRL levels in a group of female athletes and is probably not the cause of menstrual dysfunction. This group of highly trained athletes may not be typical, and exercise-induced amenorrhea in other individuals may involve opioid-induced pituitary hormone abnormalities.

▶ Although the findings of these authors are valuable and interesting, they must be confirmed using larger sample sizes. The authors recognized that with such a small group of highly trained subjects and the possibility that exercise-induced amenorrhea may be a heterogeneous disorder, a larger sample may involve opioid-induced pituitary hormone abnormalities.—Col. J.L. Anderson, PE.D.

Resting Metabolic Rate and Energy Balance in Amenorrheic and Eumenorrheic Runners
Myerson M, Gutin B, Warren MP, May MT, Contento I, Lee M, Pi-Sunyer FX, Pierson RN, Brooks-Gunn J (Columbia Univ; St Luke's-Roosevelt Hosp Ctr, New York; Educational Testing Service, Princeton, NJ)
Med Sci Sports Exerc 23:15–22, 1991   2–33

Introduction.—Low body fat is a factor frequently associated with athletic menstrual dysfunction (AMD). Other factors associated with AMD are the severity of the training regimen, energy drain, quantity and quality of diet, aberrant nutritional patterns, and chronological and gynecologic age. Metabolic and nutritional factors associated with AMD were investigated in 3 groups of women.

Methods.—Components of energy expenditure, caloric intake, body composition, and attitudes toward eating in highly trained amenorrheic and eumenorrheic runners and eumenorrheic sedentary controls were studied. The amenorrheic and eumenorrheic runners were similar in age, weight, percent body fat by hydrodensitometry, training pace and mileage, best 10-km race time, years running, and maximal oxygen consumption.

Results.—The amenorrheic group had a significantly lower resting metabolic rate and a higher score on the scale of aberrant eating patterns than the eumenorrheic or sedentary women.

Conclusion.—This is the first study to document a lower resting metabolic rate in amenorrheic runners compared with eumenorrheic runners or sedentary controls. Despite a less adequate diet than the eumenorrheic runners, the adaptive response of amenorrhea and a reduced lower resting metabolic rate in the amenorrheic runners appears to maintain energy balance and stable weight.

▶ These authors, for the first time, have shown that amenorrheic runners as subjects have a lower resting metabolic rate than do the eumenorrheic subjects. They think that this finding suggests an adaptive response in the amenorrheic runner that may reflect a physiologic mechanism to conserve energy. They also reported that the amenorrheic and eumenorrheic runners were not significantly different in percent body fat. This agrees with our studies at West Point that body fat itself is not sufficient to suggest a causal effect for amenorrhea.—Col. J.L. Anderson, PE.D.

Alterations in Dietary Carbohydrate, Protein, and Fat Intake and Mood State in Trained Female Cyclists
Keith RE, O'Keeffe KA, Blessing DL, Wilson GD (Auburn Univ, Ala)
Med Sci Sports Exerc 23:212–216, 1991   2–34

Introduction.—Carbohydrate consumption has been linked to increased athletic performance and altered mood states. However, there are few data on the effects of feeding different levels of carbohydrate, protein, and fat over longer periods of time on the mood state of athletes.

Methods.—Seven trained female cyclists consumed a low carbohydrate (LCHO), moderate carbohydrate (MCHO), and high carbohydrate (HCHO) level diet with varying protein and fat levels for 1 week each in random order. Cyclists completed a Profile of Mood States (POMS) questionnaire after each weekly diet treatment and then rode on a cycle ergometer at 80% maximal oxygen uptake until fatigued. The POMS questionnaire measured tension, depression, anger, vigor, fatigue, and confusion, and provided a total mood score.

Findings.—The subjects consuming the low carbohydrate diet had greater tension, depression, anger, and total mood scores and less vigor than subjects consuming the moderate or high carbohydrate diets. The MCHO and HCHO diet subjects showed no significant differences. The LCHO diet may result in decreased muscle glycogen or changes in hormone or substrate levels that could adversely affect training and mood state.

Conclusions.—Consumption of a low carbohydrate, high protein, high fat diet cause significant changes in the mood state of female cyclists in a training and exercise program. The LCHO diet was associated with greater tension, depression, anger, and total mood scores on the POMS questionnaire. The changes in mood were improved with the addition of more dietary carbohydrate. The MCHO and HCHO diet subjects showed no significant differences.

▶ These findings seem to agree with anecdotal evidence from men who were training for the marathon and tried the "carbohydrate loading" nutritional technique. The early phase of that technique required a very low carbohydrate intake. The men who tried this reported great swings in mood to include depression and irritability, to the point where they gave up that phase and used only the high carbohydrate intake phase. When they did this, they felt much better, and the depression and irritability subsided.—Col. J.L. Anderson, PE.D.

Effect of an Iron Supplement on Body Iron Status and Aerobic Capacity of Young Training Women
Magazanik A, Weinstein Y, Abarbanel J, Lewinski U, Shapiro Y, Inbar O, Epstein S (Wingate Institute for Physical Education and Sport, Netanya; Golda Meir Medical Center, Petah-Tikva; Tel Aviv University, Israel)
Eur J Appl Physiol 62:317–323, 1991   2–35

Introduction.—Iron deficiency occurs frequently in female athletes, but the precise effects of exercise on body iron status remain uncertain. The effects of an oral iron supplement on aerobic capacity and body iron status were studied in young women engaging in 7 weeks of intensive physical training.

Methods.—An oral iron supplement of 160 mg was used by 13 women, aged 19 years, during a 7-week program of running, climbing, jumping, and weight lifting. Training was based on the overload principle and entailed a gradual increase in intensity throughout the period. A placebo was used by 15 other women.

Results.—The women who were given iron supplements had significantly higher hemoglobin, packed cell volume, and ferritin values than placebo recipients. The hemoglobin increased 9.3% during training in women given iron and 2.4% in those given placebo. Two thirds of placebo recipients and none of the women given iron had a serum ferritin level less than 10 ng/mL at the end of training. Only those given iron had a substantial increase in maximal aerobic capacity in the first 3 weeks of training. Subsequently, aerobic capacity also increased in the placebo recipients.

Conclusion.—A daily oral iron supplement improves body iron status and hematologic variables in young women who train intensively. Supplementation also promotes a higher maximal aerobic capacity early in the course of training.

▶ This study, probably more than any I have reviewed over the years concerning iron supplements for women, is very positive and direct in saying that iron supplements are beneficial. The authors believe that women engaged in strenuous physical activity should be monitored and their body iron status should be maintained. They report a high correlation between hemoglobin concentration and $\dot{V}O_{2max}$ and they show that hemoglobin concentration can be maintained with a daily supplement of 160 mg of ferrous sulfate.—Col. J.L. Anderson, PE.D.

Menstrual Function and Eating Behavior in Female Recreational Weight Lifters and Competitive Body Builders
Walberg JL, Johnston CS (Virginia Technical Inst, Blacksburg)
Med Sci Sports Exerc 23:30–36, 1991   2–36

Background.—The combination of intensive activity, extreme dietary practices to minimize body fat while maximizing muscle mass, and low body fat may contribute to menstrual irregularities among female weight lifters and body builders. The highest rates of amenorrhea appear in ballet dancers and runners, but there are no detailed reports of menstrual dysfunction in weight lifters. Descriptive information about the eating behavior and menstrual function of females who weight train for general conditioning and a subset of women who competed in a body building competition is provided.

Subjects.—A group of 103 female weight lifters (WL) and a group of 92 female controls (C) answered a survey on eating behavior and attitudes, including the Eating Disorder Inventory, and menstrual function. The weight-lifting group was further divided into a competitive (COMP) group (12 subjects) and a noncompetitive group.

Findings.—The incidence of menstrual dysfunction was highest in the subset of 12 WL who had competed in at least 1 body-building competition and was significantly higher for the WL group than for the control group. More WL than C women reported missing at least 1 menstrual period during the last year. Fifteen percent of the WL and 9% of the C group had an excessive drive for thinness as rated by the Eating Disorders Index. Significantly more women in the WL group responded that they were terrified of becoming fat, were obsessed with food, used laxatives for weight control, and claimed they had been anorexic in the past. Responses in the COMP group were significantly higher than in the WL group for women who used to be anorexic, were terrified of becoming fat, or experienced uncontrollable urges to eat.

Conclusions.—Women who do weight lifting for general conditioning, and a subset of these women who compete in body building, have a significantly higher incidence of a history of anorexia nervosa, excessive concern about their weight and food consumption, and menstrual dysfunction than women in a control group. Self-reported menstrual dysfunction was present in almost a third of all WL and the majority of competitive body builders.

▶ These findings are not surprising. However, it would be wrong to ascribe a cause and effect relationship to them. It is just as likely that these women got involved in weight lifing because they were terrified of becoming fat. Among any group of exercising women we will probably find a subset who are involved because they are afraid of becoming fat. That is an educational problem. We need to teach people more about developing healthy life styles rather than merely teach them to lift weights, to run, or to do any other kind of exercise. Our schools need more support to be able to run quality physical education programs, which would at least partially solve the problems identified in this study.—Col. J.L. Anderson, PE.D.

Preseason Strength and Flexibility Imbalances Associated With Athletic Injuries in Female Collegiate Athletes
Knapik JJ, Bauman CL, Jones BH, Harris JMcA, Vaughan L (U S Army Research Inst of Environmental Med, Natick, Mass; Wellesley College)
Am J Sports Med 19:76–81, 1991   2–37

Background.—It has traditionally been thought that athletic injuries are associated with specific strength and flexion imbalances, although studies of this relationship have shown limited success. The association was investigated in 138 female college athletes attending a Division III institution.

Methods.—The athletes, with a mean age of 18.9 years at entry into the study, participated in 8 weight-bearing sports. Preseason strength and flexibility tests were administered to all subjects. Strength testing consisted of measurement of the maximal isokinetic torque of the right and left knee extensors at 30 and 180 degrees/second. Flexibility testing consisted of measurement of the active range of motion of several lower body joints. Some athletes were tested in more than 1 year of the 3-year study, but the analysis included only the first year of testing. The women were then followed up during their sports seasons for injuries.

Results.—One or more injuries occurred in 40% of the subjects, many of them lacrosse players. Eighty percent of injuries were to the lower extremity. More injuries were encountered when the right knee flexor was 15% stronger than the left at 180 degrees/second, when the right hip extensor was 15% more flexible than the left, and when the knee flexor knee extensor ratio was less than .75 at 180 degrees/second. Higher injury rates tended to be associated with knee flexor or hip extensor imbalances of at least 15%, on either side of the body.

Conclusions.—Specific imbalances of strength and flexibility are associated with injury of the lower extremity. Imbalances measured at 30 degrees/second do not appear to be related, but those measured at 180 degrees/second do. Studies of a larger number of subjects and fewer subjects with imbalances greater than 15% are called for.

▶ We have performed similar research at West Point in the past, but we were primarily studying knee injuries requiring surgery. It is interesting, because we found that athletes with greater than a 10% bilateral strength deficiency in knee extensor strength were more likely to sustain injury to the knee. We also found that a ratio of less than .66 for knee flexor to extensor strength was a sign of potential future knee injury. All our subjects were men. We did not, however, include flexibility of the hip extensors in our studies. This kind of work needs to be continued. At this point, it is not intuitively obvious to me why the measurements made by these researchers should have any relationship to the cause of ankle sprains.—Col. J.L. Anderson, PE.D.

Biochemical and Histochemical Adaptation to Sprint Training in Young Athletes
Cadefau J, Casademont J, Grau JM, Ferńandez J, Balaguer A, Vernet M, Cussó R, Urbano-Márquez A (University of Barcelona, Spain)
Acta Physiol Scand 140:341–351, 1990   2–38

Objective.—Muscle adaptation to physical training depends in part on the mode, intensity, and duration of the training. Whether a consistent pattern of adaptation occurs after a prolonged (8-month) period of specific, controlled sprint training was investigated.

Study Design.—Eight of 16 teenage athletes had participated in a sprint training program during the previous year. An anaerobic program was followed, and much effort was devoted to promoting muscle strength. Speed and strength were emphasized early and late in the program, whereas aerobic capacity, power, and general strength were emphasized in the middle part. Vastus lateralis biopsy specimens were compared before and after training.

Observations.—The athletes gained body weight and had an increase in arm perimeter during the training period. They also grew in height,

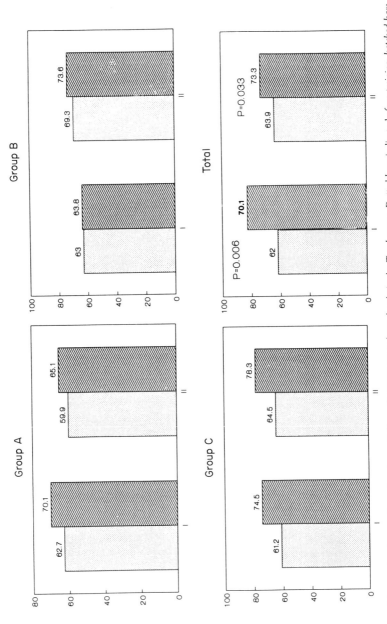

Fig 2–8.—Diameter in microns of type I and type II fibers. Statistics are indicated only in the *Total* group. *Dotted bars* indicate before training; *hatched bars*, after training. (Courtesy of Cadefau J, Casademont J, Grau JM, et al: *Acta Physiol Scand* 140:341–351, 1990.)

although not significantly. Muscle glycogen content increased, as did the activities of glycogen synthase, glycogen phosphorylase, phosphofructo-kinase, pyruvate kinase, succinate dehydrogenase, and transaminases. However, aldolase, lactate dehydrogenase, and creatine kinase activities did not change. The proportion of type I muscle fibers increased, and both fiber types increased significantly in diameter after training (Fig 2–8).

Conclusions.—Prolonged sprint training appears to lead to a bio-chemical muscular adaptation to anaerobic exercise. The morphological adaptations that occur appear to be less specific.

▶ These investigators present an excellent paper in which they attempt to document and eventually quantify the adaptive response to sprint training, with an emphasis on speed and strength training. They are fully aware of some previous research that called into question the adaptive muscle response to sprint training. However, not all of the previous work had con-trolled for number and length of training sessions, intensity of training, or pre-vious training in other disciplines that could interfere with the results. This study used both men and women as subjects. It is interesting to see, al-though the numbers are small, that women appear to adapt to this training much the same way the men adapted. It will be interesting to see whether these results can be replicated using a larger number of subjects, both men and women. I would also like to see a control group, the same age, that is involved in some other type training, perhaps aerobic training only.—Col. J.L. Anderson, PE.D.

Gender Differences in Psychological Strategies Among Talented Swimmers: An Exploratory Study
Spink K (University of Saskatchewan, Canada)
Aust J Sci Med Sport 22:68–70, 1990   2–39

Background.—The suggestion that gender affects the psychological aspects of athletic performance has not been tested, although the sexes are known to differ in their attributions for success and failure and in their use of imagery. An exploratory study to seek gender differences in certain psychological aspects of talented athletes was performed in 30 elite swimmers.

Methods.—There were 15 male and 15 female swimmers. Mean age was 16.5 years for the males and 15.3 years for the females. All subjects completed a questionnaire seeking information on the psychological fac-tors that affected their performance, both in training and competition. The data gathered were analyzed by means of t tests and stepwise dis-criminant function analyses for gender.

Results.—Female swimmers spent more time before a competitive event thinking about it, spent more hours in other types of training, and used more visual imagery both before and during competition. The females talked to themsleves more and had a more difficult time recovering from their mistakes. Males thought more about their earlier mistakes than did females.

Conclusions.—Some psychological factors differentiating male from female swimmers have been identified. Future studies in this area should include athletes in different sports with difference performance histories and should include larger samples.

▶ The intent of this study was to identify psychological differences between men and women athletes that can be replicated in future studies. Obviously the author is aware that this is but one small step in investigating these psychological differences, if there are any. For some reason, there has seemed to be a reluctance on the part of sports psychologists to want to deal with this question. Hopefully, we will see an increase in the sophistication of our studies in this arena over the next few years.—Col. J.L. Anderson, PE.D.

Vaginal Perforation Due to Jet Ski Accident
Wein P, Thompson DJ (Royal Women's Hospital, Melbourne, Australia)
Aust NZ J Obstet Gynaecol 30:384–385, 1990   2–40

Background.—Vaginal lacerations resulting from waterskiing falls have been reported. Such cases are characterized by a lack of protective clothing and a fall in a sitting position or being pulled through water in a crouching position. A similar injury resulted from a fall from a jet ski.

Case Report.—Woman, 29, fell backwards off a jet ski and struck the water in sitting position and at the same time was struck in the perineum by the water jet of a jet ski in front of her. Perineal and abdominal pain and vaginal bleeding occurred immediately. On examination, she had a small perineal tear with bleeding from high in the left vaginal fornix, which was not well seen. The tear was sutured, the vagina packed. Intravenous 3.5% polygeline colloid was administered, and the patient was transferred.

Discussion.—Speculum examination showed a large laceration of the posterior vaginal fornix extending into the left lateral fornix. Signs and blood test results suggesting early peritonitis were explained by full-thickness vaginal perforation through the pouch of Douglas, as the patient had previously had tubal ligation. Examination under anesthesia showed a 10-cm laceration in the posterior vaginal fornix and a 5-cm defect in the peritoneum of the pouch of Douglas. There were no overt signs of peritoneal soiling. The broad ligament was closed to secure hemostasis and the peritoneum, vagina, and perineal laceration were closed in layers. Intravenous antibiotics were started intraoperatively. The patient was febrile on postoperative day 1 but this resolved by day 4. The patient was discharged on day 6, and she had no complaints 4 weeks later.

Conclusions.—It is essential to recognize this type of injury in patients who have vaginal or rectal bleeding after waterskiing or jet-ski falls. Wearing of adequate protective clothing could prevent these injuries.

▶ Waterskiing has been tied to vaginal lacerations in women and to rectal tears in men, owing to high pressure douches or enemas, respectively. This is the first report of a vaginal laceration in a woman who fell off a jet-ski. Like similar water ski injuries, this jet-ski injury involved the posterior vaginal fornix, where the vagina is least supported by fascia. In a similar case, a 17-year-old girl wearing a 2-piece bathing suit and riding as a passenger slid off the back of a jet-ski and fell behind its nozzle (1). She was struck in the perineum by the full force of the jet spray, suffering a vaginal laceration that led to a retroperitoneal hematoma. Hypogastric artery ligation controlled the bleeding and avoided more extensive surgery. These injuries could be prevented if all participants in high-speed water sports wore adequate protective clothing such as wetsuits, or at least wetsuit pants.—E.R. Eichner, M.D.

Reference

1.   Haefner HK, et al: *Obstet Gynecol* 78:986, 1991.

Nonunion of a First Rib Fracture in a Gymnast
Proffer DS, Patton JJ, Jackson DW (Columbus, Ohio; Southern California Ctr for Sports Med, Long Beach, Calif)
Am J Sports Med 19:198–201, 1991   2–41

Introduction.—Isolated fractures of the first rib have been reported in athletes participating in various sports, including football, baseball, basketball, and dancing. A first rib fracture sustained without direct, violent trauma is likely to be stress induced, precipitated by muscle forces acting on the first rib. The fractures are usually asymptomatic and are found incidentally on routine chest roentgenograms. They usually heal with an adequate period of rest. A competitive gymnast sustained an isolated first rib fracture that persisted as a symptomatic nonunion 2 years after injury.

Case Report.—Girl, 12, complained of stabbing posterior right shoulder pain related to strenuous workouts of 2 years' duration. She had sustained an isolated right rib fracture 2 years previously. Roentgenograms taken at that time revealed a simple, transverse, nondisplaced right rib fracture. Discomfort persisted for 1½ years after the initial onset of pain and was exacerbated by a shove in the back 6 months before her visit. Roentgenograms revealed a typical hypertrophic nonunion. A transaxilliary resection of the right first rib was performed, and the patient had an uneventful recovery.

Conclusion.—Persistent symptomatic nonunion of an isolated fracture of the first rib has not been reported previously. Transaxilliary resection of 90% or more of the first rib is recommended if a symptomatic nonunion persists.

▶ A unique injury for a gymnast—fracture of the first rib, with nonunion. This injury is thought to arise not from direct trauma, but from muscle traction: the scalenus pulling up and the intercostals and others pulling down. Similar fractures of lower ribs have been reported in female rowers, for example. Nonunions of the first rib are often asymptomatic and are usually found incidentally on routine chest x-rays. Apparently, this is the first such nonunion to be persistently symptomatic; hence, the operation, with success.—E.R. Eichner, M.D.

Radial Growth Plate Injury in a Female Gymnast
Ruggles DL, Peterson HA, Scott SG (Mayo Clinic and Found, Rochester, Minn)
Med Sci Sports Exerc 23:393–396, 1991   2–42

Fig 2–9.—Dowel grip used by gymnasts to increase grip strength. (Courtesy of Ruggles DL, Peterson HA, Scott SG: *Med Sci Sports Exerc* 23:393–396, 1991.)

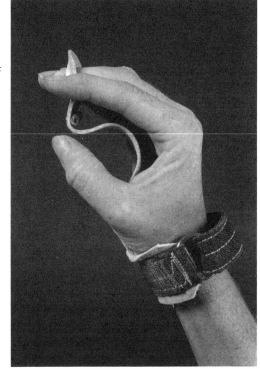

Background.—Gymnastics is the fastest-growing sport among women; training has intensified and new equipment has evolved. Chronic wrist pain from overuse is also increasing. This may be related to the increased use of dowel grips (Fig 2–9). A patient with radial growth plate injury resulting from this equipment was studied.

Case Report.—Girl, 12, an elite competitive gymnast, complained of right wrist pain. She trained for 4 hours, 5 times a week, and had relied increasingly on dowel grips for the past year. She had diffuse pain over the dorsum of the right wrist for 3 months, especially after exertion. A previous radiographic examination had shown bilateral widening of the proximal growth plates; symptoms did not respond to a 1-month trial of short arm cast and modified activity. Despite casting, the growth plate had continued to widen. She ceased gymnastics for 3 months, after which symptoms had resolved and the radiographic picture had improved. Activity was restarted progressively during 4 weeks. The radiographic picture continued to improve the next month. The patient continued to compete 15 months after the onset of symptoms.

Conclusions.—A female gymnast with growth plate injury of the wrist is examined. This injury may be related to creation of excessive loads, beyond the normal strength of the physis, by dowel grips. The injury should continue to be monitored, with early recognition and intervention.

▶ With more and more women taking up gymnastics, this report is timely in calling attention to radial growth plate injury as a possible consequence of overusing dowel grips. Dorsal wrist pain had been related to handsprings, roundoffs, and maneuvers on the uneven parallel bars; however, the diffuse dorsal wrist pain in this 12-year-old female gymnast was most likely related to her overuse of dowel grips, leather straps that act like minisplints to maintain the fingers in flexion at the metacarpophalangeal, proximal interphalangeal, and distal interphalangeal joints. By encircling the wrist and extending along the palm, the dowel grip forms a hook that aids in gripping the bar during high-speed giant loops. The cost, however, is that excessive loads may be created, beyond the normal strength of the physis. Athletes, coaches, and physicians should be alert to early signs of overuse of dowel grips.—E.R. Eichner, M.D.

3 Nutrition, Metabolism, Drugs, and Doping

Effects of Prior Exercise on the Thermic Effect of Glucose and Fructose

Balon TW, Welk GJ (Univ of Iowa, Iowa City)

J Appl Physiol 70:1463–1468, 1991

3–1

Background.—Previously, exercise has been shown to potentiate the thermic effect of a glucose load. It is unknown whether this phenomenon occurs when different carbohydrates are used, and the role of insulin is unclear. The thermic effects of glucose and fructose during control rest and postexercise trials were compared.

Methods.—Subjects were 6 endurance-trained male athletes with a mean age of 23 years. Each man ingested 100 g of fructose or glucose, either at rest or after recovery from 45 minutes of treadmill exercise at 70% of maximal consumption of O_2. The athletes performed all 4 trials in randomized order. From baseline to 3 hours after ingestion consump-

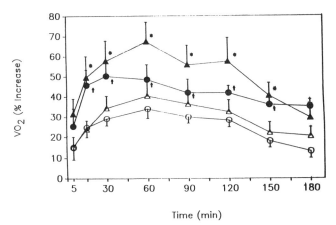

Time (min)

Fig 3–1.—Increase in consumption of O_2 ($\dot{V}O_2$) expressed as % change from baseline after ingestion of 100 g of carbohydrate. *Open circles,* rest + glucose trial; *filled circles,* exercise + glucose trial; *open triangles,* rest + fructose trial; *filled triangles,* exercise + fructose trial. *$P < .05$ between exercise + fructose and rest + fructose trials. *$P < .05$ between exercise + fructose and rest + fructose trials. †$P < .05$ between exercise + glucose and rest + glucose trials. (Courtesy of Balon TW, Welk GJ: *J Appl Physiol* 70:1463–1468, 1991.)

tion of O_2, respiratory exchange ratio, and plasma concentrations of glucose, insulin, glycerol, and lactate were measured.

Results.—Both challenges increased consumption of O_2 (Fig 3-1). Glucose increased net energy expenditure by 44 kcal and fructose increased net energy expenditure by 51 kcal over baseline during control trials. However, with exercise the thermic effect of both carbohydrate challenges was increased by 20 to 25 kcal. In both control and exercise trials ingestion of glucose increased plasma concentration of insulin to a greater extent than did ingestion of fructose.

Conclusions.—Fructose and glucose elicit a similar potentiation of thermogenesis after exercise. Because fructose, which is primarily metabolized by the liver, and glucose elicited a similar postexercise potentiation of thermogenesis, the results indicate that the thermogenic phenomenon is not limited to skeletal muscle. In addition, carbohydrate-induced thermogenesis after exercise is unrelated to incremental increases in plasma concentration of insulin.

▶ The increase in energy expenditure following a meal is referred to as dietary-induced thermogenesis and that characteristic of food is referred to as its thermic effect. In recent times exercise before a meal has been demonstrated to enhance this thermic effect (1). Insulin is thought to have a pivotal role in this thermic effect of food (2). To separate out the importance of insulin, the authors chose to study both the effects of glucose, a potent insulin stimulant, and fructose, the glucose isomer that is not quite as potent an insulin stimulant, on postexercise thermogenesis. An additional bonus of this study was the desire to separate out the sites of increased thermogenesis; fructose is primarily metabolized in the liver, whereas glucose would be oxidized primarily in muscle after exercise. All of this is particularly relevant as our society becomes obsessed with weight control. If there is a significant increased energy expenditure postprandially, then it would be wise to adopt an activity program designed to maximize exercise at exactly that time. The study was simple but nicely executed and clearly demonstrated that the thermic effect of both fructose and glucose was similar but real, and that they were insulin independent.—J.R. Sutton, M.D.

References

1. D'Alessio D, et al: *J Clin Invest* 81:1781, 1988.
2. Felig P, et al: *Am J Physiol* 244:E45, 1983.

Table of Nonprotein Respiratory Quotient: An Update
Péronnet F, Massicotte D (University of Montreal, Quebec)
Can J Sport Sci 16:23–29, 1991   3–2

Introduction.—A key step in indirect respiratory calorimetry is to determine the composition of the mixture of carbohydrates and fat that is oxidized using a table of nonprotein respiratory quotients. The table shows, for a given ratio rate of carbon dioxide produced per rate of oxygen used, both the percent of energy provided from carbohydrate vs. fat oxidation and the energy equivalent of oxygen. The respiratory exchange ratio can either be taken as a nonprotein respiratory quotient, assuming that negligible protein is oxidized, or may be corrected for protein oxidation.

The Problem.—Lusk's table, developed in 1924 and still universally used, was derived from biochemical and physical data that now are outdated.

The Solution.—A new table of nonprotein respiratory quotients was developed that is consistent with modern chemical and physical data. It is based on the average composition of human triacylglycerol stores, the energy potential of fatty acids and glucose, and the volumes occupied by 1 mole of oxygen or carbon dioxide under STPD conditions. This model takes into account 13 fatty acids that represent more than 99% of those present in human triacylglycerols. The differences between this table and that developed by Lusk are small.

▶ This paper is included because it is a small but important contribution to precision in the commonly used nonprotein respiratory quotient. The Respiratory Exchange Ratio (RER), which in steady state is assumed to be the Respiratory Quotient (RQ), has widespread use by both clinicians and physiologists to quantify the proportion of fat and carbohydrate used during exercise. More precision is welcome. I recommend this article to readers.—J.R. Sutton, M.D.

Dietary Carbohydrate, Muscle Glycogen, and Power Output During Rowing Training

Simonsen JC, Sherman WM, Lamb DR, Dernbach AR, Doyle JA, Strauss R (Ohio State Univ, Columbus)
J Appl Physiol 70:1500–1505, 1991   3–3

Introduction.—The belief that high carbohydrate diets enhance training capacity is based on studies that have varied carbohydrate intake over a few days and measured muscle glycogen, but did not assess power output during training. To determine whether a high carbohydrate diet would increase muscle glycogen and power output compared with a moderate carbohydrate diet over 4 weeks of intense training, 12 male and 10 female collegiate rowers were studied.

Methods.—The athletes were randomized to receive either a high carbohydrate diet, consisting of 10 g·kg body mass^{-1}·day^{-1}, or a moderate carbohydrate diet, consisting of 5 g·kg body mass^{-1}·day^{-1}. Protein intake was 2 g·kg body mass^{-1}·day^{-1}, with fat intake adjusted to maintain body mass. Individuals performed 4 weeks of intense, twice-daily rowing

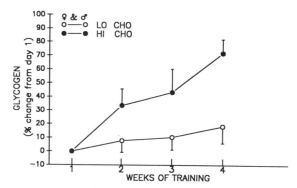

Fig 3–2.—Percent change in muscle glycogen from day 1 for moderate carbohydrate diet (MOD) (5 g carbohydrate (CHO) · kg body mass⁻¹) and high carbohydrate diet (HI) (10 g CHO · kg body mass⁻¹ · day⁻¹) groups during 4 weeks of intense twice-daily rowing training. (Courtesy of Simonsen JC, Sherman WM, Lamb DR, et al: *J Appl Physiol* 70:1500–1505, 1991.)

training, consisting of 40 minutes at 70% peak oxygen consumption (VO_2) and either 3 2,500-m time trials to assess power output or interval training at 70% to 90% peak VO_2.

Results.—The mean intensity of training was 65 minutes at 70% peak VO_2 and 38 minutes at 90% or more peak VO_2. There was an average .9-kg decrease in body weight, which was considered too small to affect power output. The high carbohydrate group had a 65% increase in mean muscle glycogen content. In the moderate carbohydrate group, muscle glycogen remained constant at 119 mmol/kg (Fig 3–2). In time trials, the mean power output increased slightly but significantly more in the high carbohydrate group (10.7% vs. 1.6% after 4 weeks).

Conclusion.—In rowers performing intense twice-daily training, a high carbohydrate diet increases muscle glycogen content and power output compared with a moderate carbohydrate diet. However, the moderate carbohydrate diet is sufficient to maintain normal muscle glycogen and power output. Variations in carbohydrate intake have more pronounced effects as training progresses.

▶ Most work in the area of dietary carbohydrate and muscle glycogen has related to the effect of changes in diet on a single bout of exercise. What is much more relevant to the coach and the athlete, however, is how diet might effect performance over a period of time, particularly during a training season leading up to major competition, which may be punctuated by several important competitions over a relatively short period of time. From this standpoint, the present contribution is important because many have felt that irrespective of the diet, substrate adaptation may well occur that does not appear to be entirely true. It is clear from this study that there is a significant difference between 10 g of carbohydrate per kilogram and 5 g of carbohydrate per kilogram on muscle glycogen throughout a 4-week intensive rowing training period where the rowers, as is customary, trained twice a day.

Not only was the muscle glycogen improvement dramatically greater in the high carbohydrate group, but there were also important implications for performance.—J.R. Sutton, M.D.

Influence of Physical Activity on Gastric Emptying of Liquids in Normal Human Subjects

Marzio L, Formica P, Fabiani F, LaPenna D, Vecchiett L, Cuccurullo F (Università "G D'Annunzio," Chieti, Italy; Ospedale Civile, Teramo, Italy)
Am J Gastroenterol 86:1433–1436, 1991 3-4

Introduction.—Gastric emptying time of ingested solids does not seem to be affected during physical stress, whereas gastric emptying time of liquids appears to be affected by the intensity of the physical stress. An earlier study found that the simultaneous measurement of gastric liquid emptying by scintigraphy and real time ultrasonography (RUS) performed under resting conditions yielded similar results. This study examined whether gastric emptying of liquids varies between mild and heavy exercise, using scintigraphy and RUS to assess liquid emptying rates.

Methods.—Seventeen normal individuals, aged 24–34 years, who did not jog or run routinely, exercised twice on a treadmill for 30 minutes. Liquid gastric emptying was evaluated 3 times, including during basal conditions, after mild exercise at 50% of predicted maximum heart rate, and after more vigorous effort at 70% of maximum heart rate. The heart rates were achieved by varying the speed and inclination of the treadmill. All study subjects drank 500 mL of mineral water within 2–3 minutes before the baseline studies and immediately after the mild and more vigorous physical stresses. Gastric emptying was evaluated by RUS in 11 persons and by scintigraphy in 6 persons.

Results.—Gastric emptying of the mineral water followed a linear relationship at rest, as well as during mild or vigorous physical stress. Compared with basal conditions, gastric emptying of water was accelerated after mild stress but it was prolonged after vigorous effort. Thus, mild physical activity accelerated the gastric emptying of water, whereas more intense physical activity delayed it. Real time ultrasonography and scintigraphy gave similar results.

Conclusion.—Mild physical exercise favors the digestive process.

▶ The impact of exercise on gastrointestinal motility is interesting from a number of perspectives, perhaps the most important being the provision of appropriate amounts of fluid to the athlete during an event. Thirst provides an inadequate gauge of fluid needs during vigorous effort, and the sports nutritionist must steer a careful line between dehydration and an excess of fluid that leads to the discomfort of a distended stomach.

The emptying process depends in part on the intensity of effort and in part on the volume of the gastric contents. Thus, with the type of protocol used in these experiments (a single relatively large drink, variously described as 400 or 500 mL over 3 minutes immediately postexercise), if emptying is indeed delayed, there may be a later "catch up" of the emptying process.

Most previous studies have been undertaken *during* exercise, and it is interesting that what the authors describe as "maximal" exercise (30 min at 70% of maximal heart rate) produces a change of gastric function that persists into the recovery period. Presumably, the stomach is continuing to respond to some change in its hormonal milieu induced by the bout of physical activity.—R.J. Shephard, M.D., Ph.D., D.P.E.

Effect of Exercise on Intestinal Motility and Transit in Trained Athletes
Soffer EE, Summers RW, Gisolfi C (Univ of Iowa, Iowa City)
Am J Physiol 260:G698–G702, 1991   3–5

Introduction.—Numerous studies have examined the effects of exercise on the cardiac, pulmonary, and endocrine systems, but little is known about its impact on the gastrointestinal tract system. The effects of exercise on duodenojejunal contractile activity, orocecal transit, and plasma concentrations of β-endorphin were investigated in 8 healthy young male cyclists.

Methods.—A new system that allows continuous ambulatory recording of gut motor activity was used. A thin flexible probe was passed transnasally and positioned under fluoroscopy so that one strain gauge transducer was in the duodenum and another in the proximal jejunum. The transducers were connected to a solid-state data logger carried in a shoulder bag. On 2 consecutive days, the cyclists exercised at 60%, 80%, and 90% peak oxygen uptake.

Results.—Although plasma β-endorphin concentrations were increased by exercise, the changes were not significant. Exercise at the 2 higher intensities interrupted intestinal postprandial activity, with its effect occurring more consistently at 90% than at 80% peak oxygen uptake. Short, intense exercise did not affect orocecal transit time, indicating that a temporary interruption of the postprandial activity pattern is not sufficient to change overall transit times. Results of an infusion of naloxone during some sessions suggest that the results of exercise on intestinal postprandial motor activity may not be mediated by opioids.

Conclusion.—Exercise intensity must be a controlled variable in studies of the effects of exercise on gut function. Ambulatory recording using a digital data logger is a suitable means of studying gut function during exercise.

▶ To this point, gastrointestinal physiologists with a penchant for exercise have mainly been interested in how rapidly the stomach empties when various carbohydrate preparations are ingested. Distance runners often complain of gastrointestinal symptoms and even diarrhea (1). However, there are also a number of other reasons to be interested in the function of the more distant reaches of the intestines, not the least of which are the impact of exercise on the recycling of cholesterol and the retention of possible carcinogens such as nitrosamines formed from meat treated with nitrites. Research has recently been facilitated by the development of a duodenal/jejunal probe that transmits pressure differentials to a solid-state data logger carried in a shoulder bag. Bouts of exercise at 80%–90% of maximal oxygen intake were here shown to interrupt the normal postprandial pattern of duodenal and jejunal movement by an activity front. There were no gastrointestinal symptoms in the present study, possibly because exercise was performed on a cycle ergometer. Mechanical bouncing of the viscera probably plays an important role in the symptoms experienced while running. In terms of the other issues of hypercholesterolemia and carcinogenesis, an increase of colonic motility is more important than changes in the movement patterns in the jejunum. There is already some evidence that exercise speeds colonic transit (2), but more data are required.—R.J. Shephard, M.D., Ph.D., D.P.E.

References

1. Moses FM, *Sports Med* 9:159, 1990.
2. Crowell MD, et al: *Gastroenterology* 98:A340, 1990.

Eating Disorders—The Role of the Athletic Trainer
Grandjean AC (International Ctr for Sports Nutrition, Omaha)
Athlet Train, JNATA 26:105–112, 1991   3–6

Background.—The increased prevalence of anorexia nervosa and bulimia nervosa has resulted in improved understanding of the cause, pathologic aspects, and treatment of these conditions. They appear to be common in athletes whose sports emphasize thinness. The risks and management of eating disorders in athletes are examined, including the athletic trainer's role.

Discussion.—Many athletes in sports that emphasize thinness (e.g., ballet, body building, cheerleading, and gymnastics), may be preoccupied with weight or have a tendency toward eating disorders. Eating disorders appear to be increasing in prevalence among female dancers, with up to 33% of university dancers being at risk. This group also has a high incidence of amenorrhea and irregular menstrual cycles, which is a diagnostic criterion for anorexia nervosa. Eating disorders also appear to be prevalent in female gymnasts and especially swimmers. Elite female distance runners may also be at risk. The presence of abnormal eating patterns and cessation of menstruation alone are not sufficient to diagnose an eating disorder—emotional lability and social withdrawal are important clues. Athletics themselves do not "cause" eating disorders, but disorders may be triggered by comments of important persons in the athlete's life (e.g., a coach, trainer, athletic director, or teammate). To prevent eating disorders, and to deal with them when they do occur, the athletic department should first ensure that all staff members are educated about the problem. A system should be created for handling eating disorders when they occur, and a total nutrition program should be devised to include nutrition counseling and assistance in suitable ways to lose or gain weight. Steps should also be taken to ensure that staff policies or behaviors do not contribute to the development of eating disorders.

Conclusions.—The risks and management of eating disorders in athletes are studied, emphasizing the athletic trainer's role. Knowledge about these disorders and preparation for managing them when they arise are important. Weigh-ins themselves, although often targeted for elimination, need not be eliminated if they are kept in perspective.

▶ Coaches and athletic trainers must be aware of the problems associated with eating disorders, and of the role that they, as coaches and trainers, play in dealing with these problems. Coaches must never make unreasonable demands on their athletes to lose weight or fit a particular "body image." An unwarranted remark or statement can be devastating to an athlete's self-esteem and may contribute to many eating disorder problems. A referral system should be in place for these athletes and used when appropriate. Please be advised that one wrong word, nickname, or simple remark can exacerbate a significant problem.—F.J. George, A.T.C., P.T.

Relation of Age and Physical Exercise Status on Metabolic Rate in Younger and Older Healthy Men
Poehlman ET, Melby CL, Badylak SF (Univ of Vermont, Burlington; Colorado State Univ; Purdue Univ, Lafayette, Ind)
J Gerontol Biol Sci 46:B54–B58, 1991   3–7

Background.—The extremes of fatness and leanness are regulated by fluctuations in energy balance and are important concerns in our aging population. Little is known about the effect on metabolic rate of regular participation in physical exercise in aging men. The effects of age and habitual physical exercise on resting metabolic rate (RMR) and the thermic effect of a meal test (TEM) were studied.

Methods.—Twenty men aged 18 to 34 and 16 men aged 50 to 78 participated. All were in excellent general health. Resting metabolic rate was measured with a ventilated hood, and TEM was measured for 180 minutes after a liquid meal was consumed.

Results.—After adjustment for fat-free weight (FFW) and percent body fat, RMR was found to be lower in sedentary older men than in older active men and younger sedentary and active men. Total and percent TEM were highest in active young men, followed by active older men,

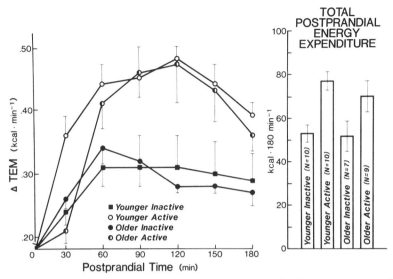

Fig 3-3.—Increase in postprandial energy expenditure for active and sedentary, younger and older men after ingestion of a liquid meal. The inset shows the total postprandial energy expenditure (kcal · 180⁻¹) in the 4 groups. (Courtesy of Poehlman ET, Melby CL, Badylak SF: *J. Gerontol Biol Sci* 46:B54–B58, 1991.)

sedentary young men, and sedentary older men. Neither age nor body composition was significantly related to TEM (Fig 3-3).

Conclusions.—Older men who lead a sedentary life may have a lower RMR, independent of FFW and percent body fat, than younger men and older men who exercise regularly. A higher TEM is associated with physical exercise, regardless of age.

▶ There is growing evidence that factors contributing to the control of obesity include a small stimulation of resting metabolism and an enhancement of the thermic effect of food brought about by involvement in an exercise program. The present data confirm such findings in young men, and also show that active elderly individuals have a similar advantage over their sedentary peers.—R.J. Shephard, M.D., Ph.D., D.P.E.

Physical Activity and Reduced Occurrence of Non-Insulin-Dependent Diabetes Mellitus
Helmrich SP, Ragland DR, Leung RW, Paffenbarger RS Jr (Univ of California, Berkeley; Stanford Univ, Stanford, Calif)
N Engl J Med 315:147–152, 1991   3–8

Introduction.—Physical activity is recommended to patients with non-insulin-dependent diabetes mellitus (NIDDM) because it increases insulin sensitivity. However, it is not known whether physical activity can prevent this disease.

Methods.—Questionnaires eliciting information on patterns of physical activity and other personal characteristics were distributed to 5,990 male alumni of the University of Pennsylvania. Follow-up data were obtained from 1962 to 1976. In 98,524 man-years of follow-up, NIDDM developed in 202 men.

Results.—The development of NIDDM was inversely related to leisure-time physical activity, expressed in kilocalories expended per week in walking, stair climbing, and sports. Incidence rates decreased as energy expenditures increased from less than 500 to 3,500 kcal. For each 500-kcal energy expenditure increment, the age-adjusted risk of NIDDM decreased by 6%. This association was unchanged after adjustment for obesity, hypertension, and a parental history of diabetes. Consideration

Age-Adjusted Rates of NIDDM Among 5,990 Men, 1962–1976,
According to Measures of Physical Activity in 1962

PHYSICAL-ACTIVITY INDEX, 1962 (kcal/wk)	PREVA-LENCE*	MEN WITH NIDDM	RATE PER 10,000 MAN-YEARS	RELATIVE RISK	P VALUE FOR TREND
All activities†					
<500	17	42	26.3	1.00‡	
500–999	22	51	24.7	0.94	
1000–1499	15	30	20.7	0.79	
1500–1999	9	18	20.7	0.78	0.01
2000–2499	7	12	17.8	0.68	
2500–2999	7	15	23.7	0.90	
3000–3499	5	11	22.6	0.86	
≥3500	18	23	13.7	0.52	
All activities except vigorous sports					
<500	21	46	23.8	1.00‡	
500–999	26	56	23.0	0.97	
1000–1499	16	31	20.8	0.87	
1500–1999	9	18	21.8	0.92	0.07
2000–2499	7	11	17.8	0.75	
2500–2999	6	16	30.7	1.29	
3000–3499	4	10	24.4	1.03	
≥3500	13	14	11.4	0.48	
Vigorous sports only					
<500	84	182	22.6	1.00‡	
500–999	7	10	15.7	0.69	
1000–1499	1	0	0	—	
1500–1999	1	1	12.0	0.53	0.05
2000–2499	3	5	19.5	0.86	
2500–2999	1	1	12.6	0.56	
3000–3499	1	1	9.0	0.40	
≥3500	2	2	10.3	0.46	

*Expressed as the number of man-years assigned to each subcategory divided by the number of man-years for the entire study population.
†Includes walking, climbing stairs, and playing sports.
‡Reference category.
(Courtesy of Helmrich SP, Ragland DR, Leung RW, et al: *N Engl J Med* 325:147–152, 1991.)

of weight gain between time of college attendance and 1962 weakened the association. The protective effect of physical activity was strongest in men at highest risk for NIDDM (table).

Conclusion.—Increased physical activity is effective in preventing NIDDM. The protective benefit of exercise is especially marked in men at highest risk for the disease.

▶ This is one further piece of evidence on the benefits of habitual physical activity, gleaned from the very productive long-term follow-up of University of Pennsylvania alumni. It is important to stress that the primary measure of obesity available to these authors was the relatively crude body mass index (BMI, weight/height^2). In the North American population as a whole, a high average BMI undoubtedly reflects obesity, but in the individual patient, a high BMI may reflect a muscular body build rather than an accumulation of fat. On the other hand, the weight gained by an individual since leaving university is almost always fat. I suspect that this may be why control of the data for the BMI did not weaken the association between habitual physical activity and protection against diabetes, but adjustment for the weight gained since university did weaken the association. If the BMI is used as an index of body composition, exercise has no protective effect against diabetes unless the BMI is greater than 24 kg/m^2. All of these findings seem in keeping with the view that the protective effect of regular physical activity is due in large measure to the control of obesity. In those with a high risk of diabetes, the protective effect seems proportional to the energy expended, over the range 500–2,000 kcal/week. To set this information in perspective, it may be worth emphasizing that 2,000 kcal/week is a substantial exercise commitment, amounting to about an hour of vigorous physical activity 7 days/week. In another analysis of the same data, Paffenbarger and associates demonstrated that activity of this order would extend the lifespan by about 2 years, but it would be necessary to spend much of the added 2 years in exercising; thus, the therapeutic value of the exercise (in terms of an increased quality-adjusted life expectancy) was strongly influenced by whether the person was enjoying the exercise or not.—R.J. Shephard, M.D., Ph.D., D.P.E.

The Relation of Physical Activity to Cardiovascular Disease Risk Factors in Mauritians
Zimmet PZ, Collins VR, Dowse GK, Alberti KGMM, Tuomilehto J, Gareeboo H, Chitson P (International Diabetes Institute, Melbourne; University of Newcastle Upon Tyne, England; National Public Health Institute, Helsinki; Ministry of Health, Port Louis, Mauritius)
Am J Epidemiol 134:862–875, 1991   3–9

Background.—Some cross-sectional studies have shown that physical activity lowers the prevalence of abnormal glucose tolerance and other cardiovascular disease risk factors. The population of Mauritius in the Indian Ocean has a high prevalence of abnormal glucose tolerance and other cardiovascular disease risk factors. The impact of physical activity on the risk of abnormal glucose tolerance and other cardiovascular disease risk factors was examined.

Study Design.—The survey sample included 4,658 Asian Indian, Creole, and Chinese adults, aged 25–74 years, who had been randomly selected on the basis of census divisions. The sample was considered representative of the total population and of each ethnic group. Persons with known diabetes were excluded from the study. Study participants were classified as active or inactive based on a combined leisure and occupational physical activity score determined at the interview. All participants were given a 2-hour oral glucose tolerance test. Plasma total cholesterol, triglycerides, high density lipoprotein cholesterol, and uric acid levels were measured from fasting blood specimens. Resting 12-lead ECGs were performed only on persons aged 35–74 years.

Results.—Active individuals had significantly lower 2-hour plasma glucose concentrations, significantly lower fasting and 2-hour serum insulin concentrations, and significantly higher high density lipoprotein cholesterol levels than inactive persons. Plasma uric acid and fasting triglyceride levels were also reduced in active persons, but the differences were significant only in women. Mean body mass index and waist:hip ratio were nearly identical in active and inactive men, but they were significantly increased in inactive women. However, the magnitude of the differences was small. Multiple linear regression analyses identified a positive association between physical inactivity and the prevalence of noninsulin-dependent diabetes mellitus and impaired glucose tolerance.

Conclusion.—The promotion of physical activity and exercise should become an important strategy in the prevention of cardiovascular disease and glucose intolerance in Mauritians and other susceptible populations.

▶ Many governments are increasingly aware of the problem of diabetes mellitus among indigenous populations. The epidemic of diabetes has been associated with a rapid acculturation of indigenous populations to the lifestyle of "Western" society, with a decrease of physical activity and an increase of body fat. The present study unfortunately does not quantitate activity very closely—for instance, it is possible to do a lot of walking and gardening, and yet be classed as having an "inactive" leisure. However, this may not be too important, as the main source of energy expenditure for the Mauritians seems to have been occupational (active groups such as construction workers and sugar cane cutters being contrasted with unemployed, shop workers and office workers). Further, the activity index, despite any limitations it may have had, was related to glucose tolerance and insulin levels. This finding is the more interesting, because even the inactive group were not very obese (body mass index 22 kg/m² in men and 24.8 kg/m² in women).

Plainly, it seems important to the health of populations to encourage an increase of physical activity as they move from a life of hunting or subsistence agriculture to city life.—R.J. Shephard, M.D., Ph.D., D.P.E.

Strength Training Does Not Improve Lipoprotein-Lipid Profiles in Men at Risk for CHD

Kokkinos PF, Hurley BF, Smutok MA, Farmer C, Reece C, Shulman R, Charabogos C, Patterson J, Will S, Devane-Bell J, Goldberg AP (Univ of Maryland, College Park; Johns Hopkins Univ, Baltimore)
Med Sci Sports Exerc 23:1134–1139, 1991   3–10

Background.—Many researchers have found that strength training improves lipoprotein-lipid profiles. However, their research had methodologic limitations that makes interpreting the findings difficult. The effects of 2 different strength training programs on lipoprotein-lipid profiles were explored further.

Methods.—Sixteen untrained men (mean age, 46 years) were enrolled in a 20-week study of the effect of strength training on lipoprotein-lipid profiles and postheparin lipase activities. The participants had abnormal lipoprotein-lipid profiles and 2 or more other risk factors for coronary heart disease (CHD). Daily variations in blood lipoprotein levels were controlled for by establishing baseline values in at least 2 blood samples obtained from the training and control groups on separate days.

Results.—Training increased upper body strength by 50% and lower body strength by 37% as measured by the 1-repetition maximum test. The control group had no changes in test results. No significant changes in maximal aerobic power were associated with training, nor were there any significant changes in plasma levels of triglycerides, total cholesterol, high-density-lipoprotein cholesterol, or low-density-lipoprotein choles-

Plasma Lipid and Lipoprotein Concentrations in the Training and Control Groups

	Training Group			Control Group	
	PRE	POST (Day 1)	POST (Day 2)	Initial	Final
TG	193 ± 96	171 ± 101	178 ± 98	199 ± 91	181 ± 97
TC	213 ± 22	210 ± 22	200 ± 23	202 ± 35	207 ± 30
HDL–C	35 ± 6	36 ± 8	35 ± 7	39 ± 11	40 ± 11
LDL–C	139 ± 16	139 ± 21	131 ± 21	123 ± 33	131 ± 29
TC/HDL–C	6 ± 1	6 ± 1	6 ± 1	5 ± 2	5 ± 2

Note: Values are means ± 1 SD. All lipid values are expressed in mg/dL. None of the differences was significant.
Abbreviations: TG, triglycerides; TC, total cholesterol; HDL-C, high-density-lipoprotein cholesterol; LDL-C, low-density-lipoprotein cholesterol.
(Courtesy of Kokkinos PF, Hurley BF, Smutok MA, et al: *Med Sci Sports Exerc* 23:1134–1139, 1991.)

terol. Training did not affect the activities of postheparin lipoprotein lipase or hepatic lipase (table).

Conclusions.—Twenty weeks of strength training apparently does not change plasma lipoprotein-lipid profiles or the regulatory enzymes of triglyceride and high-density-lipoprotein cholesterol in men at risk for CHD. The inability of strength training to improve lipid profiles does not seem to be a result of inadequate training stimulus or methodologic flaws. Methodologic problems in past studies may have led to the belief that strength training improves these profiles.

▶ There have recently been several papers suggesting that a strength training program is as effective as endurance activity in optimizing lipid profiles. This is inherently surprising, because a substantial quantity of work must be performed to induce a response through aerobic training (1), and the total energy cost of most muscle building programs is quite low. The present paper makes a useful contribution, both by demonstrating the absence of effect from a strength training regimen and by offering an explanation of earlier apparently positive findings. Defects in earlier research included the absence of a control group, lack of adequate baseline values, and failure to distinguish the acute response to exercise from the long-term status of the individual. However, the most important difference between the present study and earlier research was probably the absence of any change in body fat in the present investigation. In studies where body fat has decreased, it seems probable that the muscle-building has been accompanied by a negative energy balance, and that the improvement of lipid profile is a response to the dietary restriction rather than the muscle hypertrophy.—R.J. Shephard, M.D., Ph.D., D.P.E.

Reference

1. Williams PT, et al: *JAMA* 247:2672, 1982.

Increased Blood Antioxidant Systems of Runners in Response to Training Load
Robertson JD, Maughan RJ, Duthie GG, Morrice PC (Rowett Research Institute Aberdeen; University Medical School, Aberdeen, Scotland)
Clin Sci 80:611–618, 1991   3–11

Introduction.—There is evidence that the antioxidant system can adapt to chronic oxidative stress, such as physical training. The magnitude of the increase in the serum activity of muscle-specific enzymes after exercise appears to rely on physical conditioning. The relationship between regular physical training and antioxidant defense mechanisms in men was studied.

Methods.—Antioxidants were measured in venous blood samples from 20 male runners and 6 sedentary men, aged 20–40 years. Individual body weight and physical activity patterns were in steady state. Their di-

Concentrations of Intermediates and Activities of Antioxidant Enzymes in Blood Cells From the 3 Groups of Persons: Sedentary Persons (N = 6), Low-Training Runners (16–43 km per Week, N = 6) and High-Training Runners (80–147 km per Week, N = 6)

	Sedentary subjects	Low-training runners	High-training runners
Erythrocyte glutathione content (mg/g of Hb)			
Total	0.86	1.24*	1.20*
	(0.38–1.18)	(0.97–1.68)	(0.91–1.49)
GSH	0.57	0.92**	0.82*
	(0.16–0.84)	(0.71–1.22)	(0.55–0.99)
GSSG	0.14	0.15	0.21*
	(0.10–0.18)	(0.09–0.23)	(0.16–0.26)
Erythrocyte GSHPx activity (units/g of Hb)	77.1	93.9	98.5*
	(60.7–110.8)	(64.9–100.9)	(80.3–126.5)
Erythrocyte CAT activity (arbitrary units/g of Hb)	817	1009	1122
	(346–2017)	(894–1574)	(581–2971)
SOD activity (units/g of Hb)	1.63	1.47	1.65
	(1.15–2.21)	(0.96–1.89)	(1.08–2.53)
Erythrocyte Se content (μg/g of Hb)	0.27	0.37	0.45*
	(0.22–0.42)	(0.26–0.67)	(0.35–0.69)
Erythrocyte vitamin E content (μg/g of Hb)	4.4	15.2*	14.3*
	(1.2–15.2)	(12.8–29.8)	(9.7–27.0)
Lymphocyte ascorbic acid concn. (μmol/g of protein)	24.6	24.3	38.2[a]
	(16.7–66.3)	(16.3–28.3)	(13.2–79.5)

Note: A Mann-Whitney U-test was used for comparison of: (1) the groups of runners with the sedentary group: asterisk indicates P < .05; *double asterisk*, P < .01; (2) the high-training group with the low-training group: [a]indicates P < .01. The data are expressed as medians with the range in parentheses.
(Courtesy of Robertson JD, Maughan RJ, Duthie GG, et al: *Clin Sci* 80:611–618, 1991.)

ets were also analyzed. Six runners participated in low weekly training, 16–43 km, and 6 participated in high weekly training, 80–147 km.

Results.—Body weight and percentage body fat negatively correlated with weekly training distance. Energy intake and maximum oxygen uptake also correlated with weekly training. Plasma creatine kinase activity, an indicator of muscle damage, was significantly associated with weekly training distance. Plasma concentration of thiobarbituric acid-reactive substances, indicators of free-radical-mediated lipid peroxidation, decreased with increased maximum oxygen uptake. Erythrocyte α-tocopherol content was higher in the runners than in the sedentary men. Lymphocyte ascorbic acid levels were significantly increased in the high-training group compared with those in the low training group. Weekly training distance was significantly, positively correlated with erythrocyte activities of the antioxidant enzymes, glutathione peroxidase, and catalase. Total erythrocyte glutathione content was increased in the high- and low-training groups, a result of an increase in reduced glutathione content (table).

Conclusion.—The protective antioxidant capacity of blood is enhanced in endurance runners. Despite these changes, habitual physical exercise may still result in some muscle damage. Except for erythrocyte α-tocopherol, the improvements in blood antioxidants were related to the amount of training. Improved blood antioxidant potential may be associated with both the physical activity and dietary intakes of antioxidant vitamins and trace-element cofactors of antioxidant enzymes.

▶ Small quantities of free radicals such as superoxide and hydrogen peroxide are formed as normal byproducts during metabolism (1). If the overall rate of metabolism is increased by a bout of vigorous exercise, the production of such compounds is proportionately augmented. The risk of tissue damage is then correspondingly enhanced, because any substantial concentration of such compounds can cause alterations in the structure of key proteins and peroxidation of lipid cell membranes.

At first inspection, the potential accumulation of free radicals might seem a solid argument for avoiding exercise. Fortunately, the body also contains enzymes (peroxidases and catalases) that break down the harmful peroxides, and there is growing evidence that regular physical activity induces an increase in the activity of such enzymes that is more than sufficient to compensate for any increase in peroxide formation.

The study of Robertson and associates is cross-sectional in nature. Probably because of the increase in tissue peroxidases, plasma indicators of lipid peroxidation were lowest in subjects with the largest aerobic power, and such subjects also made less use of their dietary antioxidants, as shown by higher tocopherol and ascorbic acid levels. This finding is all the more significant, because unlike many runners, the present sample were not taking supplements of vitamin C or vitamin E. Despite the enhanced antioxidant status, some muscle damage apparently occurred (as indicated by creatine kinase leakage).—R.J. Shephard, M.D., Ph.D., D.P.E.

Reference

1. Sjodin B, et al: *Sports Med* 10:236, 1990.

Smoking Cessation and Severity of Weight Gain in a National Cohort
Williamson DF, Madans J, Anda RF, Kleinman JC, Giovino GA, Byers T (Centers for Disease Control, Atlanta; Natl Ctr for Health Statistics, Hyattsvillle, Md)
N Engl J Med 324:739–745, 1991   3–12

Introduction.—Although the detrimental health effects of cigarette smoking have been greatly publicized, more than 25% of adults in the United States continue to smoke. The recent Surgeon General's report noted that individuals tend to gain 1.8 kg (about 4 pounds) after stopping smoking. Weight gain was analyzed in a large group of patients weighed in the First National Health and Nutrition Examination Survey (NHANES I) between 1971 and 1975.

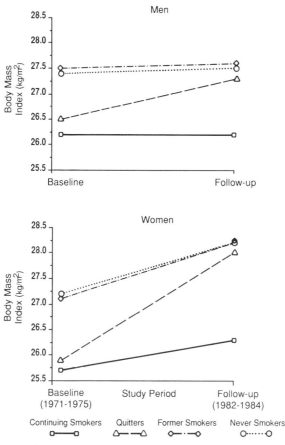

Fig 3–4.—Mean body mass index at baseline and follow-up according to smoking status. *Squares* indicate continuing smokers; *triangles*, quitters; *circles*, former smokers; and *diamonds*, never smokers. (Courtesy of Williamson DF, Madans J, Anda RF, et al: N *Engl J Med* 324:739-745, 1991.)

Methods.—Data from the 1982 to 1984 NHANES Epidemiologic Follow-Up Study was analyzed prospectively. From 1982 to 1984, 14,407 adults between the ages of 25 and 75 were included and divided into 6 mutually exclusive groups: never smokers, former smokers, intermittent smokers, continuing smokers, sustained quitters, and recent quitters. Weight change was recorded, as were age and body mass index.

Results.—Compared with continuing smokers, sustained quitters appeared older and better educated at baseline. Irrespective of their smoking group, women tended to gain about 1 to 2 kg more than men during follow-up; the sustained quitters increased their weight the most overall. The mean weight gain associated with stopping smoking was 1 kg greater in women (3.8 kg) than in men (2.8 kg). Sex-specific mean measurements of body mass index at baseline for sustained quitters were significantly different from those of never smokers (Fig 3-4). Black quitters demonstrated higher weight gain than did their nonblack counterparts. Underweight female sustained quitters had a fourfold greater chance of gaining 13 kg than their heavier counterparts had. Women who were sustained quitters also demonstrated a higher risk of weight gain if they performed low amounts of recreational physical activity, were younger than 55 or had had 1 or more live births.

Conclusions.—Major weight gain often accompanies the cessation of smoking, but this occurs in a minority of the individuals who stop cigarette use. Weight gain may cosmetically inhibit a person from stopping smoking. Effective weight control methods are needed to aid smokers attempting to quit.

▶ The impact of smoking cessation on body mass, as seen in this large study, is in keeping with much previous experience. The average increase of body mass (1–2 kg) is small, and the negative impact of this change on health is much smaller than other positive health benefits that result from smoking cessation. Nevertheless, the vanity of some women may be offended by even a small increase of fat around the thighs and hips, with a risk of smoking recidivism, particularly if smoking was originally perceived as a means of controlling weight. It is thus important that any smoking cessation program be part of an overall lifestyle package that includes dietary advice and a prescription for an increase of physical activity.—R.J. Shephard, M.D., Ph.D., D.P.E.

Exercise-Induced Hyperkalaemia Can Be Reduced in Human Subjects by Moderate Training Without Change in Skeletal Muscle Na,K-ATPase Concentration
Kjeldsen K, Nørgaard A, Hau C (University of Copenhagen; Aarhus University Hospital, Skejby, Denmark; Military Infirmary, Nørresundby, Denmark)
Eur J Clin Invest 20:642–647, 1990   3–13

Background.—Research has suggested that capacity for muscle performance and skeletal muscle concentration of Na,K-ATPase are related. Plasma concentration of potassium was evaluated during exercise before and after training and this finding was related to skeletal muscle Na,K-ATPase.

Methods.—The subjects were 15 male conscripts with a mean age of 20 years, who were undergoing a 10-week program of moderate physical conditioning for military service. Before and after training, the venous plasma level of potassium was measured as the subjects performed bicycle exercise. To assess Na,K-ATPase, ^{3}H-ouabain binding studies were done. The putative relationship between plasma level of potassium and skeletal muscle Na,K-ATPase was then evaluated.

Results.—At exhaustion the peak plasma level of potassium was decreased from 6.1 mmol/L^{-1} before training to 5.6 mmol/L^{-1} after train-

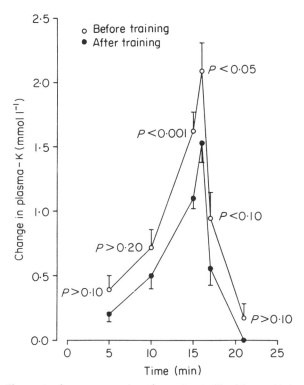

Fig 3–5.—Changes in plasma concentration of potassium in blood from cubital arm vein during exercise before and after training. Values are means with bars denoting standard error of mean. Each point represents values from 15 subjects except the value of time at 16 minutes, which represents only 14 subjects because subject 14 stopped at end of exercise period from 10 to 15 minutes because of exhaustion before as well as after training. His value at exhaustion is given at time 15 minutes and his values obtained after 1 and 5 minutes of rest are given at times 17 and 21 minutes, respectively. P values for differences between values before and after training are given. (Courtesy of Kjeldsen K, Nørgaard A. Hau C: *Eur J Clin Invest* 20:642–647, 1990.)

ing. Plasma level of potassium was .2 to .5 mmol/L^{-1} higher after training, throughout the exercise period, and within the first minutes of rest (Fig 3–5). There was no correlation between peak values or increases in plasma concentrations of potassium and ^{3}H-ouabain binding sites in the vastus lateralis muscle, either before or after training.

Conclusions.—Training appears to reduce the net loss of potassium from the skeletal muscle pool during exercise. In addition, training may expose the heart to a smaller rise in plasma level of potassium and moderately improve capacity to clear extracellular potassium during exercise. The latter finding may result from increased activity of existing Na,K -pumps in resting skeletal muscle fibers. This may explain the observation that the risk of cardiac events is decreased after training, despite the increase in catecholamine response.

▶ This is an interesting study that examines the effects of training on venous potassium after exhaustive exercise. It is true that the authors actually found that following training the plasma potassium increase on exercise was less but the magnitude of the potassium rise was relatively modest (a peak of 6.1 mmol/L). Why this is important is that there is more and more concern that with short-term high-intensity exercise, changes in electrolytes, especially potassium and acid-base, may well be casually related to sudden death particularly in such sports as squash. In such very vigorous exercise in middle aged persons who may well have established coronary artery narrowing, the combination of marked increases in myocardial oxygen demands with increases in serum potassium may well be fatal. A much more extreme example was the study of Kowalchuk et al. (1) who showed that femoral venous potassium rose as high as 78 mmol/L after 30 seconds of supramaximal exercise. Repeated bouts of short-term exercise of a supramaximal intensity will result in similar levels or even higher serum concentrations of potassium and also major acid-base disturbances. For a review of the role of ionic processes in muscular fatigue during intense exercise, the reader is referred to the recent review by McKenna (2).—J.R. Sutton, M.D.

References

1. Kowalchuk JM, et al: *J Appl Physiol* 65:280, 1988.
2. McKenna MJ: *Sports Med* 13:134, 1992.

On the Role of Actomyosin ATPases in Regulation of ATP Turnover Rates During Intense Exercise
Hochachka PW, Bianconcini MSC, Rarkhouse WS, Dobson GP (University of British Columbia, Vancouver; Simon Fraser University, Burnaby, BC; Natl Inst on Alcohol Abuse and Alcoholism, Rockville, Md)
Proc Natl Acad Sci USA 88:5764–5768, 1991   3–14

Introduction.—Actomyosin ATPase is the dominant ATP sink during muscular work. Its catalytic capacity in fast-twitch oxidative glycolytic fibers exceeds that in slow-twitch oxidative fibers by about threefold. However, the relative contributions of these 2 actomyosin ATPases to the control of the metabolic rate during exercise are uncertain. In the present study fast- and slow-twitch fibers with similar mitochondrial densities were compared in running-trained adult male rats.

Findings.—In the setting of short-term near-maximal aerobic exercise, fast-twitch oxidative glycolytic (fast red) muscle fibers had ATP turnover rates 2 to 4 times greater than those for slow-twitch oxidative (slow red) fibers. Fluxes through the $ATP \rightleftharpoons ADP + P_i$ cycle were well regulated. At the lower limit forward flux exceeded backward flux by only .06%. At the upper limit ATPase rates exceeded rates of ATP synthesis by .12%.

Discussion.—There appears to be a substantial difference in the in vivo ATP turnover rates sustained by fat red and slow red muscle fibers. The very high precision of energy coupling that is observed may be analogous to what is found in insect flight muscles. These muscles can sustain a 2 to 3 order-of-magnitude increase in flux through the glycolytic pathway during flight with only a modest change in the concentration of pathway intermediates. This degree of regulatory precision depends not on mass action-regulated enzymic mechanisms, but rather on finely tuned allosteric regulation or the covalent modification of key enzymes. Similar mechanisms may operate in the regulation of oxidative metabolism in working mammalian muscles.

▶ The reason for including this animal study is not so much for the importance in rodents but for the elegance of the work and the ability of the authors to quantify ATP turnover rates and to demonstrate that there is a 2- to 4-times greater ATP turnover rate in the fast when compared with the slow-twitch oxidative fibers.—J.R. Sutton, M.D.

Interaction of Exercise and Insulin Action in Humans
Wasserman DH, Geer RJ, Rice DE, Bracy D, Flakoll PJ, Brown LL, Hill JO, Abumrad NN (Vanderbilt Univ, Nashville)
Am J Physiol 260:E37–E45, 1991   3–15

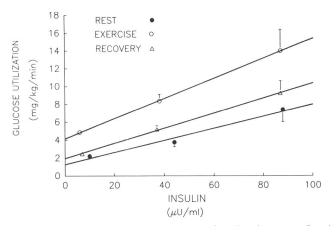

Fig 3–6.—Glucose uptake vs. insulin concentrations over low physiologic range (less than 90 μU/ mL) during rest, exercise, and recovery. y-intercept was used to estimate glucose uptake, which occurs at insulin concentration of zero (insulin-independent). Data are means ± standard error; $n = 5$ at each point. (Courtesy of Wasserman DH, Geer RJ, Rice DE, et al: *Am J Physiol* 260:E37–E45, 1991.)

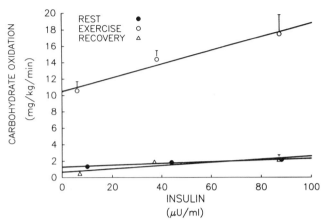

Fig 3–7.—Carbohydrate oxidation vs. insulin concentrations over low physiologic range (less than 90 μU/mL) during rest, exercise, and recovery. y-Intercept was used to estimate carbohydrate oxidation, which occurs at insulin concentration of zero (insulin-independent). Data are means ± standard error; $n = 5$ at each point. (Courtesy of Wasserman DH, Geer RJ, Rice DE, et al: *Am J Physiol* 260:E37–E45, 1991.)

Background.—The interaction between exercise and insulin can be investigated by assessing the specificity of this interaction on the metabolism of other substrates. Little is known about the action of exercise and insulin on fat metabolism. The effect of exercise on insulin-mediated glucose uptake, on the route of glucose disposal, and on insulin-independent glucose mechanism was studied, as well as the combined effect of exercise and insulin on fat and amino acid metabolism.

Methods.—Twenty-five healthy male volunteers were studied. Five controls received insulin infusion. The others received a hyperin-

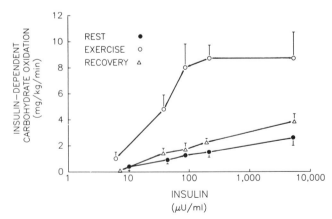

Fig 3–8.—Insulin-dependent carbohydrate oxidation (total carbohydrate oxidation − insulin-independent carbohydrate oxidation) at each respective insulin concentration during rest, exercise, and recovery. Data are means ± standard error; $n = 5$ at each point. (Courtesy of Wasserman DH, Geer RJ, Rice DE, et al: *Am J Physiol* 260:E37–E45, 1991.)

sulinemic euglycemic clamp at a dose of .5, 1, 2, or 15 mU/kg/min. All subjects were studied for 40 minutes at rest, for 100 minutes of moderate intensity bicycle exercise, and for 100 minutes of recovery. Isotopic methods and indirect calorimetry were used to evaluate metabolism.

Results.—From rest to recovery there was no change in plasma level of glucose. Total use of glucose began at 2.4 mg/kg/min, increased to 4.9 mg/kg/min during exercise, and decreased to 2.6 mg/kg/min during recovery (Fig 3–6). Carbohydrate oxidation (CHO OX) values were 1.4, 10.6, and .5 mg/kg/min (Fig 3–7). Together, exercise and insulin clamps resulted in a synergistic increase in infusion of glucose, insulin-dependent R_d, and CHO OX. Half-maximal doses of insulin-dependent R_d and CHO OX decreased and maximal responses increased in response to exercise. During rest, exercise, and recovery, insulin-dependent R_d was estimated at 1.3, 4.1, and 1.9 mg/kg/min and insulin-independent CHO OX at 1.2, 10.4, and .6 mg/kg/min (Fig 3–8). Exercise increased total suppression of free fatty acids and oxidation of fat by insulin.

Conclusions.—There appears to be a synergistic interaction by exercise and insulin to stimulate R_d and CHO OX. Most of these effects are independent of the action of insulin. Exercise increases the magnitude of insulin's suppressive effect on levels of free fatty acid and fat oxidation.

▶ One of the apparent paradoxes in exercise metabolism is the increasing glucose use in the presence of failing plasma concentration of insulin. It has therefore been assumed that exercise will increase the insulin action or stimulate glucose uptake by some insulin-independent mechanism. In vitro studies have suggested an increased insulin action on glucose uptake (1); however, even the complete absence of insulin glucose uptake will be stimulated (2). Studies of depancreatised dogs show that exercise will increase glucose uptake in the absence of insulin, but this is extremely small—approximately 15% of that found in the intact dogs (3). Thus the authors felt the need to conduct some whole body studies, and their experimental design was indeed complex and well executed. It was important to study rest and exercise, because the primary route of insulin-mediated glucose used at rest is usually by nonoxidative pathways, whereas with exercise almost all the glucose is oxidized. The authors also questioned whether oxidated processes may be sensitized to insulin action. The experimental design chosen is rather complex; the authors use tritiated glucose and the hyperinsulinemic euglycemic clamp at 4 different insulin infusion rates during rest and moderate exercise. The findings are of interest. They do show an insulin-independent action, but my reason for including the study is because of the particularly elegant nature of the questions asked and the experimental model used to explore mechanisms.—J.R. Sutton, M.D.

References

1. Vranic M, et al: *J Clin Invest* 57:245, 1976.
2. James DE, et al: *Am J Physiol* 248:E575, 1985.
3. Bjorkman O, et al: *J Clin Invest* 81:1759, 1988.

Hypothalamic-Pituitary-Adrenal Axis Function in Elderly Endurance Athletes

Heuser IJE, Wark H-J, Keul J, Holsboer F (Clinical Institute, Munich, Germany; University of Freiburg, Germany)
J Clin Endocrinol Metab 73:485–488, 1991   3–16

Background.—Repeated activation of the hypothalamic-pituitary-adrenal (HPA) axis in response to stress can reduce the ability of the axis to terminate such activation. This is reflected by continuously elevated plasma levels of cortisol after exposure to stress has ceased. The functional integrity of the HPT axis was evaluated in mentally healthy older subjects who were endurance trained and thus had been subjected to frequent periods of excessive HPA activation.

Methods.—The subjects were 10 male runners with a mean age 57 years, who ran an average of 70 km/week. All had been running for at least 10 years. Thirteen sedentary volunteers of the same age served as controls. All subjects were pretreated with dexamethasone, 1.5 mg, and then were challenged with human CRH, 100 µg.

Results.—The 2 groups had similar basal levels of cortisol and ACTH. However, the athletes had significantly higher cortisol responses to CRH, and their ACTH responses tended to be higher as well (Figs 3–9 and 3–10). The athlete's test results were then compared to those of 9 age-matched previously studied patients with depression; the responses to the CRH challenge were similar. Postchallenge levels of cortisol were 44 nmol/L in controls, 149 nmol/L in the runners, and 157 nmol/L in the depressed patients.

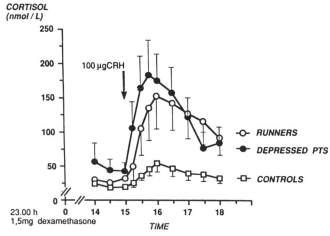

Fig 3–9.—Response of cortisol to hCRH challenge after pretreatment with dexamethasone in 10 runners, 9 patients with depression, and 13 sedentary controls. (Courtesy of Heuser IJE, Wark H-J, Keul J, et al: *J Clin Endocrinol Metab* 73:485–488, 1991.)

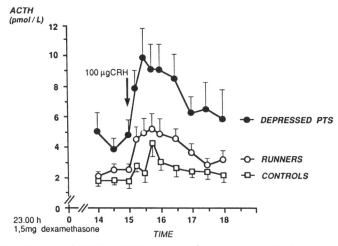

Fig 3–10.—Response of ACTH to hCRH challenge after pretreatment with dexamethasone in 10 runners, 6 patients with depression, and 13 sedentary controls. (Courtesy of Heuser IJE, Wark H-J, Keul J, et al: *J Clin Endocrinol Metab* 73:485–488, 1991.)

Conclusions.—Physiology of the HPA appears to be determined by previous exposure to stress associated with hypercortisolism, regardless of causes. The observed alterations may result from a stepwise decrease in corticotropic sensitivity to the negative feedback signal, which results in a switch to positive glucocorticoid feedback. Alternatively, the changes may result from enhanced cosecretion of ACTH secretagogues such as vasopressin, or they may result from a combination of these mechanisms.

▶ Examining the similarities in various pathologic and supraphysiologic states may help unravel common mechanisms in health and disease. This study is one such example. In it the authors explore the hypothalamic-pituitary-adrenal similarity between endurance trained runners and patients with depression to test the hypothesis that both groups have somewhat similar endocrine disturbances. At first sight this hypothesis might seem to be paradoxical in that most exercise enthusiasts would exclaim that exercise makes one happy and not depressed and certainly acute bouts are said to alleviate depression. The authors also chose elderly subjects for their study although they do not explicitly state why this is so but presumably it is because of the relatively large number of the elderly with endogenous depression. I found the endocrine methodology fascinating because the authors not only measured basal concentrations of ACTH and cortisol, but they also suppressed the hypothalamic-pituitary axis with dexamethasone the day prior to the study by means of corticotropin-releasing hormone stimulation of the hypothalamus. If chronic stimulation was present, then this may already be observed from the basal samples because the elderly runners had almost double the cortisol concentration of the controls but almost half that of the depressed patients. There were similarities and differences as can be seen by the figures between the runners and the depressed patients. I would have also liked to have seen the use of exercise as a stimulant to examine the physiologic integrity of the hypothalamic-pituitary axis in all 3 groups. Some time ago a study of elderly or masters athletes was done to determine whether there was a decline in hypothalamic-pituitary-adrenal reserve in the elderly. The study showed that immediately before exercise these runners had double the normal basal concentration of cortisol and that there was a brisk response following a 1,500 meter run and an even brisker response following a 5,000 meter run. However, those authors did not consider the possibility of a state of overstimulation (1).—J.R. Sutton, M.D.

Reference

1. Sutton JR, Casey JH: *J Clin Endocrinol Metab* 40:135, 1975.

Corticotropin-Releasing Hormone Is Not the Sole Factor Mediating Exercise-Induced Adrenocorticotropin Release in Humans
Smoak B, Deuster P, Rabin D, Chrousos G (Uniformed Services Univ of the Health Sciences; NIH, Bethesda, Md)
J Clin Endocrinol Metab 73:302–306, 1991   3–17

Introduction.—Although corticotropin-releasing hormone (CRH) is the main stimulator of adrenocorticotropic hormone (ACTH), other factors may modulate its release. Exercise causes reproducible changes in the pituitary-adrenal axis, with changes in hormone concentrations being proportional to the intensity of the exercise. To determine whether CRH is the sole mediator of ACTH release, exercise was used as a physiologic stimulus in 5 men and 5 women, aged 24–39 years.

Methods.—In a randomized manner on separate visits, each person received a 6-hour infusion of ovine CRH, 1 μg/kg·h, or a placebo saline infusion. Plasma concentrations of ovine CRH where high enough to saturate the capacity of the corticotroph to respond further to CRH at the fourth hour of each infusion. At this time, individuals performed a high-intensity intermittent run. Blood was drawn after exercise for hormonal analyses.

Results.—During CRH infusion, the mean plasma ACTH level increased from 4.6 to 8.6 pmol/L and the mean cortisol level increased from 361 to 662 mmol/L. The mean ACTH level increased to 32 pmol/L after exercise, despite the increase in the cortisol level. On placebo infusion, ACTH increased from 3.4 to 18.1 pmol/L after exercise (Fig 3–11). Infusion of CRH was associated with higher time-integrated responses for postexercise values of ACTH and cortisol. Heart rate and plasma lactate, epinephrine, and norepinephrine concentrations were not significantly different between the tests.

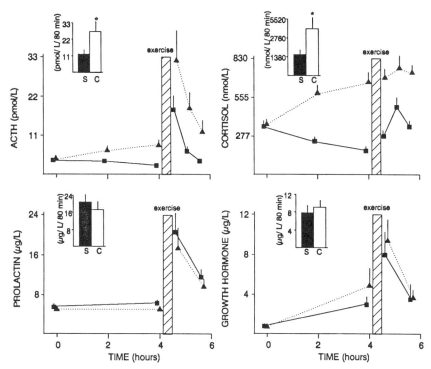

Fig 3–11.—Mean (± SE) ACTH, growth hormone, prolactin, and cortisol plasma concentrations during a 6-hour infusion of ovine CRH (*slashed line* or C) or saline (*solid line* or S) before and after an intense exercise bout. The *insets* show the postexercise area under the curve for each substance. *Stars* indicate significant differences (P < .05). (Courtesy of Smoak B, Deuster P, Rabin D, et al: *J Clin Endocrinol Metab* 73:302-306, 1991.)

Conclusion.—Some factor in addition to CRH appears to evoke ACTH release during exercise. One possibility is vasopressin, which is produced by the magnocellular and/or parvocellular neurons of the hypothalamus.

▶ I have included this paper simply because it brings out the increasing complexity of hypothalamic mediation of adrenocorticotropin release. Although CRH is probably the main one, other factors are clearly also involved.—J.R. Sutton, M.D.

Endurance Training Decreases Serum Testosterone Levels in Men Without Change in Luteinizing Hormone Pulsatile Release
Wheeler GD, Singh M, Pierce WD, Epling WF, Cumming DC (University of Alberta, Edmonton)
J Clin Endocrinol Metab 72:422–425, 1991   3–18

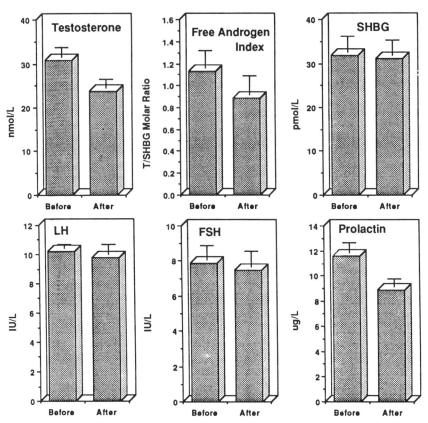

Fig 3–12.—Mean (± standard error of mean) total levels of testosterone, free androgen index (FAI), sex hormone-binding globulin (SHBG) capacity, and levels of LH, FSH, and PRL before and after 6 months of supervised running training. Total levels of testosterone, FAI, and serum levels of PRL declined significantly. (Courtesy of Wheeler GD, Singh M, Pierce WD, et al: *J Clin Endocrinol Metab* 72:422–425, 1991.)

Background.—Total and bioavailable levels of testosterone appear to be reduced in some highly trained male athletes. These alterations may result from weight loss, increased serum level of cortisol, changes in luteinizing hormone (LH) pulsatile release, or all of these. The effect of endurance training on levels of androgen was studied in 15 previously sedentary men.

Methods.—The subjects were placed on a 6-month program of supervised running, with mileage being increased to a mean of 56 km/week. Before and after training total testosterone, sex hormone-binding globulin, free androgen index, weight, and levels of LH, FSH, prolactin, and cortisol were measured. In addition, LH pulsatile release was evaluated in 5 of the men.

Results.—Total testosterone, free androgen index, and level of prolactin decreased significantly. Levels of both LH and FSH were unchanged

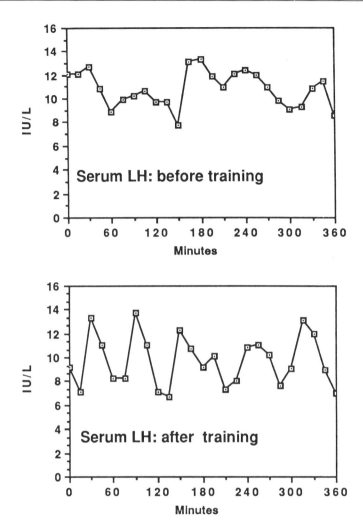

Fig 3–13.—Pretraining and posttraining serum levels of LH in single runner before and after training. Samples were obtained at 15-minute intervals over 6 hours. (Courtesy of Wheeler GD, Singh M, Pierce WD, et al: *J Clin Endocrinol Metab* 72:422-425, 1991.)

(Fig 3–12). Mean weight decreased from 76.9 to 74.2 kg, but this was not correlated with changes in serum level of testosterone. There was no significant change in LH pulsatile release (Fig 3–13).

Conclusions.—Endurance training reduces serum levels of testosterone and prolactin, as reported previously. The decrease in testosterone is unrelated to changes in LH pulsatile release, weight, or increased serum level of cortisol. Rather, changes in level of testosterone appear to result from peripheral mechanisms, such as increased tissue use or hepatic clearance.

▶ The effect of exercise and physical activity status on reproductive endocrine function is clearly very complex in females and in males. It has been known for more than 2 decades that serum testosterone increases with acute exercise in young males (1). Furthermore, this increase is largely the result of an increase in the metabolic clearance of the hormone rather than an increased secretion (2). However, in older endurance trained athletes, there is increasing evidence that a reduction in serum testosterone may be found (3), and there may be a male equivalent of the athletic amenorrhea. In fact, MacConnie et al. (4) demonstrated a subtle hypothalamic defect in athletes who were not quite as well trained as the previous group but yet had subtle hypothalamic pituitary defects but normal testosterone levels. When given injections of GnRH, this group of athletes had a decreased LH responsiveness when compared with their matched nonrunning controls. Now Cummings et al. have returned to the field with yet another study in the area but where the training mileage of the subjects was more modest—only 56 kilometers per week. Not surprisingly, accompanying hormonal changes were also modest, but they did show a decrease in serum testosterone and free androgen index [the molar ratio of testosterone to sex hormone binding globulin (SHBG)] but no changes in LH pulsatile release. This raised further questions about the possible control mechanisms for the decreased testosterone in such a modest training program. The hypothalamic pituitary function may be effected in a manner not quantitatively measurable by current techniques but resulting in a lower set point for serum testosterone without changing serum LH or LH pulsatility. One of the authors goes on to speculate about possible changes in the clearance of testosterone as a possible mechanism. To test such a hypothesis, more detailed studies of testosterone clearance rates, previously performed during exercise (2), may well be worth repeating in these various groups, but at rest.—J.R. Sutton, M.D.

References

1. Sutton JR, et al: *BMJ* 1:520, 1973.
2. Sutton JR, et al: Testosterone production rate during exercise, in Landry F, Orban WAR (eds): *3rd International Symposium on Biochemistry of Exercise.* Miami: Symposia Specialists Inc., 1978, pp 227–234.
3. Wheeler GD, et al: *JAMA* 252:514, 1984.
4. MacConnie SE, et al: *N Engl J Med* 315:411, 1986.

Autosomal Dominant Erythrocytosis Caused by Increased Sensitivity to Erythropoietin
Juvonen E, Ikkala E, Fyhriquist F, Ruutu T (University of Helsinki, Finland)
Blood 78:3066–3069, 1991   3–19

Background.—Familial erythrocytosis is a group of various disorders in which the total red cell volume is abnormally high. This condition is usually caused by an abnormal hemoglobin molecule, but it can also result from abnormal metabolism of 2,3-diphosphoglycerate or other causes. In 1 family with familial erythrocytosis caused by excessive sensitivity of erythroid progenitors to erythropoietin 1 affected member has been an Olympic cross-country skiing champion, despite levels of hemoglobin of 200 g/L or more since childhood.

Methods.—The family was known to have high levels of red blood cells, but the cause was not known. Hemoglobin seemed structurally and functionally normal. Erythroid progenitors from bone marrow and blood were studied in vitro. A family pedigree was determined, based on levels of hemoglobin.

Results.—Pedigree analysis showed autosomal dominant inheritance of erythrocytosis. Affected family members had low or low normal serum concentrations of erythropoietin. In culture, cells from these members formed higher numbers of erythroid colonies than controls in a methyl cellulose assay when levels of erythropoietin were lower than usual. Usually with increased levels of erythropoietin, the increased formation of erythroid colonies was enhanced, compared to controls. In contrast to any controls some erythroid colony growth was seen with cells from family members even when cultured in the absence of added erythropoietin.

Conclusions.—In this family erythrocytosis seems to be inherited as an autosomal dominant trait, caused by increased sensitivity to erythropoietin. This condition appears to be compatible with long life, good health, and even exceptional physical fitness. However, this does not imply that levels of red blood cells should be artificially increased to improve physical performance: life-long adaption to this condition may have been protective for the affected Olympic athlete.

▶ The success of one member of this family in Olympic cross-country ski competition is further evidence that endurance performance is enhanced by a high hemoglobin level, whether achieved fortuitously (by a genetic abnormality), or dishonestly (by autotransfusion or administration of recombinant erythropoietin). It would technically be possible to distinguish competitors with this sort of inherited trait by plotting erythroid colony formation against erythropoietin levels, as demonstrated in this paper.—R.J. Shephard, M.D., Ph.D., D.P.E.

Exercise in Hemodialysis Patients After Treatment With Recombinant Human Erythropoietin

Lundin AP, Akerman MJH, Chesler RM, Delano BG, Goldberg N, Stein RA, Friedman EA (State Univ of New York, Brooklyn)
Nephron 58:315–319, 1991   3–20

Background.—Recombinant human erythropoietin (rhEPO) can raise hemoglobin and hematocrit to normal levels in patients requiring chronic hemodialysis. This treatment offers the potential of an increased exercise capacity in these anemic patients, as delivery of oxygen to working muscles is enhanced. The effect of substantial increases in blood hemoglobin from rhEPO treatment on exercise capacity was studied in 10 patients receiving maintenance hemodialysis.

Methods.—Seven men and 3 women (mean age, 44.3 years) had been receiving maintenance hemodialysis for a mean of 29.7 months. All were tested by treadmill exercise to exhaustion before rhEPO administration and after a minimum rise of 1g/dL in hemoglobin.

Results.—With a change in hemoglobin from 7.1 g/dL to 9.8 g/dL, peak oxygen consumption with exercise rose by 50.3%. The respiratory exchange ratio at a given level of submaximal exercise dropped significantly (Fig 3–14).

Conclusions.—Administration of rhEPO to anemic patients with end-stage renal failure who are receiving chronic hemodialysis significantly increases hemoglobin levels, hematocrit, and maximal exercise capacity. The rhEPO-induced increase in hemoglobin levels also reduces the respiratory exchange ratio and, in turn, anaerobiosis during submaximal exercise.

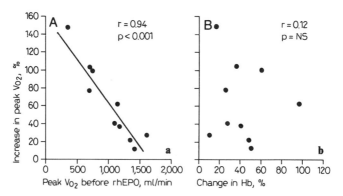

Fig 3–14.—**A,** inverse correlation between baseline peak oxygen uptake (Vo$_2$) with percent increase in peak Vo$_2$ after rhEPO; **B,** no correlation between percent change in hemoglobin and percent change in peak Vo$_2$ with rhEPO. (Courtesy of Lundin AP, Akerman MJH, Chesler RM, et al: *Nephron* 58:315–319, 1991.)

▶ Recombinant erythropoietin is a legitimate form of therapy in patients with anemia resulting from hemodialysis. Unfortunately, the existence of this new therapeutic resource is going to be a temptation to endurance athletes who wish to boost their blood hemoglobin levels, and recombinant erythropoietin will be one more substance of concern to the doping experts. In the present study, a 12-week course of 150 U/kg, given intravenously after dialysis, increased the average hemoglobin by 38% and the hematocrit by 51%, with a dramatic 50% improvement of aerobic power. Gains might be smaller in a person who began treatment with a normal hemoglobin level, but nevertheless it seems likely that erythropoietin doping could have a large influence on race outcome. Presumably, detection of the abuse would require demonstration of a disproportionate ratio between levels of erythropoietin and the renal erythropoietin factor.—R.J. Shephard, M.D., Ph.D., D.P.E.

Anabolic Steroid Education and Adolescents: Do Scare Tactics Work?
Goldberg L, Bents R, Bosworth E, Trevisan L, Elliot DL (Oregon Health Sciences Univ, Portland)
Pediatrics 87:283–286, 1991   3–21

Background.—Adolescent athletes may be susceptible to an education program that deemphasizes the benefits of anabolic androgenic steroids and emphasizes their adverse effects. Adolescent athletes' opinions before and after a balanced education program or a "scare tactics" program were compared.

Methods.—One hundred ninety-two matched pairs of preintervention and postintervention surveys were completed. The 65 subjects in group 1 attended the balanced presentation; 70 in group 2 attended the adverse effects-only program; and 57 in group 3 served as controls.

Results.—Adolescents in group 1 significantly increased their agreement with 5 of 10 targeted adverse effects. By contrast, the adolescents in group 2 did not change their level of agreement with any of the risks.

Conclusions.—A teaching approach that stresses only the untoward consequences of anabolic steroids is ineffective, even in the short-term. A more balanced presentation of the risks and benefits may improve understanding of the potential adverse effects of these drugs. Additional strategies may also be needed to change teenage athletes' attitudes toward anabolic androgenic steroid use.

▶ Given the limits of a questionnaire study, this research suggests that high school football players, when apprised on anabolic steroids by medical students who were previous local high school and/or college athletes, respond less to "scare tactics" than to a "balanced approach" that does not deny the potential ergogenic "benefits" of the drugs. Other tactics that may help curb anabolic steroid abuse include: (1) educating children on alternatives to drug use, such as good nutrition and strength training; (2) an environment in which teachers, coaches, parents, and students work together to create a "drug-free" approach to sports; and (3) channeling preadolescents into sports predicted to coincide with projected adult body size, so they don't need to "bulk up" to make the team.—E.R. Eichner, M.D.

Effects of Anabolic-Androgenic Steroids on Muscular Strength
Elashoff JD, Jacknow AD, Shain SG, Braunstein GD (Cedars-Sinai Med Ctr-University of California at Los Angeles)
Ann Intern Med 115:387–393, 1991   3–22

Introduction.—The literature from January 1966 to April 1990 was searched for topics relating to subjects who received more than 1 dose of anabolic-androgenic steroids and in whom changes in muscular strength were measured. The existence and effect of anabolic-androgenic steroid effects on strength were assessed in trained athletes and untrained healthy young men.

Methods.—Only 16 of the 30 studies found were included in the data summary because of insufficient study design in the other 14. Tabulations were made of study design, reporting of results, and adequacy and correctness of statistical methods. Percentage of strength improvement for the largest muscle group studied was calculated by comparing the difference between the control and steroid-treated groups.

Results.—The data summarized showed very slight strength improvement in previously trained athletes taking anabolic-androgenic steroids as compared to the placebo group. No firm conclusions could be drawn concerning the efficacy of anabolic steroids in enhancing overall athletic performance.

Discussion.—Much of the data were insufficient to draw firm conclusions. Steroids are often taken in megadoses, and several different types may be taken at 1 time. Therefore, it is not possible to focus on results taken only from studies using anecdotal usage reports, or those where steroids were administered only in small, controlled doses.

▶ This review on anabolic steroids and muscular strength is similar in scope and balance to that on anabolic steroids and serum lipids (see Abstract 3–23). It also has the same limitations, the main one being that the studies in print may not closely relate to how athletes use the drugs in real life. This review suggests that anabolic steroids do not seem to increase strength in previously untrained subjects; that is, the median percent strength increase in both the placebo and the steroid group was about 10%. In contrast, the 9 valid studies of trained athletes, taken at face value, support the claim that anabolic steroids improve strength in trained athletes, because in all 9 studies, slightly greater increments in strength were found in the steroid group compared with the placebo group; the median difference was 5% across all

9 studies. Even this conclusion, however, is largely restricted to the effects of methandrostenolone on bench press results. Most authorities now agree that, alas, anabolic steroids do improve strength in athletes who train hard. However, as the authors state, no firm conclusion is yet possible on whether anabolic steroids enhance overall athletic performance. Meanwhile, sadly, untold thousands of American kids are rashly taking anabolic steroids to make the team and/or look good on the beach (see also Abstract 3–21).—E.R. Eichner, M.D.

Atherogenic Effects of Anabolic Steroids on Serum Lipid Levels: A Literature Review
Glazer G (Highland Hosp, Rochester, NY)
Arch Intern Med 151:1925–1933, 1991   3–23

Objective.—Approximately 1 million Americans are using anabolic steroids (AS). Since the first data on the effects of AS on plasma lipid levels were published in 1975, the literature on the adverse effects of AS has been growing. The current body of literature linking AS to atherogenic alterations in plasma lipid levels was studied, and then the cardiac risk of AS use was calculated.

Findings.—A review of 15 mostly prospective cohort studies of weight lifters self-administering large doses of AS revealed that AS produces a dramatic and remarkably consistent depression of high-density lipoprotein (HDL) levels and severe depression of HDL_2 levels, while raising low-density lipoprotein levels. The weighted average decrease in HDL levels was 52%, the weighted average decrease in HDL_2 levels was 78%, and the weighted average increase in low-density lipoprotein levels was 36%. There is minimal to no dose relationship in AS-induced HDL level depression, and a maximal or near-maximal HDL level decrement results even from therapeutic doses of orally administered AS. Furthermore, AS-induced HDL level depression occurs early, approaching its nadir within 1 week of initiation of AS use, and returns to pretreatment levels 3–5 weeks after cessation of AS use with no significant residual HDL level depression. Using the Framingham cohort data as a basis for calculating the magnitude of the low-density lipoprotein-based increased risk for coronary heart disease associated with the use of AS, the adverse effects of AS on serum lipid levels increased the coronary heart disease risk 3–6 times, on the average. Limited data suggest that the cardiac risk-increasing effects of AS on serum lipid levels do not occur with parenterally administered AS, but this finding obviously cannot be confirmed by controlled studies for ethical reasons.

Comment.—The actual incidence of coronary heart disease among AS users is currently underreported in the medical literature because young patients with coronary heart disease are not routinely queried on AS use.

Moreover, many of these patients would likely conceal their AS use if questioned.

▶ A comprehensive, thoughtful review of the literature on anabolic steroid use and serum lipid levels. Taken as a whole, the key studies suggest that anabolic steroids rapidly (within a week or so of beginning their use) cut HDL levels in half and increase low-density lipoprotein levels by one third. The fall in HDL is mainly in the HDL2 subfraction. Among the possible mechanisms for the fall in serum HDL level, the favored one is the induction, by anabolic steroids, of postheparin plasma hepatic triglyceride lipase (HTGL), an enzyme situated in the luminal surface of hepatic endothelium that is thought to catabolize HDL by means of its phospholipase activity, thus removing HDL from plasma. Although no dose effect was apparent in this review, one should remember, as noted in another reveiw (see Abstract 3–22) that the dosage range was relatively narrow in the various studies and that these studies may not relate to how athletes actually use anabolic steroids. Athletes tend to use weird combinations of drugs, as well as doses 10 to more than 100 times greater than those used in the studies. One careful study indicates that an injectable anabolic steroid, testosterone enanthate, does not especially impair the serum lipid profile, at least as compared to the oral preparation, stanozolol (1). Fortunately, at least as suggested by the studies, when athletes stop using anabolic steroids, their HDL levels return to baseline within a month or so, and the author knows of only 4 cases of myocardial infarction in such athletes at young ages. Such complications may be underreported, however, and this area remains a critical health concern.—E.R. Eichner, M.D.

Reference

1. 1990 YEAR BOOK OF SPORTS MEDICINE, pp 194-196.

Influence of Anabolic Steroids on Body Composition, Blood Pressure, Lipid Profile and Liver Functions in Body Builders
Kuipers H, Wijnen JAG, Hartgens F, Willems SMM (University of Limburg, Maastricht, The Netherlands)
Int J Sports Med 12:413–418, 1991   3–24

Background.—The use of anabolic steroids in body building is widespread. To date, the effects of anabolic steroids on muscle mass and body composition in body builders have not been definitively established. Although authors agree on the detrimental effects of these drugs, knowledge of the relationship between the different types, doses, effects, and side effects is fragmentary. The effects of anabolic steroids on body composition, muscle fiber dimensions, liver function, and risk factors for cardiovascular disease were studied in 26 experienced body builders.

Results Before and After Placebo or Drug Administration (Steroid) in Double-Blind Cross-Over Group (N = 5)

	placebo before	after	steroid before	after
BPsys	122.0 ± 9.8	119.0 ± 5.0	120.4 ± 9.1	118.4 ± 13.5
BPdia	70.4 ± 5.0	69.8 ± 3.1	72.8 ± 5.1	67.8 ± 9.0
TotC	4.8 ± 0.7	4.9 ± 0.6	4.8 ± 0.5	4.9 ± 0.5
HDL-C	1.24 ± 0.15	1.28 ± 0.22	1.34 ± 0.15	1.00 ± 0.32*
TG	1.0 ± 0.6	1.1 ± 0.5	0.9 ± 0.5	1.4 ± 0.7
GGT	21.0 ± 5.6	18.6 ± 6.7	22.2 ± 8.8	24.6 ± 14.5
ALT	39.7 ± 10.1	41.0 ± 7.2	28.0 ± 0.1	40.0 ± 7.1
APH	81.0 ± 14.1	82.0 ± 15.1	78.6 ± 14.1	70.4 ± 23.7

Note: *Values* are means ± 1 SD. Listed are systolic (*BPsys*) and diastolic blood pressure (*BPdia*) in mm Hg, total cholesterol (*TotC*) in mmol/L, HDL cholesterol (*HDL-C*) in mmol/L, triglycerides (TG) in mmol/L, gamma-glutamyl transpeptidase (*GGT*) in units/L, alanine transaminase (*ALT*) in units/L, and alkaline phosphatase (*APH*) in units/L.
° Indicates P < .05 comparing pretreatment and posttreatment values.
(Courtesy of Kuipers H, Wijnen JAG, Hartgens F, et al: *Int J Sports Med* 12:413–418, 1991.)

Methods.—The participants were divided into 3 groups. The first consisted of 7 men who self-administered anabolic drugs for 8 to 10 weeks. Those subjects were studied at the beginning and end of steroid administration. The second group, composed of 14 men, received intramuscular injections of either placebo or nandrolone-decanoate in a double-blind fashion for 8 weeks. The third group, a double-blind cross-over group, consisted of 5 men who received a weekly intramuscular injection for 2 periods of 8 weeks each, interspersed by a 12-week washout period. The weekly injections contained either placebo or nandrolone-decanoate.

Results.—Anabolic steroids induced a 25% to 27% reduction in high-density-lipoprotein cholesterol, which was virtually reversed 6 weeks after drug use was stopped. In the self-administering group, there was a rise in diastolic blood pressure, which returned to preanabolic values about 6 weeks after drug administration was stopped. There were no adverse effects on plasma activity of liver enzymes. Increased lean body mass was noted in all groups, although the increase in the men receiving anabolic steroids was superior to that of the placebo-treated subjects. The increased lean body mass suggests muscle mass increase (table).

Conclusions.—Anabolic steroid use in experienced body builders enhances muscle development more than training alone. Girth gains can be maintained for at least 3 months after drug use is stopped. Deleterious effects on blood lipid profile and blood pressure are transient. Anabolic steroid use appears to have a mild effect on liver function and does not seem to jeopardize health.

▶ Body builders are among the more notorious users of anabolic steroids, and because they often operate with little or no advice and have little concern other than to enhance their muscle mass, they are inclined to take even larger doses than athletes who presumably have some concerns about the overall functioning of their bodies. The dose used in the present double-blind experiments, 100 mg/week, is 4–8 times the Canadian pharmaceutically recommended dose, but still does not match the very large doses that are sometimes administered without supervision (one subject was injecting 2,000 mg once a week for 10 weeks). The substantial and persistent gains of lean mass that occur with both the supervised and the unsupervised use of steroids are in keeping with previous observations. The absence of any change in muscle water seems to rule out one previously suggested explanation of the associated increase in muscle bulk (greater tissue hydration). However, it is puzzling that the muscles showed no change in the average diameter of either type I or type II fibers. Possibly, the lean mass was increased by a retention of water in the plasma and/or the extracellular space. It would have been interesting to know whether there were any changes of muscular strength, but unfortunately this was not recorded. There have been suggestions that oral 17-α alkylated androgens are particularly prone to have adverse effects on the liver. However, caution must be shown in giving nandrolone decanoate a clean bill of health, because the only measure of hepatic function available was the plasma level of 3 hepatic enzymes, and hepatic disorders are not always clearly indicated by such tests.—R.J. Shephard, M.D., Ph.D., D.P.E.

Athletes' Projections of Anabolic Steroid Use
Yesalis CE, Buckley WE, Anderson WA, Wang MQ, Norwig JA, Ott G, Puffer JC, Strauss RH (Pennsylvania State Univ, University Park; Michigan State Univ, East Lansing; Vanderbilt Univ, Nashville; West Virginia Univ, Morgantown; Univ of California, Los Angeles; et al)
Clin Sports Med 2:155–171, 1990   3–25

Introduction.—Self-reports on the use of anabolic steroids by athletes point to increased steroid use in the past 4 decades. Self-reporting, however, is likely to represent the lower boundary of use because of presumed underreporting. An attempt was made to define an upper boundary of steroid use by using projected response survey techniques and indirect questions asked of collegiate athletes. Respondents were asked to estimate the level of their competitors' steroid use.

Methods.—Male and female athletes at 5 National Collegiate Athletic Association (NCAA) division I institutions responded to a voluntary, self-administered survey. The overall response rate was 74%, with a total

Projected Anabolic Steriod Use by Sport for Males

Sport	Percentage									Don't know	Total	Weighted mean
	None	1–5%	6–10%	11–15%	16–25%	26–35%	36–50%	51–75%	>75%			
Gymnastics	46.34	34.15	7.32	4.88	—	—	—	—	—	10.53	100.00	2.42
Basketball	18.33	28.33	13.33	10.00	6.67	1.67	3.33	—	—	18.67	100.00	7.99
Track and field	4.24	11.86	11.02	13.51	13.56	14.41	8.47	4.24	—	23.26	100.00	20.50
Lacrosse	10.81	45.95	16.22	—	8.11	2.70	—	—	—	7.32	100.00	7.11
Football	2.57	4.57	7.43	8.57	14.57	22.00	16.86	7.71	1.71	14.92	100.00	29.25
Swimming/diving	8.99	41.57	19.10	15.73	4.49	—	—	2.25	—	9.17	100.00	7.77
Baseball	16.22	31.76	16.89	10.14	9.46	3.38	2.03	—	—	12.26	100.00	8.30
Volleyball	5.00	35.00	20.00	5.00	10.00	—	—	—	—	20.69	100.00	7.13
Wrestling	15.22	41.30	8.70	8.70	4.35	4.35	4.35	—	—	15.38	100.00	8.23
Other	39.09	39.09	7.11	2.54	—	4.35	0.51	—	—	12.44	100.00	2.59
All sports												14.65

Note: Percentages were based on the answers to the question: What percentage of competitors in your sport at the division I level do you believe have ever used anabolic steriods?
(Courtesy of Yesalis CE, Buckley WE, Anderson WA, et al: *Clin Sports Med* 2:155–171, 1990.)

of 1,638 participants. The indirect survey method relies on hearsay and projection, which may result in overestimating the behavior.

Findings.—The mean overall projected rate of use of anabolic steroids across all sports surveyed was 14.7% for male and 5.9% for female athletes. The highest projected anabolic steroid use rates among men's sports were among football players (29.3%) and track and field athletes (20.6%) (table). In women's sports, the greatest projected anabolic steroid use rate was among track and field athletes (16.3%). These rates are at least 3 times as high as those obtained from self-reports in previous NCAA surveys.

Conclusions.—Data on the use of anabolic steroids have generally been obtained in self-reports from athletes. Here, respondents were asked to report on their estimates of competitors' levels of steroid use. The true figure of use may lie between the lower-level estimates from self-reports and the upper-level estimates obtained from the projective response technique used in this study.

▶ This report suggests that despite the Ben Johnson scandal and the resulting Dubin Commission Enquiry (1), there is a frighteningly large use of anabolic steroids by university level athletes. Two points emerge. One is that all of the stringent measures taken to restrict doping in recent years seem merely to have convinced competitors that the use of anabolic steroids give a substantial competitive advantage. Second, many competitors indicate that they would be willing to abandon their doping practices, but only if they are convinced that their opponents have also renounced such abuse. The high rate of perceived use by opponents is thus a major obstacle to eradication of steroid abuse.—R.J. Shephard, M.D., Ph.D., D.P.E.

Reference

1. Dubin C: *Commission of Inquiry Into the Use of Drugs and Banned Practices Intended to Increase Athletic Performance,* Catalogue CP32–56/1990E. Canadian Government Publishing Center, 1990.

Doping Control of Testosterone and Human Chorionic Gonadotropin: A Case Study
de Boer D, De Jong EG, van Rossum JM, Maes RAA (University of Utrecht, The Netherlands)
Int J Sports Med 12:46–51, 1991   3–26

Introduction.—Both testosterone (T) and human chorionic gonadotropin (hCG) are used by athletes to improve their performance, examples of a practice known as doping. Doping control now requires a distinction between anabolic substances of endogenous and exogenous origins. The ratio of T to epitestosterone glucuronide (T/E) has been an acceptable indicator of exogenous testosterone administration. Use of a sandwich-type specific assay rather than a competitive hCG/hCGβ assay for urinary hCG was assessed.

Study.—Both the T/E ratio and the urinary hCG concentration were followed during the course of self-administration of T and hCG by an athlete before competition. The athlete used Sustanon 100 (testosterone esters), Pregnyl (hCG), and Synacthen-Depot (an ACTH analogue).

Observations.—The T/E ratio increased after each dose of testosterone esters was taken. The ratio of T to luteinizing hormone rose slightly

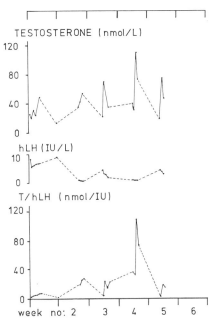

Fig 3–15.—Serum testosterone (nmol/L) and hLH levels (U/L) and the ratio of testosterone to hLH (nmol/L) reconstructed from occasionally taken serum samples. *Dotted lines* indicate an unknown value. (Courtesy of de Boer D, De Jong EG, van Rossum JM, et al: *Int J Sports Med* 12:46–51, 1991.)

after initial T administration and again after combined administration of T and hCG (Fig 3–15). The urine was negative for exogenous T just after competition, but hCG was present.

Discussion.—Testosterone supplementation is not recommended because of the unfairness of the practice and the possible health risks. In addition, evidence favoring the effectiveness of the practice is lacking.

▶ After many years of protesting that anabolic steroids had no effect on performance, sports physicians have finally had to admit that massive doses of compounds such as stanozolol can induce muscle hypertrophy, resulting in the dramatic gains of sprint performance exemplified by the Ben Johnson scandal. At the same time, the introduction of random "doping" tests and advances in gas chromatographic/mass spectroscopic techniques have allowed the controlling laboratories to detect competitors who have used even small quantities of exogenous stimulants of anabolism. Unfortunately, instead of renouncing the practice of doping, some athletes have now resorted to the administration of endogenous stimulants of anabolism. Because these compounds are already present in the bloodstream of all competitors, it is much more difficult to detect their external administration.

In many instances, a testosterone ester has been injected intramuscularly, and if a blood sample could be obtained, this treatment could be detected by gas chromatography/mass spectroscopy. Usually, however, the athlete provides only a urine specimen. When testosterone is excreted, it is converted to a glucuronide. A high ratio of testosterone glucuronide to the other endogenous excretion product, episterone glucuronide, is indicative of doping. The ratio of testosterone to the human luteinizing hormone (HLH) is also increased after the external administration of testosterone esters, although to date hLH measurements have not yet been used to detect doping.

Human chorionic gonadotrophin (HCG) can be detected by the method proposed here, but an exogenous origin cannot be inferred simply from a high HCG level. In women, the source could be a normal or an abnormal pregnancy, and in men a variety of tumors can also lead to a secretion of this substance. Simultaneous suppression of FSH concentrations may offer a means of excluding women with a high HCG due to early pregnancy. But always, it seems that the dishonest athlete is one step ahead of the "doping police."—R.J. Shephard, M.D., Ph.D., D.P.E.

Criteria to Indicate Testosterone Administration
Kicman AT, Brooks RV, Collyer SC, Cowan DA, Nanjee MN, Southan GJ, Wheeler MJ (London University)
Br J Sports Med 24:253–264, 1990   3–27

Introduction.—Detecting testosterone presents a new problem for drug control in sports. A method for such detection using radioimmunoassay was developed.

Methods.—The radioimmunoassay is used to measure the urinary ratios of testosterone (T) to epitestosterone (E) and luteinizing hormone (LH). The effect of a single intramuscular injection of testosterone followed by stimulation with human chorionic gonadotrophin (HCG) on these ratios was determined in 3 normal men, using commercially available epitestosterone antiserum.

Results.—Both the T/E and T/LH ratios could be used to detect testosterone administration. The latter ratio also served as an indicator of HCG use because of the cross-reactivity with the LH antiserum. Exercise affected these ratios insignificantly. An intramuscular injection of combined T/E heptanoates increased ratios of T/LH, but not of T/E (Fig 3–16).

Conclusion.—Both T/E and T/LH ratios can be used to detect testosterone use in men. Because of the high incidence of testosterone positives in sports in recent years, it seems prudent to use the T/LH test as a primary screening technique.

▶ This paper points out one more trick that can be used in doping. The testosterone/episterone ratio can be normalized if both of these compounds are administered in an appropriate ratio. However, the testosterone/luteinizing hormone (LH) ratio is then increased. Presumably, doping laboratories will

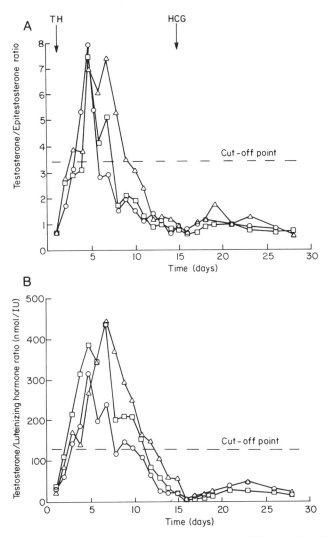

Fig 3–16.—The effects of administration of testosterone heptanoate (TH) followed by HCG stimulation on **(A)** urinary T/E and **(B)** T/LH ratios for persons 1 (*squares*), 2 (*circles*) and 3 (*triangles*). (Courtesy of Kicman AT, Brooks RV, Collyer SC, et al: *Br J Sports Med* 24:253–264, 1990.)

need to develop standard methods to determine LH if combined testosterone/episterone abuse is not to be undetected.—R.J. Shephard, M.D., Ph.D., D.P.E.

The Effects of Muscle-Building Exercise on Forearm Bone Mineral Content and Osteoblast Activity in Drug-Free and Anabolic Steroids Self-Administering Young Men
Fiore CE, Cottini E, Fargetta C, Di Salvo G, Foti R, Raspagliesi M (University of Catania, Catania, Italy)
Bone Miner 13:77–83, 1991   3–28

Introduction.—Weight bearing appears to be essential for the beneficial effects of exercise on bone. To determine the effects of power lifting on peripheral bone mass and bone metabolism, athletes engaged in competitive body building were evaluated. Because some of the men were taking androgens to increase muscle mass, it was also possible to investigate the possible additional stimulus of anabolic steroids on bone formation.

Methods.—The 18 male body builders had been exercising with weights for at least 2 years. Of these individuals, 8 were self-administering androgens according to an 8 weeks on and 2 weeks off schedule. Controls were 14 weight- and age-matched nonexercisers. Bone mineral content (BMC) and bone density (BD) were measured at appendicular sites by single photon absorptiometry. Serum levels of bone Gla-protein (BGP) were also measured.

Results.—Muscle-building exercise was associated with increased BMC and BD at the distal radius, which contains both cortical and trabecular bone. Serum BGP levels were also significantly higher in body builders than in controls. The body builders who were taking androgens did not have significantly higher BMC, BD, or BGP serum levels than individuals who were not taking androgens.

Conclusion.—Because androgens play a definite role in the maintenance of bone mass, some additive stimulus for osteoblast activity was expected in the men treated with anabolic steroids; however, these findings suggest that exercise is the major determinant of bone density increase.

▶ There have been previous reports that the administration of anabolic steroids stimulates an increase of bone mineral content (1, 2), although for some reason this occurs mainly in the first year of treatment. The lack of response seen here could have 2 possible explanations. First, steroids had been administered for more than 2 years, and it may be that the osteoblasts were no longer responding to this stimulus. Alternatively, the response previously described could have been an indirect one, associated with an increase of muscle strength, and in the present cross-sectional comparison, muscle strength was developed rather equally in those who were abusing steroids and those who were not.—R.J. Shephard, M.D., Ph.D., D.P.E.

References

1. Chesnut CH III, et al: *Metabolism* 26:267, 1977.
2. Geusens P, Dequeker J: *Bone Miner Res* 1:347, 1986.

Performance and Metabolic Responses to a High Caffeine Dose During Prolonged Exercise
Graham TE, Spriet LL (Univ of Guelph, Ontario)
J Appl Physiol 71:2292–2298, 1991   3–29

Background.—It has been proposed that caffeine ingestion during endurance exercise elevates catecholamines, enhancing fat oxidation, which would spare muscle glycogen and prolong time to exhaustion. This hypothesis is unproven, and the metabolic effects of caffeine ingestion are uncertain.

Objective and Methods.—High doses of caffeine were given to trained runners to determine whether the caffeine would raise epinephrine levels at rest and during exercise but not alter substrate use or enhance endurance performance. Seven competitive distance runners, 6 men and 1 woman, ran and cycled to exhaustion at approximately 85% maximum oxygen uptake ($\dot{V}O_{2max}$) during 2 trials each, 1 hour after ingestion of either 9 mg of caffeine per kg or a placebo. Expired gas samples and blood samples were taken before and during exercise for analysis, and preexercise and postexercise urine samples were also analyzed.

Findings.—The average endurance time running and cycling was significantly increased by caffeine, as were the times to exhaustion of all individual subjects (Fig 3–17). Caffeine ingestion significantly increased plasma epinephrine concentrations before exercise, from .22 to .44 nM, and also significantly increased epinephrine levels during running and cycling and at exhaustion. In contrast, caffeine ingestion had no effect on norepinephrine levels at rest or during exercise. Further effects of caffeine ingestion included elevation of plasma glycerol concentrations, but no changes in respiratory exchange ratios or plasma free fatty acid levels during exercise.

Conclusions.—Caffeine in high doses that do not result in urinary levels greater than those accepted by the International Olympic Committee seem to dramatically enhance endurance performance and increase epinephrine concentrations of elite runners during running and cycling. Further study is required to determine whether the performance effect is due to carbohydrate sparing.

▶ This will be a benchmark study in the long-running debate on caffeine and athletics. For a concise discussion of the "state of the art" leading up to this

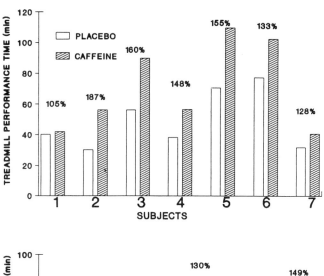

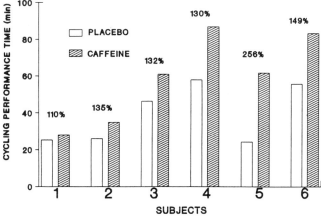

Fig 3–17.—Individual performance times of subjects running (*top*) and cycling (*bottom*) to exhaustion after placebo or caffeine ingestion. Subjects 4 and 6 were caffeine users (450–720 mg/day); subjects 1, 2, and 7 were light users (120–150 mg/day); and subjects 3 and 5 were nonusers (< 20 mg/day). (Courtesy of Graham TE, Spriet LL: *J Appl Physiol* 71:2292–2298, 1991.)

study, see reference (1). The design of the current study controls for many of the variables that have yielded mixed results in past studies on caffeine and exercise. Elite runners were the subjects, and they prepared for the exercise trials as if they were competitions, by consuming pretrial diets high in carbohydrates, by refraining from caffeine intake for 48 hours before each trial, and by incorporating the exercise trials into their training as heavy workouts. The caffeine dose was high, and its effect was astonishing. Running time to exhaustion increased from 49 to 71 minutes, and cycling time to exhaustion increased from 39 to 59 minutes. Every subject increased his or her exercise time to exhaustion, both running and cycling, during the caffeine trial. Caffeine ingestion dramatically increased plasma epinephrine levels at rest and during exercise but had no effect on norepinephrine responses. The high dose of caffeine and the elevated epinephrine levels were associated with elevated plasma glyercol levels but there were no significant changes in levels of plasma free fatty acids or in the respiratory exchange ratio during exercise. Hence, more research will be needed to conclusively determine whether the ergogenic effects of caffeine ingestion stem from a shift toward greater fat use and a sparing of carbohydrate use, the mechanism these authors seem to favor.—E.R. Eichner, M.D.

Reference

1. 1991 Year Book of Sports Medicine, pp 174–176.

Failure of Caffeine to Affect Metabolism During 60 Min Submaximal Exercise

Titlow LW, Ishee JH, Riggs CE (Univ of Central Arkansas, Conway; Univ of Arkansas, Fayetteville)
J Sports Sci 9:15–22, 1991   3–30

Background.—Recent research on the effect of caffeine on athletic performance suggests that its effect is specific to individuals, mode of exercise, and/or diet. The caffeine dosage used in these studies, however, appears to be significantly higher than the 200 mg typically consumed before athletic performance. The effects of 200 mg caffeine on metabolism during submaximal exercise performance were studied.

Methods.—Five men, mean age 25 years, performed 2 60-minute monitored treadmill workouts at 60% maximal heart rate during 2 weeks. By random assignment, the men took a caffeine or placebo capsule 60 minutes before exercising. Testing was done in the afternoon after a midnight fast. Venous blood was drawn before exercise, every 15 minutes during exercise, and 10 minutes after recovery and analyzed for free fatty acid, triglycerides, glucose, lactic acid, hemoglobin, and hematocrit. The respiratory exchange ratio, perceived exertion, and oxygen uptake were also recorded every 4 minutes while the men exercised.

Results.—There were no significant differences in heart rate or blood pressure between groups before or after exercise except for blood pressure before exercise, which appeared to be significantly increased in the men taking caffeine. There were no significant differences in the way the men perceived level of exertion or in trials for respiratory exchange ratio or maximum oxygen uptake. There were also no significant between-group differences in hematocrit, hemoglobin, or glucose response. Lactic acid, triglyceride, and free fatty acid response changes did not differ significantly (Fig 3–18).

Conclusions.—In a dose of 200 mg, caffeine offers no real metabolic advantage during 60 minutes of submaximal exercise. This dose of caf-

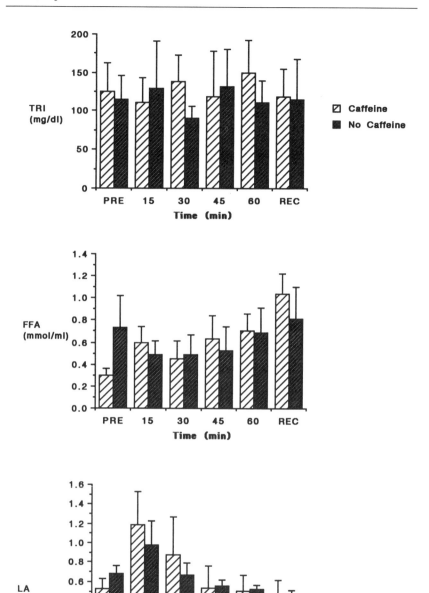

Fig 3–18.—Lactic acid (LA), free fatty acid (FFA), and triglyceride (TRI) responses. (Courtesy of Titlow LW, Ishee JH, Riggs CE: *J Sports Sci* 9:15-22, 1991.)

feine apparently did not change performance or substrate metabolism significantly.

▶ In this study, caffeine appears to have little or no value as a means of modifying responses to exercise. The dose (200 mg) is somewhat smaller than that used by Graham et al. (Abstract 4–9) of 5 mg/kg, and this may account for the lack of effect on either metabolism or perceptions of effort. Certainly, larger doses do produce a shift to lipid metabolism (1).—R.J. Shephard, M.D., Ph.D., D.P.E.

Reference

1. Costill DL, et al: *Med Sci Sports Exerc* 10:155, 1978.

Anaerobic Work and Power Output During Cycle Ergometer Exercise: Effects of Bicarbonate Loading

McNaughton L, Curtin R, Goodman G, Perry D, Turner B, Showell C (Tasmanian State Institute of Technology, Tasmania, Australia)
J Sports Sci 9:151–160, 1991   3–31

Background.—The use of ergogenic aids has become widespread. The effects of induced metabolic alkalosis during cycle ergometer performance of 60 seconds were studied to further validate the use of bicarbonate as an ergogenic aid.

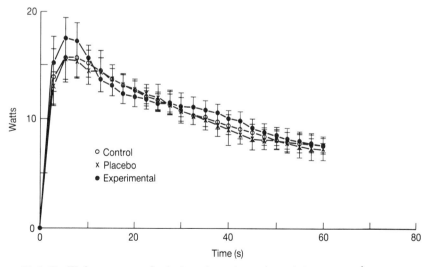

Fig 3–19.—Work output curves for the 3 conditions (mean ± 1 SD). (Courtesy of McNaughton L, Curtin R, Goodman G, et al: *J Sports Sci* 9:151-160, 1991.)

Methods.—Eight trained male cyclists regularly competing in track races were assessed under control, alkalotic, and placebo conditions. Basal, preexercise and postexercise blood samples in each condition were examined for pH, partial pressure of carbon dioxide (PCO_2), partial pressure of oxygen, bicarbonate, base excess, and lactate.

Results.—At basal levels, all blood gas measurements were within normal limits. When compared with control and placebo conditions, there were significant differences in the amount of work produced and maximal power output in the experimental condition. Postexercise pH declined in all 3 conditions. Postexercise PCO_2 rose significantly in the alkalosis trial. The preexercise base excess and bicarbonate levels were both higher in the alkalotic condition than at basal levels, suggesting that bicarbonate ingestion significantly increases the buffering ability of the blood. Postexercise lactate levels were significantly higher after the alkalotic trial compared with the control and placebo conditions just after exercise and for 3 minutes thereafter. Postexercise lactate values were greater than basal or preexercise values immediately after exercise and for the next 5 minutes (Fig 3–19).

Conclusions.—Bicarbonate appears to be an effective ergogenic aid when used for anaerobic exercise such as that described in this study. Its ergogenic property is probably attributable to the accelerated efflux of H^+ ions from the muscle tissue resulting from increased extracellular bicarbonate buffering.

▶ It is already widely accepted that administration of an appropriate dose of bicarbonate immediately before a short distance race can boost performance by about 3% (1). This is a small gain in absolute terms, but is nevertheless very significant in terms of athletic records. The present authors show an even larger (7.3%) gain of work output over a 1-minute all-out cycle ergometer test. The dose of bicarbonate (400 mg/kg, much as in earlier studies) was administered 1 hour before the exercise bout. The suggested explanation of the enhanced performance is similar to that offered previously—a speeding of lactate efflux from the active muscles because of increased extracellular buffering. Some support for this hypothesis can be found in higher blood lactate readings at the immediate end of exercise (although the extra lactate is not much in excess of the extra work performed after bicarbonate administration). Given that in the absence of bicarbonate doping, blood lactates do not peak until 2–4 minues after a bout of anaerobic exercise, accelerated lactate efflux may not be the total explanation of the phenomenon. I was some what discouraged by the final conclusion of the paper . . . "The use of bicarbonate as a buffering substance . . . is well warranted." Certainly, bicarbonate cannot be detected because it is a normal body constituent, but the artificial manipulation of bicarbonate levels is hardly consistent with the ethics of athletic competition.—R.J. Shephard, M.D., Ph.D., D.P.E.

Reference

1. Wilkes D, et al: *Med Sci Sports Exerc* 15:277, 1983.

Effect of Antihypertensive Medication on Endurance Exercise Capacity in Hypertensive Sportsmen

Vanhees L, Fagard R, Lijnen P, Amery A (University of Leuven, Belgium)
J Hypertens 9:1063–1068, 1991   3–32

Background.—It has previously been shown that β-adrenergic blockers can depress exercise capacity, but little is known about the effects on endurance exercise capacity of calcium blockers, and nothing has been reported on the effects on endurance exercise of converting enzyme inhibitors. All 3 types of antihypertensive medications were tested for their effects on endurance exercise capacity and on some metabolic factors.

Methods.—Fourteen male patients with a mean age of 39 years who had mild hypertension were enrolled in the study. Twelve of these men ran or rode bicycles, or both, and 2 engaged in competitive soccer or judo for a mean of 5 hours per week. The men received 240 mg/day of slow-release verapamil, 50 mg/day of atenolol, 10 mg/day of enalapril, or placebo for a 3-week period according to a randomized double-blind crossover design. Their exercise endurance at 70% capacity was then determined on a cycle ergometer and compared with their performance before receiving a drug or placebo. Blood samples were taken before and after exercise.

Results.—Atenolol alone affected exercise endurance, resulting in a significant mean decrease of 38%. Atenolol alone affected blood chemistry, decreasing plasma levels of free fatty acids before and after exercise, and increasing concentrations of potassium after exercise. Atenolol alone significantly reduced systolic blood pressure and heart rate during exercise. All drugs tested reduced diastolic blood pressure during exercise, especially enalapril.

Conclusions.—In mildly hypertensive sportsmen atenolol seems to significantly reduce endurance exercise capacity and can affect metabolic factors. Enalapril and verapamil do not have these effects.

▶ Atenolol induced a small (10%) decrease of oxygen intake relative to the other 2 types of antihypertensive medication, but the main explanations of the substantial decrease in exercise endurance seem not cardiac, but rather a reduction in lipolysis both at rest and during exercise, and a fatiguing rise of plasma potassium concentration. Before becoming too enthusiastic for the alternatives (calcium-channel blockers or converting enzyme inhibitors), it is nevertheless important to stress that with the doses chosen, the atenolol was the most effective of the 3 medications in reducing blood pressures (particularly the systolic reading). It is conceivable that if the dose of the other 2 drugs had been increased to match the change of blood pressure induced by atenolol, then they also might have induced fatigue (although the deterioration of performance during atenolol treatment was not related to the change of blood pressure).—R.J. Shephard, M.D., Ph.D., D.P.E.

Influence of Physical Exercise on Serum Digoxin Concentration and Heart Rate in Patients With Atrial Fibrillation
Bøtker HE, Toft P, Klitgaard NA, Simonsen EE (Haderslev Hospital, Haderslev; Odense University Hospital, Odense, Denmark)
Br Heart J 65:337–341, 1991   3–33

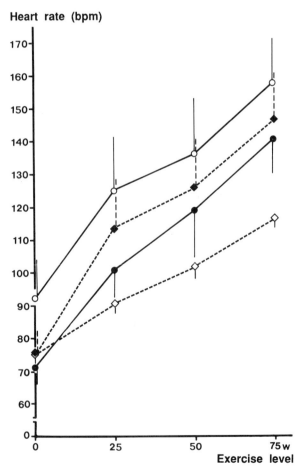

Fig 3–20.—Heart rates (mean [SEM]) at rest and during exercise in patients with atrial fibrillation at 0, low, and high digoxin concentration. Heart rates from control patients in sinus rhythm are shown for comparison. (Courtesy of Bøtker HE, Toft P, Klitgaard NA, et al: *Br Heart J* 65:337–341, 1991.)

Introduction.—Digoxin may fail to prevent an excessive increase in heart rate during exercise in patients with atrial fibrillation, possibly because of altered pharmacokinetics. Most digoxin is bound to skeletal muscle, and redistribution during exercise therefore could alter the amount present in other tissues.

Methods.—Heart rate and the serum digoxin concentrations were monitored at rest and on exercise in 8 men with atrial fibrillation and in 8 others with ischemic heart disease who were in sinus rhythm. Serum digoxin levels were 0, low, and high within the therapeutic range of .6–2.6 ng/mL. Patients performed cycle exercise for 20 minutes at work-rates of 25, 50, and 75 W.

Results.—Serum digoxin levels decreased significantly at each work-rate in the patients with and also in those without atrial fibrillation. Baseline levels returned after 1 hour of rest. In the patients with fibrillation, the absolute reduction in heart rate with increments in digoxin dosage were similar at rest and on exercise (Fig 3-20). Digoxin did not affect the changes in mean blood pressure occurring on exercise.

Conclusion.—An increased dose of digoxin during exercise would bring only slight improvement while increasing the risk of toxicity. Patients with an excessive increase in pulse rate on exercise might be given a calcium channel blocker, but exercise endurance is not increased and there also is a risk of toxicity with these drugs. Use of a β-blocker is another alternative.

▶ Much of current pharmacology is based on the response of anesthetized animals, and it is fairly obvious that vigorous exercise will lead to drastic alterations in many aspects of pharmacokinetics, including the absorption, metabolism, and excretion of various drugs.

The present report looks at the influence of commonly used intensities of cycle ergometer exercise on serum digoxin concentrations. In confirmation of several earlier studies, digoxin levels decreased by about a third, during exercise presumably because digoxin was being bound to sites in the active skeletal muscle. The exercise-induced increase of heart rate was 20–30 beats/min greater in patients with atrial fibrillation than in control subjects, and whereas the prescribed dose of digoxin normalized resting heart rate, it proved inadequate for this purpose during exercise. On the other hand, the decrease of heart rate induced by digoxin was similar in rest and exercise, suggesting that the supposed inadequate control of exercise heart rate may reflect the influence of the underlying disease process rather than a more specific exercise-induced alteration of pharmacokinetics. The authors suggest that exercise-induced alterations of autonomic balance reduce the ability of the atrioventricular node to screen out the excessive number of impulses arriving from the atrium, although it is also possible that the higher exercise heart rate in those with atrial fibrillation reflects a poor physical condition, with a small stroke volume. Whereas there is empiric evidence that calcium channel blockers give a "better" control of exercise heart rate (1), such drugs fail to increase the overall well-being of the patient (2). It is equally unclear whether use of β-blockers to reduce the heart rate to a "normal" value improves well-being (3, 4). As the population ages, an ever-increasing number of people will be affected by atrial fibrillation, and it will be important to determine whether attempts at normalizing the exercise heart rate are a beneficial component of therapy, or meddlesome interference in what would otherwise be a normal adaptation to a poor level of physical condition.—R.J. Shephard, M.D., Ph.D., D.P.E.

References

1. Klein HO, Kaplinsky E: *Am J Cardiol* 50:894, 1982.
2. Lewis R, et al: *Eur Heart J* 8:148, 1987.
3. Brown RW, Goble AJ: *BMJ* ii:279, 1969.
4. David D, et al: *Am J Cardiol* 44:1379, 1979.

4 Environment, Hematology, Immune Function

Optimal Practice Times for the Reduction of the Risk of Heat Illness During Fall Football Practice in the Southeastern United States
Francis K, Feinstein R, Brasher J (Univ of Alabama at Birmingham)
Athlet Train, JNATA 26:76–80, 1991   4–1

Background.—Fall football practice usually begins in early August when the weather is often very hot and humid in the southeastern United States. This places athletes at risk of heat illness, even more so when they practice in a padded football uniform. The best times in August and September to conduct football practice in the southeastern United States were defined, and guidelines to reduce the risk of heat illness were offered.

Methods.—Three-year climatologic data for the months of August and September were obtained from the regional weather stations of 10 southeastern cities in the United States. The relative severity of the climactic conditions was ranked according to the *Football Weather Guide*, giving a graphic depiction of temperature and humidity relative to the risk of exertional heat illness developing in football players. Daily 3-year averages for each 3-hour time period were superimposed on the *Football Weather Guide.*

Results.—In August, no environmental combinations at any time in any of the 10 cities would be considered safe for outdoor football practice in full uniform. In September, results were similar for 8 of the 10 cities. The exceptions, 3 pm and 6 pm for Columbia, South Carolina, and 3 pm for Jackson, Mississippi, were outside the "danger" zone but still within the "cautionary" zone, in which there is still increased risk of heat illness.

Conclusions.—In the southeastern United States, there appears to be no environmentally safe time for football practice in August and September without running the risk of heat injury. As the time of the beginning of the season cannot be changed, coaches should implement precautionary measures. The least environmental heat load appears to occur between 3 and 9 pm, but this is still a danger period. Measures to prevent heat injury are studied.

▶ Because of the time of year that football is played, many games in August, September, and occasionally October, will be played in environmentally unsafe conditions. Hopefully, by the time these games are played, athletes will have participated in a proper program of practice and conditioning that will acclimate them to the unsafe conditions of heat and humidity. Much of the danger occurs during practice sessions early in the season when many of the athletes are in poor condition and not acclimated to doing intense physical exertion in high heat and humidity. Another complicating factor that must be considered is that at the beginning of the season, teams often practice twice a day in the hot humid weather. There is not enough time between practice sessions to allow athletes to rehydrate themselves, and the problem is accumulative.

The authors offer suggestions to prevent heat illness. These safety measures include practicing during the coolest time of day, using fishnet jerseys and light colored uniforms to reflect the sun's rays, taking frequent and compulsory rest breaks, consuming adequate amounts of water *before* and during practice, measuring body weight before and after practice, instituting a progressive acclimatization program, and monitoring of players carefully for signs of heat stress. These guidelines hold true for all parts of the country where the combination of heat and humidity are a problem. Please read Abstract 4–2, which also addresses this problem.—F.J. George, A.T.C., P.T.

Team Sports in Hot Weather: Guidelines for Modifying Youth Soccer
Elias SR, Roberts WO, Thorson DC (Group Health, Inc, St Paul; Minn Health PA, White Bear Lake, Minn)
Phys Sportsmed 19:67–80, 1991   4–2

Background.—Athletes, particularly children and adolescents, are at risk of morbidity and mortality when playing competitive sports during hot, humid weather. At a USA Cup youth soccer tournament played in such conditions, 18 of about 4,000 athletes collapsed by the middle of the second day of play, necessitating immediate modifications of play.

Game Modifications.—Depending on age group, the games were shortened by 3 to 5 minutes per half. Thus, the under-12 group, which usually played 25-minute halves, played 22-minute halves, and the under-19 group, which usually played 40-minute halves, played 35-minute halves. This additional time was added to the half-time breaks, lengthening them by 6 to 10 minutes. In addition, a 2-minute quarter break was given in each half and unlimited substitutions were allowed. The number of heat injuries decreased immediately except in the 13- and 14-year-old boys, probably because they tended to ignore the safety recommendations.

Guidelines to Prevent Heat Injury.—Game modifications are suggested according to wet bulb globe temperature (WBGT), with quarterly fluid breaks at WBGT over 65°F, shortened game times or unlimited substitutions at WBGT over 73°F, and moving midday games to earlier or later times at WBGT over 82°F. Events should not be scheduled at the hottest time of the day or year, and the insidious nature of dehydration should be recognized. Presenting symptoms usually include dizziness, light-headedness, weakness, headache, mild disorientation, nausea, and syncope. Players should be allowed to rest in an air-conditioned area, with ice packs applied to the groin, neck, and axillae; and oral hydration should be begun. Intravenous hydration is occasionally required.

Conclusions.—Game modifications for soccer played in extremely hot weather to prevent heat injury have been developed. The modifications could be adapted for use in other sports. Players, coaches, officials, and parents need to be made aware of the potential for heat injury.

▶ The game must go on. Abstract 4–1 and 4–2 establish guidelines to prevent heat illness during athletic events. The authors of Abstract 4–2 have made suggestions for games and tournaments that should be beneficial to all sports. Games were shortened in length, the length of half-time was increased, 2-minute compulsory water breaks were taken each quarter, and unlimited substitutions were allowed. A big part of a coach's game plan on a hot, humid day should be regularly scheduled substitutions. At the end of the game, if the better players are not exhausted from the heat, a victory may be ensured. *Water, water, water:* athletes practicing and playing on hot, humid days cannot get too much of it, *before*, during, and after the competition.—F.J. George, A.T.C., P.T.

Collapsed Runners: Blood Biochemical Changes After IV Fluid Therapy

Noakes TD, Berlinski N, Solomon E, Weight L (University of Cape Town, South Africa)

Phys Sportsmed 19:70–81, 1991   4–3

Background.—It is not known why some athletes collapse after long-distance races or triathlon events. To date, no one has studied the effects of routine intravenous administration of fluids on blood biochemical values in these runners. Serum sodium concentrations and other indicators of fluid status were measured in collapsed and noncollapsed runners.

Methods.—The study was conducted among 32 collapsed and 16 noncollapsed runners seen in the medical tent at the finish line of a 56-K race run annually in Cape Town. At the discretion of the attending physician, the collapsed runners were randomly assigned to intravenous treatment consisting of 1–2 L of .9% sodium chloride with 5% glucose or no treatment. The 20 given no treatment received a placebo infusion

Initial and Final Postrace Hematologic and Blood Biochemical Measurements for
Collapsed Ultramarathon Runners in Groups Receiving or Not Receiving Treatment With
Intravenous Fluid

	Treatment (N = 26)		Nontreatment (N = 6)	
	Initial	Final	Initial	Final
Hemoglobin (g/L)	16.3 ± 1.4	13.7 ± 1.3	15.7 ± 1.2	14.9 ± 1.1
Hematocrit (%)	49 ± 4	42 ± 4	47 ± 3	46 ± 3
Increase in plasma volume (%)		19.6 ± 6.4		5.3 ± 8.0
Serum sodium (mmol/L)	139 ± 5	126 ± 11	133 ± 13	133 ± 7
Serum potassium (mmol/L)	4.0 ± 0.5	3.5 ± 0.6	3.9 ± 0.7	4.1 ± 0.3
Blood glucose (mmol/L)	5.2 ± 1.7	16.4 ± 4.5	4.5 ± 1.2	5.4 ± 2.2
Serum osmolaty (mmol/kg)	278 ± 9	265 ± 20	267 ± 25	268 ± 12

Mean ± SD.
(Courtesy of Noakes TD, Berlinski N, Solomon E, et al: *Phys Sportsmed* 19:70–81, 1991.)

and free access to oral fluids. Fourteen runners in the latter group were
eventually crossed over to treatment at the physician's discretion.

Findings.—Profound hyperglycemia developed in the 26 collapsed
runners who were given fluid intravenously. Marked hyponatremia developed in 14 of these. Blood glucose and serum sodium values remained
within the normal range in the 6 collapsed runners who did not receive
fluids intravenously (table).

Conclusions.—Most collapsed runners are probably not sufficiently
dehydrated to warrant intravenous therapy with fluids. Such treatment
should be reserved for collapsed runners with clear biochemical or other
signs of dehydration. These findings argue against the notion that dehydration is the sole cause of exercise-associated collapse.

▶ This report would be a little easier to interpret if more details had been
given about the run. In particular, what did the runners drink over the 56-km
distance, and what was the change in their body mass during the period of
competition? The situation is further confused by a reversal of colors in one
of the attractively colored graphs in the original article. However, in essence,
this seems an extension of earlier observations that runners who are provided with fluids ad libitum can become overhydrated during a long race
(particularly if conditions are cool) (1). If this basic premise is accepted, it is
evident that administering a large quantity of .9% saline solution is going to
lead to hyponatremia. Further, given that the blood glucose was 5.2 mmol/L
at the end of the event, there seems no reason to administer 5% glucose intravenously. It is particularly interesting that despite subsequent proof that
they had taken the wrong approach, the supervising physicians insisted on

administering fluid to 14 of the 20 individuals who had been selected as a "no-treatment" control group. Plainly, there is a need for a critical audit of much of the emergency room treatment given to athletes.—R.J. Shephard, M.D., Ph.D.

Reference

1. Noakes TD, et al: *Med Sci Sports Exerc* 17:370, 1985.

Endotoxemia and Release of Tumor Necrosis Factor and Interleukin 1α in Acute Heatstroke

Bouchama A, Parhar RS, El-Yazigi A, Sheth K, Al-Sedairy S (King Faisal Specialist Hospital and Research Centre, Riyadh, Saudi Arabia)
J Appl Physiol 70:2640–2644, 1991   4–4

Introduction.—Heatstroke produces a syndrome resembling sepsis or endotoxemia. Shock occurs with increased cardiac output and reduced systemic vascular resistance. Adult respiratory distress syndrome ensues, ending in multiorgan system failure and death.

Methods.—To determine whether heatstroke is associated with endotoxemia and the release of tumor necrosis factor (TNF-α) and/or interleukin-1α (IL-1α), 17 adult patients with classic heatstroke were studied. Their mean rectal temperature was 42.1°C. Blood samples taken at admission and after cooling were examined for TNF-α and IL-1α by an enzyme-linked immunosorbent assay.

Results.—All patients initially had increased levels of TNF-α, IL-1α, and lipopolysaccharide. Values did not correlate significantly with body temperature. All values were significantly lower after cooling, but they remained above control values.

Conclusions.—Heatstroke is associated with endotoxemia as well as with the release of TNF-α and IL-1α. These mediators may well have a role in the pathogenesis of heatstroke.

▶ This study is one of an increasing number that bring to the clinician's attention that heatstroke and the multisystem organ involvement that follows very much resemble septic shock. Previously held ideas of the pathogenesis of heatstroke were related to the cellular toxicity of the heat and/or other simple reflex cardiovascular changes that might be derived from poor cardiac filling pressure in dehydrated subjects. There is, however, more and more evidence that endotoxin is the initial trigger in the cascade of events leading to the pathologic entity we know as heatstroke (1). These endotoxins, which are lipopolysaccharide-protein complexes and come from the cell wall of gram-negative bacteria, are an extremely potent stimulus to (TNF and IL-1α (2). These latter two substances are endogenous pyrogens, which result in fever and are responsible for the shock and tissue injury associated with endotoxemia (3). In this paper, patients with classic (not exertional) heatstroke had measurements made of a number of important mediators such as TNF and IL-1α. Although no control measurements were made, there was an interesting relationship with increasing temperature in these patients with heatstroke and the plasma concentration of these mediators. Furthermore, although these were not exercising patients, the lessons almost certainly apply, perhaps even more so, to exertional heatstroke.

Even in those who do not have heatstroke, evidence is accumulating that during exercise, and particularly if exercise is associated with significant hyperthermia, there will be bacterial translocation in the gut and increases in the concentration of lipopolysaccharide, IL-1α, and TNF. These important mediators then can stimulate a cascade of varying biological responses, stimulating the complement pathways, coagulation pathways, numerous cytokines, colony stimulating factor, and interferon. Of all these, however, most evidence suggests that TNF and interleukin I are the primary mediators of endotoxic shock. An additional family of proteins may also be important. In response to heatstroke, these are the so called heatshock proteins or proteins that respond to stress and may actually help protect the organism against some of the destruction mediators. In particular, heatshock proteins 28 and 70 are important in the acquired tolerance of mammalian cells to hyperthermia.

Thus, under most circumstances during exercise, mild elevation of some of these trigger mediators might occur, but it has been shown by Brock-Utne and colleagues that the increase in some of these mediators in persons who subsequently develop heatstroke is much greater (4). Of all the pathologic features of heatstroke, it is the development of disseminated intravascular coagulation, together with rhabdomyolysis, that are responsible secondarily for the multiorgan pathology seen in heatstroke that results in significant morbidity and mortality.—J.R. Sutton, M.D.

References

1. Gathiram P, et al: *Circ Shock* 25:223, 1988.
2. Old LJ: *Nature* 330:602, 1987.
3. Tracey KJ, et al: *Science* 234:470, 1986.
4. Brock-Utne JG, et al: *S Afr Med J* 73:533, 1988.

Are Psoriatic Patients at Risk of Heat Intolerance?

Leibowitz E, Seidman DS, Laor A, Shapiro Y, Epstein Y (Tel-Aviv University, Israel)
Br J Dermatol 124:439–442, 1991
                                          4–5

Background.—Body surface area that is capable of secreting and evaporating sweat is decreased in patients with widespread psoriasis. Thermoregulation may be compromised, and the patients may suffer excessive heat accumulation during physical training. Sixteen young patients with psoriasis were studied to determine whether they were at increased risk of heat intolerance.

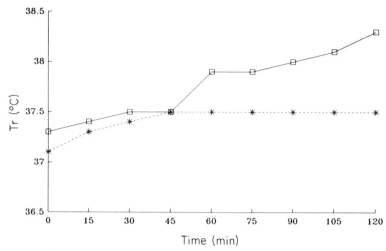

Fig 4–1.—Changes in rectal temperature (°C) in subjects during 2 hours of exercise in heat. *Squares,* subjects with psoriasis; *asterisks,* controls. (Courtesy of Leibowitz E, Seidman DS, Laor A, et al: *Br J Dermatol* 124:439-442, 1991.)

Methods.—The subjects were all male with a mean age of 20.4 years. All had varying degrees of psoriatic skin involvement, with a mean of 4.9% of skin surface area being affected. A group of healthy volunteers were studied as controls. All subjects performed a 2-hour treadmill exercise test in conditions of 40° C and relative humidity of 40%. During this

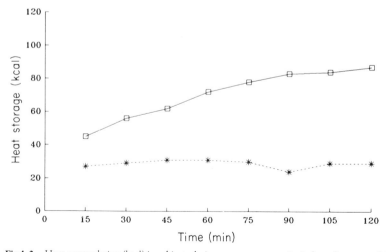

Fig 4–2.—Heat accumulation (kcal) in subjects during exposure to exercise in heat. *Squares,* subjects with psoriasis; *asterisks,* controls. (Courtesy of Leibowitz E, Seidman DS, Laor A, et al: *Br J Dermatol* 124:439-442, 1991.)

exercise rectal temperature (Tr), mean skin temperature, heart rate, and calculated heat storage (dS) were measured.

Results.—All parameters rose more sharply in psoriatic patients than in controls. At 60 minutes and at the end of exercise, Tr was significantly higher in the psoriatic patients (Fig 4–1); dS was 78 kcal in the psoriatic patients vs. 30 kcal in controls at 60 minutes; at 120 minutes dS had risen to 87 kcal in psoriatic patients but stayed at 30 kcal in controls (Fig 4–2). Psoriatic patients had a sweat rate of 590 g/hr compared to 691 g/hr for controls; this difference remained significant even when corrected for healthy skin area: 337 g/hr/m² in psoriatic patients vs. 370 g/hr/m² in controls.

Conclusions.—Patients with psoriasis appear to have decreased ability to dissipate extra heat when performing exercise in the heat. Psoriatic patients should be carefully monitored before and during exercise, because their disease is a risk factor for heat intolerance.

▶ I included this study because it highlights another group of patients who may be at risk for heatstroke, although careful scrutiny of the data does not allow this conclusion to be made. The matching of the control group with the psoriatic patients is not actually given (i.e., for $\dot{V}O_{2max}$ and the percentage of $\dot{V}O_{2max}$ at which each group was exercising). However, it can be assumed from the heart rate data, which showed a much higher heart rate in the psoriatic subjects compared with the "control" group at 60 minutes (128±4 vs. 115±4 beats/min) and 120 minutes (137±7 vs. 120±6 beats/minute), respectively, that the patients were exercising at a higher percentage of their $\dot{V}O_{2max}$. Therefore they might be expected to have a greater heat storage and greater absolute rectal temperature, as they did. Thus, the study is flawed in this regard, and I would like to see a repeated study using a control group with similar cardiorespiratory fitness or, if not, where both groups were exercised at the same relative percentage of their $\dot{V}O_{2max}$. Only then will we know that such psoriatic patients are biologically different from their unfit counterparts in terms of their risks of developing heatstroke. In the meantime, clinicians beware!—J.R. Sutton, M.D.

Is Dantrolene Effective in Heat Stroke Patients?
Channa AB, Seraj MA, Saddique AA, Kadiwal GH, Shaikh MH, Samarkandi AH (King Saud University, Riyadh, Saudi Arabia)
Crit Care Med 18:290–292, 1990   4–6

Background.—Heatstroke (HS) caused by environmental heat injury is a life-threatening emergency that is characterized by a body core temperature $> 40°$ C, altered mental status, and anhydrosis. Dantrolene sodium is the treatment of choice for both prophylaxis and the treatment of thermic distress resulting from neuroleptic malignant syndrome and malignant hyperthermia. Dantrolene may also be effective in HS patients.

Management.—Twenty patients with HS were randomized either to receive dantrolene (8 patients) or to a control group (12 patients). All the patients had rectal temperatures of $\geq 41.9°$ C on admission, and patients in both groups were cooled either by conventional methods or by the Makkah Al-Mukkaramah body-cooling unit to a rectal core temperature of 39° C. The patients in the dantrolene group were given 2–4 mg of intravenous dantrolene sodium per kg of body weight.

Methods.—Six study patients and all of the controls had central venous pressure (CVP) cannulas inserted. The CVP was monitored at 5-minute intervals, and intravenous fluids were given to maintain the CVP between 5 cm and H_2O and 10 cm H_2O. The rectal, thigh, chest, and upper-limb body temperatures were recorded continuously. In addition, all patients received Foley catheters in the urinary bladder. Blood samples were taken for analysis. Some of the patients received oxygen, whereas restless, uncooperative patients received diazepam. All patients underwent chest radiography.

Findings.—There was a significant difference in cooling time between the groups: the mean cooling time in the dantrolene group was 49.7 minutes, whereas in controls it was 69.2 minutes. Treatment with dantrolene did not affect metabolic acidosis or the creatine phosphatase values, which were high on admission and continued to increase in both groups during the cooling period. The dantrolene group had significant diuresis, with a mean volume of excreted urine of 1.2 L. The mean volume of excreted urine in the controls was 570 mL. All patients survived and were discharged within 3 days with minor neurological symptoms. There was no difference in the incidence of neurological sequelae between the 2 groups.

Conclusions.—Although the use of dantrolene in conjunction with conventional cooling was significantly effective in hastening cooling in HS patients, the outcome was no different than in controls. Because the drug is expensive, further trials are warranted to justify its use in the setting of HS resulting from environmental heat injury.

▶ Heatstroke is important because it can maim and kill. It is also preventable. Furthermore, it is increasingly common in events where most clinicians would feel such an outcome was unlikely (i.e., short distance fun runs on days when the environmental conditions seem moderate). Therefore, anything that might reduce the morbidity and mortality needs to be pursued. This study of the use of dantrolene, a substance used to treat malignant hyperthermia and patients with the neuroleptic malignant syndrome was investigated in patients with heatstroke in a prospective, randomized trial and was not shown to be effective. Although there may have been a type 2 error because of small patient numbers in this study, it is nevertheless an opportunity to reinforce the crucial issue about heatstroke; that is, that recognition of the potential for heatstroke needs to be on the mind of every clinician involved in providing care for athletic events and, most importantly, the diagnosis and treatment begin on site and immediately. It is the delay from the time of onset of hyperthermia and the institution of rehydrating and cooling measures that is probably the single most important factor within the physician's reach that will make a difference in the outcome. In a way, it is heartening to know that if dantrolene is yet to be proven of value in the treatment of heatstroke the physician need not be distracted from the simple and well-trialed approaches of rehydration and cooling, which are still the treatments of first choice (1) and should commence without delay.—J.R. Sutton, M.D.

Reference

1. Sutton JR: Heat illness, in Strauss RH (ed): *Sports Medicine*. Philadelphia: WB Saunders Publ, 1991, pp 221–358.

Poikilothermia in Man: Pathophysiology and Clinical Implications
MacKenzie MA, Hermus ARMM, Wollersheim HCH, Pieters GFFM, Smals AGH, Binkhorst RA, Thien T, Kloppenborg PWC (University Hospital Nijmegen, Nijmegen, The Netherlands)
Medicine 70:257–268, 1991   4–7

Background.—Poikilothermia, defined as inability to maintain constant core temperature independent of ambient temperature, is thought to be the most common abnormality of heat regulation. It has definite effects on mental and physical function, and prolonged hypothermia may result in many complications. The thermoregulatory defenses against both cold and heat stress were studied in 4 patients with poikilothermia to determine which effector mechanisms are affected.

Methods.—The subjects were 4 women, aged 29–38 years, with acquired poikilothermia, and 9 age-, height-, and weight-matched controls. One patient had had a tumor near the corpus callosum, 1 had an unknown diagnosis with seizures and clouded consciousness, 1 had panhypopituitarism, and 1 had traumatic cerebral contusions with bilateral thalamic lesions. Each subject was studied in a thermoneutral chamber, followed by sudden exposure to cold and heat stress on 2 different days. Parameters measured included rectal and skin temperature at various sites, skin blood flow, local evaporation rate, total evaporative heat loss, changes in body weight, degree of shivering, and metabolic rate.

Results.—In the thermoneutral environment, the patients with poikilothermia had a significantly lower rectal temperature than controls—35.3° C vs. 37° C. Resting metabolic rate was also significantly lower. None of the patients had peripheral vasoconstriction or shivering. On exposure to cold stress, 3 of the patients had markedly reduced peripheral vasoconstriction and 2 had no metabolic response. Shivering was seen in the controls but not the patients. All patients had severely reduced heat-dissipation capacity on exposure to heat challenge, leading to progressive hyperthermia.

Conclusions.—Patients with poikilothermia have serious attenuations in their mechanisms of heat conservation and dissipation. These patients need careful monitoring of core temperature and sufficient measures to maintain normothermia. Patients with suspected lesions of the hypothalamic-pituitary region should be tested early for poikilothermia.

▶ I have included this paper in my selection for the YEAR BOOK because of its clear clinical interest and unusual nature. Basically, the authors describe 4 patients who have a variety of problems including seizure disorders, a tumor, panhypopituitarism, and traumatic cerebral contusion with bilateral thalamic lesions. All of them had impaired thermoregulation and tended to be influenced very much by the thermal environment. Although this is interesting in its own right, it is important to realize that there is another group of young women, those who are anorexic and bulimic, who similarly have impairment in their ability to regulate their thermal environment, and they too are at the mercy of the environment and therefore are likely to suffer problems from both heat and cold. I recommend this article in full to the clinician interested in thermoregulation.—J.R. Sutton, M.D.

Effect of Cold Air on the Bronchial Response to Inhaled Histamine in Patients With Asthma
Dosman JA, Hodgson WC, Cockcroft DW (University of Saskatchewan, Saskatoon, Saskatchewan)
Am Rev Respir Dis 144:45–50, 1991   4–8

Background.—In earlier work, it was demonstrated that the degree of bronchoconstriction induced by breathing cold air at rest in patients with asthma correlated with the degree of preexisting nonspecific bronchial hyperreactivity to inhaled histamine. This study determined whether airway response to inhaled histamine was altered when patients with asthma breathed cold air at rest.

Methods.—The concentration of inhaled histamine required to reduce the forced expiratory volume in 1 second (FEV_1) by 20% was measured in 7 patients with asthma immediately after the inhalation of warm air or cold air. Patients breathed either warm or cold air for 10 minutes before 30-second challenges with doubling concentrations of aerosolized histamine that were nebulized while the subject breathed warm air.

Results.—When histamine was inhaled after cold air breathing, the percentage decrease in FEV_1 was consistently greater than when histamine was inhaled after warm air breathing (Fig 4–3). The provocation concentration, which reduced the FEV_1 by 20% after cold air breathing, was lower than that after warm air breathing.

Conclusions.—Breathing cold air increased the bronchial reactivity to inhaled histamine in patients with asthma. Cold air appears to alter the bronchial response to inhaled histamine in patients with asthma. Patients

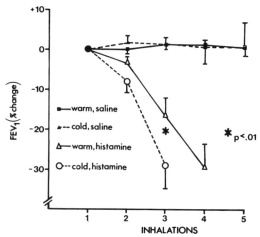

Fig 4–3.—Group mean data showing percentage change in FEV₁ after 30-second periods of nebulization with either saline or histamine under conditions of prior warm or cold air breathing. Percentage change in FEV_1 (*vertical axis*). Successive inhalations (*horizontal axis*). The first inhalation was always saline. The second inhalation was saline or the appropriate dose of histamine. The third inhalation was a doubling concentration of histamine for a given individual or saline according to a double-blind protocol. Within individual subjects, the dose of histamine at a given inhalation under both temperature conditions was virtually identical. During the third inhalation, the group mean percentage decrease in FEV_1 ($\pm$ 1 SEM) following histamine after cold challenge was significantly greater than after warm challenges. *Asterisk indicates P < .01. Filled squares* = warm saline; *filled triangles* = cold saline; *open triangles* = warm histamine; *open circles* = cold histamine. (Courtesy of Dosman JA, Hodgson WC, Cockcroft DW: *Am Rev Respir Dis* 144:45–50, 1991.)

with asthma respond to cold air like normal subjects except that they are more sensitive.

▶ Amariv and Pitt previously demonstrated that exposure to cold air increases the sensitivity of normal airways to histamine aerosols (1). The present report shows that the response in patients with asthma is similar to that of normal individuals. The mechanism for the increased response may be an increased affinity of the tracheal smooth muscle for histamine, or an increased sensitivity of the receptors to this stimulant. Another intriguing possibility is that the cold air may slow ciliary movement, thus slowing clearance of histamine from the receptors. Changes of mucosal permeability or altered vagal tone seem less likely, but it would also be interesting to test the involvement of the mast cells by experiments where cromolyn sodium was administered.—R.J. Shephard, M.D., Ph.D.

Reference

1. Amariv I, Plit M: *Am Rev Resp Dis* 140-1416, 1989.

Influence of Cold, Exercise, and Caffeine on Catecholamines and Metabolism in Men

Graham TE, Sathasivam P, MacNaughton KW (University of Guelph, Ontario)
J Appl Physiol 70:2052–2058, 1991   4–9

Background.—Recent research indicates that caffeine ingestion does not enhance thermal or fat metabolic responses to resting in cold air, despite increased plasma epinephrine and free fatty acids. Theophylline has been found to be effective during exercise but not at rest during cold stress. A study was done to test the hypothesis that caffeine ingestion before exercise in cold air would have a thermal-metabolic effect by raising fat metabolism and increasing oxygen consumption.

Methods.—Six young men who did not normally have caffeine in their diets were enrolled in 4 double-blind trials. They ingested placebo or caffeine, waited 30 minutes, then either exercised or rested for 2 hours in 5° C air.

Results.—Cold increased plasma norepinephrine. Both caffeine and exercise increased epinephrine. Serum free fatty acids and glycerol were also raised, but the difference between rest and exercise or placebo and caffeine was not significant. Caffeine did not affect either respiratory exchange ratio or oxygen consumption at rest or during exercise. The exercise trials, which did not significantly warm the body, resulted in higher plasma norepinephrine levels and lower mean skin temperatures for the first 30 minutes (Fig 4-4).

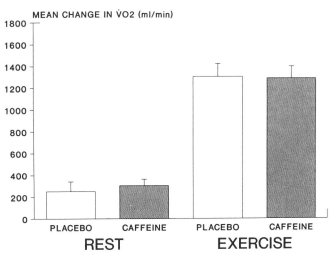

Fig 4–4.—Metabolic response during cold exposure: change in O_2 consumption ($\dot{V}o_2$) above resting level during 2 hour at 5°C. Values are means ± SE (Courtesy of Graham TE, Sathasivam P, MacNaughton KW: *J Appl Physiol* 70:2052–2058, 1991.)

Conclusions.—Skin temperature appears to stimulate plasma norepinephrine, whereas caffeine has little effect. Caffeine and exercise, however, stimulate plasma epinephrine, while cold has little effect. In this study, caffeine provided no thermal or metabolic advantage during a cold stress.

▶ Coffee is often drunk by those exercising in a cold environment with the thought that it may help in meeting the challenge of cold. Caffeine is thought to increase the output of catecholamines, and thus mobilizes fatty acids. The present experiments suffer a little from an inadequate number of subjects. Thus, caffeine gave a 250% increase of free fatty acids relative to placebo under resting conditions, but this was found to be statistically insignificant! Given the problem of small sample size and thus a lack of statistical power, the data are probably best interpreted qualitatively. They then show, in addition to the substantial mobilization of lipid by caffeine (greater in rest than in exercise), an increase of epinephrine (but not norepinephrine) under both resting and exercise conditions. This probably helps in meeting the challenge of a cold environment, because the body can metabolize either fat or glycogen during shivering.—R.J. Shephard, M.D., Ph.D.

Frusemide Antagonises Exercise-Induced But Not Histamine-Induced Bronchospasm

Feather IR, Olson LG (Southampton General Hospital, Southampton; University of Newcastle, Newcastle, England)
Aust NZ J Med 21:7–10, 1991   4–10

Introduction.—Recent research has shown that frusemide antagonizes exercise-induced bronchospasm, which has been attributed to blockade of chloride channels in the bronchial epithelium.

Methods.—To determine whether frusemide nonspecifically antagonizes bronchospasm, 10 volunteers, aged 22–35 years, were studied. Bronchial reactivity to inhaled histamine was tested after nebulizing frusemide, 30 mg, and the frusemide vehicle.

Results.—The geometric mean PD_{20} (the dose causing a 20% decrease of forced expiratory volume in 1 second) was .6 μmol after inhalation of the solution and .45 μmol after frusemide. The mean difference in PD_{20} between frusemide and vehicle was $-.50$ μmol, which was not significant (Fig 4–5).

Conclusion.—Nebulized frusemide does not antagonize histamine-induced bronchoconstriction despite its ability to block exercise-induced bronchoconstriction. The ability of frusemide to block exercise-induced bronchospasm may be specific to that stimulus.

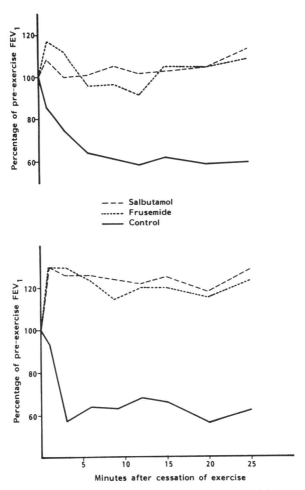

Fig 4–5.—The effect of frusemide on exercise-induced asthma. Each panel shows 3 exercise tests in a single person. (Courtesy of Feather IR, Olson LG: *Aust NZ J Med* 21:7-10, 1991.)

Altitude Diuresis: Endocrine and Renal Responses to Acute Hypoxia of Acclimatized and Non-Acclimatized Subjects

Koller EA, Bührer A, Felder L, Schopen M, Vallotton MB (University of Zurich, Switzerland, University Hospital, Geneva)
Eur J Appl Physiol 62:228–234, 1991   4–11

Background.—Recent reports suggest that altitude diuresis that occurs as a result of hypoxic stimulation of the arterial chemoreceptors decreases cardiac volume overload. Cardiovascular, renal, and endocrine responses to simulated altitude were compared in acclimatized and nonacclimatized subjects.

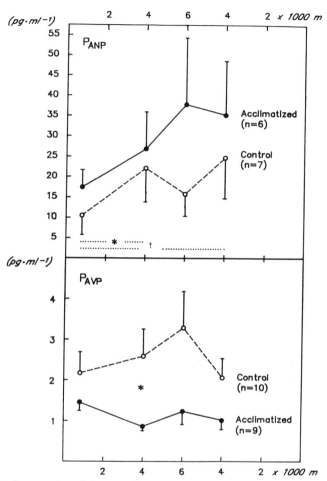

Fig 4–6.—Concentrations of plasma atrial natriuretic peptide (P_{ANP}) and arginine vasopressin (P_{AVP}) (means and standard error of means) of acclimatized and nonacclimatized subjects (controls) during stepwise, acute ascent to 6,000 m and descent to 4,000 m. Significance of altitude-induced changes in P_{ANP} refers to both groups. $^*P < .05$; $\dagger P < .01$. (Courtesy of Koller EA, Bührer A, Felder L, et al: *J Appl Physiol* 62:228–234, 1991.)

Methods.—The acclimatized subjects were male mountaineers with a mean age of 37.9 years who were exposed to acute hypoxic hypoxia for a mean of 24 days after descending from Himalayan altitudes of at least 4,000 m. Controls were healthy volunteers with a mean age 23 years. All subjects were subjected to stepwise acute exposure to simulated altitude, culminating in an altitude of 6,000 m. All testing was done with the subjects in a recumbent position.

Results.—In the acclimatized group, only moderate stimulation of the cardiovascular system was seen above 4,000 m, whereas controls showed significant changes above 2,000 m. In both groups the renal response was characterized by natriuresis and diuresis, as long as the altitude was well tolerated (Fig 4–6). Plasma level of arginine-vasopressin (AVP) decreased slightly in the acclimatized subjects, but it increased in controls, especially at above 4,000 m.

Conclusions.—The renal effects of altitude appear to be mediated by atrial natriuretic peptide release and slight suppression secretion of AVP. At altitude the increase in urine flow offsets the cardiac overload caused by hypoxic stimulation of arterial chemoreceptors. There is an association between enhanced secretion of AVP in nonacclimatized subjects and the subjective and objective signs of distress; this is because of insufficient chemoreflex effects and central hypoxia.

▶ In altitude folklore, one of the important predictors of altitude tolerance is whether there is a development of "hoendiurese." Those who failed to develop a diuresis on ascent of altitude were then thought to be more likely to suffer the ravages of altitude, particularly those of acute mountain sickness and high altitude pulmonary and cerebral edema. Although this has been in the folk literature for years, the link between fluid and water retention and the ventilatory response to altitude is of more recent origin. The use of ventilatory response to test hypoxia as a predictor of acute mountain sickness was first tested by King and Robinson (1), and in a later study (2) it was found that those persons doing well at altitude were initially those who on initial exposure had the lowest PCO_2. In this latter study, the authors found that those subjects with the worst cerebral symptoms also had the poorest pulmonary gas exchange. This led to the hypothesis that ventilatory response to hypoxia was a predictor of the susceptibility to acute mountain sickness and that both the cerebral and the pulmonary manifestations of altitude intolerance occurred more often together than separately, and that there was probably a common pathogenic mechanism linking them (3). A field study that looked at the simple indices of salt and water retention measured by weight changes and resting ventilation was performed by Hackett and colleagues (4) and showed a nice link between them. For a review of this topic, the reader is referred to the paper by Heyes and Sutton (5). The present paper adds some understanding to the mechanism linking the hypoxic stimulation of the arterial chemoreceptors, potential volume receptor stimulation, and the secretion of antidiuretic hormone (arginine vasopressin).—J.R. Sutton, M.D.

References

1. King AV, Robinson SM: *Aerospace Med* 43:419, 1972.
2. Sutton JR, et al: *Aviat Space Environ Med* 47:1032, 1976.
3. Sutton JR, Lassen N: *Bull Eur Physiopath Respir* 15:1045, 1979.
4. Hackett P, et al: *Respiration* 43:321, 1982.
5. Heyes MP, Sutton JR: *Semin Respir Med* 5:207, 1983.

Heimlich Maneuver for Near Drowning: Getting Water Out of Victims' Airways

Heimlich HJ (Heimlich Inst, Cincinnati)
Physician Sportsmed 19:105–112, 1991   4–12

Introduction.—The Heimlich maneuver has frequently been used to rid near-drowning victims' airways of water, saving their lives. Several examples of how the procedure is used were reviewed.

Expelling Water First.—If mouth-to-mouth respiration is tried before at least some water is expelled from the airway and lungs, air will not reach the alveoli. Substantial amounts of water can fill the air passages of near-drowning victims. In fresh or salt water drownings, death results from hypoxia as the water flooding the lungs blocks the trachea, bronchi, or alveoli.

Saving Wet-Drowning Victims.—Most drowning victims are victims of wet drownings, in which water flows down the trachea and floods the bronchi and lungs. Water can usually be expelled from the air passages by pressing inward and upward on the upper abdomen, which elevates the diaphragm and compresses the lungs. The Heimlich maneuver can be performed in positions other than from behind, which can be advantageous when trying to rescue a drowning victim. When the water is not too deep, the rescuer may stand in the water behind the victim, using the buoyancy of the water to lighten the victim. The rescuer repeats the inward and upward motion until water stops coming out of the victim's mouth. When a large, unconscious victim is brought out of the water, he or she should be placed in the supine position with his or her face turned sideways to let the water drain from the mouth. The rescuer faces the victim, kneeling astride one of both of the victim's thighs, and places one hand on top of the other with the heel of the bottom hand between the victim's navel and rib cage. The inward and upward motions create quick upward thrusts until water stops coming out of the victim's mouth. Infants and children can be saved by a gentler application of the Heimlich maneuver.

Conclusion.—Before mouth-to-mouth resuscitation became widely used, the Schafer method of artificial respiration, in which the rescuer performed Heimlich-like actions, was the recommended method for near-drowning victims. When mouth-to-mouth resuscitation became popular, the Schafer method was lost. Many rescuers have reported using the Heimlich maneuver successfully in near-drowning victims. In some reports, the Heimlich maneuver resulted in spontaneous breathing after cardiopulmonary resuscitation was unsuccessful.

► Cardiopulmonary resuscitation (CPR) has become an accepted emergency procedure for use with drowning victims. Performing the Heimlich maneuver before attempting CPR is not time-consuming and should assist with clearing water from the lungs. The more water that is removed from the lungs, the more effective CPR will be. The use of this maneuver is a definite adjunct to CPR for drowning victims and should be performed.—F.J. George, A.T.C., P.T.

Maximal Oxygen Uptake and Erythropoietic Responses After Training at Moderate Altitude

Klausen T, Mohr T, Ghisler U, Nielsen OJ (University Hospital of Fredriksberg, Denmark, County Hospital of Hillerød, Denmark; University Hospital of Gentofte, Denmark)
Eur J Appl Physiol 62:376–379, 1991   4–13

Background.—Altitude training to enhance maximal oxygen uptake is popular, but it is unknown whether altitude training itself or altitude-induced erythropoiesis improves maximal oxygen uptake at sea level. Erythropoietin concentrations and other indices of erythropoiesis in training were studied, including their influence on maximal oxygen uptake after altitude training.

Methods.—Subjects were 6 trained male cross-country skiers. After 3 weeks of training at 9 h/week^{-1}, the athletes train 4 h/day^{-1} for 7 days at 2,700 m above sea level. Accommodation was at 1,695 m. Before, during, and after altitude exposure, blood samples were taken for measurement of hemoglobin, erythropoietin concentration (EPO), and reticulocyte count. Comparisons before and after altitude exposure were also made of packed cell volume (PCV), transferrin-iron saturation, mean red cell volume (MCV), mean corpuscular hemoglobin concentration (MCHC), maximal oxygen uptake, maximal achieved ventilation, and heart rate.

Results.—The EPO increased from 36 mU/mL^{-1} to 47 mU/mL^{-1} at maximal altitude value. Hemoglobin increased from 8.8 mmol/L^{-1} prealtitude to 9.1 on day 2, 9.4 on day 7, and 9.2 on day 4, postaltitude. Significant increases in reticulocyte count were noted on day 3 at altitude and day 4, postaltitude. By the day 4, postaltitude, red blood cell counts had increased. Transferrin-iron saturation decreased on day 4 and increased on day 11, postaltitude; MCV, MCHC, PCV, maximal oxygen uptake, maximal achieved ventilation, and heart rate were not significantly affected.

Conclusions.—The erythropoietic response seen with altitude training appears insufficient to increase maximal oxygen uptake after altitude exposure. Changes in transferrin saturation could be signs of both altitude-induced erythropoiesis and training-induced iron deficiency. The potential benefits of erythropoiesis could be overshadowed by decreased training intensity at altitude in this study.

▶ In my opinion, this period of "altitude training"—only 1 week at moderate altitude, 2,700 m—is far too brief to be expected to improve maximal oxygen uptake, so it is no surprise to see the "negative" results here. The various changes shown in hematocrit and hemoglobin level probably resulted in large part from altitude-induced and/or exercise-induced changes in plasma volume. There was, of course, the expected increase in blood erythropoietin level, and the consequent reticulocytosis and fall in transferring saturation were markers of early acceleration of erythropoiesis in adaptation to the relative hypoxemia. For more on exercise, hypoxia, and erythropoietin, see Abstracts 4–19 and 4–20.—E.R. Eichner, M.D.

Enhanced Exercise-Induced Rise of Aldosterone and Vasopressin Preceding Mountain Sickness
Bärtsch P, Maggiorini M, Schobersberger W, Shaw S, Rascher W, Girard J, Weidmann P, Oelz O (Inselspital, Bern, Switzerland; Kinderspital, Basel, Switzerland; University Hospital, Zurich; Institute of Physiology, Innsbruck, Austria; Universitätskinderklinik, Essen, Germany)
J Appl Physiol 71:136–143, 1991   4–14

Background.—Acute mountain sickness (AMS) is associated with fluid retention, weight gain, proteinuria, and peripheral edema. Increased plasma aldosterone and antidiuretic hormone (ADH) levels at rest in persons with AMS have been reported. To investigate the hormonal responses and the possible contribution of exercise to the fluid retention of AMS, 17 mountaineers were subjected to an exercise test at low altitude and after rapid ascent to a high altitude.

Methods.—The mountaineers underwent a 30-minute exercise test on a bicycle ergometer at low altitude and after arrival at high altitude. The work load was comparable to the physical efforts associated with mountaineering.

Findings.—During a 3-day sojourn at high altitude, 8 men remained well and AMS developed in 9. The exercise-induced rise in plasma atrial natriuretic factor and changes of hematocrit, potassium, and osmolality in plasma were similar in both groups (Figs 4-7 and 4-8). At high altitude, O_2 saturation before and during exercise was lower, the exercise-induced increases in plasma aldosterone and plasma ADH were greater, and there was a fall in mean blood pressure in the AMS group. The greater rise of plasma norepinephrine and adrenocorticotropic hormone in the AMS group most likely accounted for the higher plasma aldosterone and ADH levels after exercise.

Conclusions.—The mountaineers with AMS had a hormonal constellation that favored greater water and salt retention than that of those who stayed well.

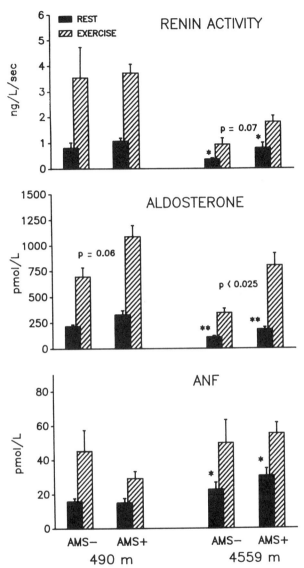

Fig 4–7.—Plasma levels of renin activity, aldosterone, and atrial natriuretic factor (ANF) before and during exercise at low and high altitude. The P values compare exercise-induced increases between groups. An *asterisk* indicates P < .01; a *double asterisk*, P < .005. (Courtesy of Bärtsch P, Maggiorini M, Schobersberger W, et al: *J Appl Physiol* 71:136–143, 1991.)

▶ This study shows that an exercise level corresponding to the efforts of mountaineering elicits a constellation of hormonal changes favoring enhanced renal sodium and water retention in subjects susceptible to acute mountain sickness (AMS). In other words, 30 minutes of exercise on a cycle ergometer at 4,559 m led to a greater increase of aldosterone and ADH

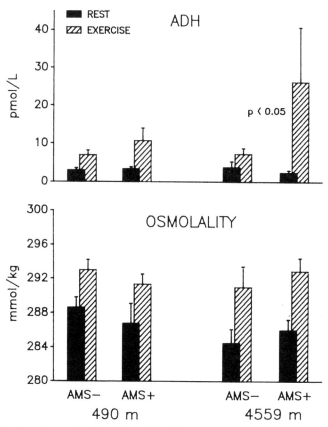

Fig 4–8.—Plasma levels of ADH and osmolality before and during exercise at low and high altitude. The P values compare exercise-induced increases between groups. $P < .05$ compared with corresponding values at low altitude. (Courtesy of Bärtsch P Maggiorini M, Schobersberger W, et al: *J Appl Physiol* 71:136–143, 1991.)

plasma levels in mountaineers who subsequently developed AMS than in those who stayed well during a sojourn of 3 days at this altitude. Stress hormone changes were also greater in those who developed AMS. Anecdotally, physical exercise is thought to facilitate the development AMS, and it seems likely that this exaggerated exercise-linked hormonal response contributes to the early fluid retention, increased capillary permeability, and subsequent edema formation that play key roles in the pathophysiology of AMS, including the cerebral edema and high-altitude pulmonary edema that go along with AMS. It is not yet clear whether these hormonal changes are a consequence or a cause of the decreased hypoxic ventilatory response that is considered to be a marker of susceptibility to AMS. In this regard, it has recently been shown that the prophylactic administration of nifedipine lowers pulmonary-artery pressure and helps prevent high-altitude pulmonary edema (1).—E.R. Eichner, M.D.

Reference

1. Bartsch P, et al: N Engl J Med 325:1284, 1991.

Acute Pulmonary Effects of Nitrogen Dioxide Exposure During Exercise in Competitive Athletes
Kim SU, Koenig JQ, Pierson WE, Hanley QS (Univ of Washington, Seattle)
Chest 99:815–819, 1991   4–15

Background.—Nitrogen dioxide (NO_2), a persistent combustion emission, is regulated by the EPA as a criteria pollutant. The pulmonary response of performance athletes after NO_2 exposure has apparently not been studied. Such data may provide valuable information on the short-term effects of NO_2 at ambient levels and may help establish a safe short-term ambient air quality standard for this pollutant.

Methods.—Nine competitive athletes were exposed to filtered air and .18 and .30 ppm NO_2 during heavy exercise in a dose-response study. The subjects were healthy intercollegiate male athletes, aged 18 to 23, who had been screened for history of cardiac disease, respiratory disease, allergic conditions, and extensive exposure to pollutants. Exposures to filtered air and NO_2 lasted for 30 minutes and were done on different days while the men exercised on a treadmill.

Results.—There were no significant changes in forced expiratory volume in 1 second in the athletes after exposure to either dose of NO_2. There were also no significant changes in total respiratory resistance, peak expiratory flow rate, or maximal expiratory flow at 50% volume of forced vital capacity (table).

Pulmonary Function Change for .30 ppm NO_2 Treatment

Subject	$\dot{V}E$ * (L/min)	ΔFEV (L)	ΔRT (cm H_2O/L/s)	$\Delta PEFR$ (L/min)	$\Delta \dot{V}max50\%$ (L/s)
1	71.9	0.26	0.07	−18	0.15
2	79.1	−0.02	−0.30	0	−0.22
3	76.0	−0.05	−0.27	20	−0.41
4	72.7	−0.05	−0.78	−43	−0.03
5	74.9	0.05	−0.07	−7	−0.78
6	58.5	−0.10	0.00	−8	−0.43
7	68.5	−0.03	0.16	−18	0.05
8	75.7	−0.02	1.10	−22	−0.05
9	71.5	0.00	−0.35	5	0.10
Mean ± SD	72.1 ± 6.0	0.00 ± 0.10	−0.05 ± 0.51	−10 ± 18	−0.18 ± 0.31

* During the final 3 minutes of running.
(Courtesy of Kim SU, Koenig JQ, Pierson WE, et al: *Chest* 99:815–819, 1991.)

Conclusions.—Short-term exposure to ambient NO$_2$ levels during heavy exercise did not adversely affect the pulmonary function of the athletes. Yet, pulmonary effects may occur in high-endurance athletes exposed to similar levels for a longer time during more vigorous exercise. Further research is needed to assess the threshold for pulmonary effects from ambient levels of NO$_2$.

▶ The athlete is at increased risk from a number of air pollutants, in part because of the location of exercise (for example, jogging at the side of a busy highway), and in part because the dose of the toxic compound is increased by mouth-breathing at a large respiratory minute volume. One pollutant commonly measured by air pollution laboratories is NO$_x$ a complex of nitrogen oxides derived largely from vehicle exhaust. It is quickly converted to ozone under the action of sunlight.

The initial effect of exposure to high concentrations of NO$_x$ is a diminution of pulmonary diffusing capacity (1). Under resting conditions, this response is seen at a concentration of .6 ppm. Effects on the airways of a resting subject are first detected at 1.5–2 ppm. It is thus a little surprising that the present authors used the less sensitive spirometric indices to look for a disturbance of function in those who were exercising. The subjects were also healthy, and there have been recent suggestions that in asthmatics, low concentrations of NO$_2$ can increase the sensitivity of the airways to SO$_2$ (2). Observations should be thus repeated, using measurements of pulmonary diffusing capacity to look for pulmonary responses, and the subjects should include not only healthy individuals, but also those with a history of asthma.—R.J. Shephard, M.D., Ph.D.

References

1. *Medical and Biological Effects of Environmental Pollutants.* National Academy of Sciences, 1977.
2. Folinsbee W, in Shephard RJ, Astrand PO (eds): *Endurance in Sport.* Oxford, Blackwell Scientific, 1992.

The Effects of Sequential Exposure to Acidic Fog and Ozone on Pulmonary Function in Exercising Subjects
Aris R, Christian D, Sheppard D, Balmes JR (Northern California Occupational Health Ctr; San Francisco Gen Hosp, Univ of California, San Francisco)
Am Rev Respir Dis 143:85–91, 1991   4–16

Introduction.—Morning fog is often acidified by nitric acid (HNO$_3$) in the coastal regions of southern California. Peak exposure to ozone (O$_3$) typically occurs after the fog has dissipated in the afternoon and evening.

Methods.—To determine whether fog containing HNO$_3$ may enhance pulmonary responses to O$_3$, 39 healthy, athletic volunteers, aged 21–39 years, were studied for lung function sensitivity to O$_3$. Selected O$_3$-sensi-

Methacholine Responsiveness of O_3-Sensitive
and Nonsensitive Persons

O_3-sensitive		O_3-nonsensitive	
Subjects	PC_{100}*	Subjects	PC_{100}*
1	4.00	11	41.50
2	2.57	12	17.70
3	2.00	13	32.00
4	0.84	14	33.90
5	1.04	15	27.86
6	4.00	16	3.25
7	8.52	17	2.83
8	1.63	18	16.00
9	0.52	19	3.61
10	4.38	20	8.00
Mean	2.95		18.67
SEM	0.80		4.54

* The concentration in milligrams per milliliter of methacholine required to produce a 100% increase in specific airway resistance above baseline.
(Courtesy of Aris R, Christian D, Sheppard D, et al: *Am Rev Respir Dis* 14:85-91, 1991.)

tive individuals exercised on 3 separate days in atmospheres containing HNO_3 fog, H_2O fog, or clean filtered air. After a 1-hour break, the exercise was continued for 3 hours in an atmosphere containing .20 ppm O_3.

Results.—Unexpectedly, the mean O_3-induced decrements in forced expiratory volume in 1 second (FEV_1) and forced vital capacity (FVC) were lower after exercise in the fog-containing conditions than in the clean filtered air condition. The mean O_3-induced decrements in FEV_1 were 26.4% after air, 17.1% after H_2O fog, and 18% after HNO_3 fog; in FVC, they were 19.9% after air, 13.6% after H_2O fog, and 13.6% after HNO_3 fog. As a group, these healthy O_3-sensitive individuals were significantly more responsive to methacholine than a group previously studied. The former group was also significantly more responsive to methacholine than healthy volunteers not sensitive to O_3 (table).

Conclusion.—Preexposure to fog lessens the effects of a subsequent O_3 exposure on pulmonary function. Nitric-acid–containing fog alone did not significantly change pulmonary function or symptoms. In addition, healthy persons with increased methacholine responsiveness may have increased O_3 sensitivity.

▶ I was perhaps a little less surprised by these findings than the authors appear to have been. It is well recognized that a second exposure to ozone induces a smaller response than the first, probably because the secretion of mucus invoked by the first exposure dilutes the irritant and offers some protection to the airway. In the same fashion, exposure to the ozone precursor may coat the airways with a film of mucus, particularly if the exposure occurs under humid conditions. As Aris and associates point out, the amount of water derived from the fog is in itself very small (probably less than 2 g), and coating of the airway by an enhanced secretion of mucus is a more reasonable explanation. As in Abstract 4–15, the NO_x/HNO_3 in itself produced no effect on static or dynamic lung volumes, despite the use of concentrations that exceeded ambient levels by one order of magnitude.—R.J. Shephard, M.D., Ph.D.

Circadian Rhythm in Anaerobic Power and Capacity
Hill DW, Smith JC (Univ of North Texas)
Can J Sport Sci 16:30–32, 1991   4–17

Background.—Characteristic circadian rhythms exist in many responses to exercise and performance measures, such as in cardiorespiratory, metabolic, and perceptual responses to submaximal exercise. The possibility of a circadian rhythm existing in anaerobic power and capacity has apparently not been explored.

Methods.—Anaerobic power and capacity in 9 college-aged men were measured at 3, 9, 15, and 21 hours. The men performed modified Wingate tests against a common resistance of 5.5 kg. Peak power was defined as the highest power output in a 5-second period during the test. Anaerobic capacity was defined as the total external work during the 30-second test.

Results.—Peak power tended to differ among testing times. The mean at 21 hours was about 8% higher than that at 3 hours. Anaerobic capacity also differed among times of day. The means at 15 and 21 hours were about 5% higher than at 3 and 9 hours (table).

Conclusions.—These findings suggest that there is a circadian rhythm in anaerobic capacity, as measured by work performed during a modified Wingate anaerobic test. There also appears to be a similar rhythm in peak anaerobic power. The amplitudes of the rhythms were 6% and 9%.

Anaerobic Power (W) and Capacity (kJ) at Different Times of Day		
	Peak power	Anaerobic capacity
03.00 h	788 ± 63	17.9 ± 1.0
09.00 h	788 ± 76	17.7 ± 1.1
15.00 h	842 ± 58	18.6 ± 1.0* †
21.00 h	863 ± 67*	18.8 ± 0.8* †

* vs 3.00 hours, $p < 0.05$
† vs 9.00 hours, $p < 0.05$
(Courtesy of Hill DW, Smith JC: *Can J Sport Sci* 16:30–32, 1991.)

Researchers must consider the effect of time of day on anaerobic power and capacity in studies involving repeated anaerobic tests.

▶ Given a circadian variation in performance, the timing of competition is very important to an athlete's success. Even if the hour that is chosen suits the local competitors, it may be quite unsuitable for those who have traveled from a different part of the world, and have not yet had the opportunity to adjust their circadian rhythms to the local situation. Several previous authors have noted a progressive improvement of brief athletic performances over the course of a normal waking day (1), but this is claimed to be the first attempt to make circadian laboratory measurements of anaerobic power and capacity, using the familiar Wingate test. In keeping with the earlier studies of athletic performance, the best scores were obtained in the afternoon and evening. Moreover, the differences were large enough to have a major impact on athletic performances. Other factors being equal, competitions should thus be organized in the early evening, and those traveling from other time zones should allow the necessary time (at least 1 day for each time zone over 3 hours) to realign their personal circadian rhythms to this schedule.—R.J. Shephard, M.D., Ph.D.

Reference

1. Shephard RJ: *Sports Med* 1:11, 1984.

Hematological Comparison of Iron Status in Trained Top-Level Soccer Players and Control Subjects

Resina A, Gatteschi L, Giamberardino MA, Imreh F, Rubenni MG, Vecchiet L (Chair of Sports Medicine, Florence, Italy; Institute of Medical Pathophysiology, Chieti, Italy)
Int J Sports Med 12:453–456, 1991   4–18

Background.—Recent studies have found that iron stores, evaluated by serum ferritin measurements, were lower in athletes. This condition has been associated with iron cost related to the load of exercise. Iron deficiency may compromise work capacity. However, its role in athletes who may have low iron scores but who are not yet anemic is controversial. Soccer is a running sport, but little is known about changes in iron status of soccer players. The iron status of 19 top-level soccer players was compared with that of 20 male controls.

Subjects.—The soccer players and controls had no impairment of physical performance and had a dietary intake adequate to cover the iron losses. Serum iron and serum total iron-binding capacity (TIBC) were measured in blood samples spectrophotometrically by the colorimetric method.

Findings.—There were no significant differences between the values of the 2 groups for serum iron, TIBC, % transferrin saturation, and serum ferritin. Seventeen of 19 soccer players had individual haptoglobin levels below the normal range and, as a group, the soccer players had serum haptoglobin levels significantly lower than the controls. This may indicate the existence of continuous hemolysis, even long after hard exercise. Increased intravascular hemolysis could lead to a shift of the red cells' catabolic pathway and cause a redistribution of iron stores among tissue compartments.

Conclusion.—Hematologic monitoring is necessary in athletes to detect subjects at risk of real iron deficiency. However, the results show no basis for routine pharmacologic iron treatment in soccer players. Iron supplementation should be used only when there is clinical evidence of reduced tissue iron supply.

▶ This cross-sectional comparison of 19 elite male soccer players with 20 male control subjects extends the concept of "exertional hemolysis," recently described in runners, swimmers, rowers, and aerobic dancers, to soccer players (1, 2). Surely, however, the degree of intravascular hemolysis here was trivial. Although the mean serum haptoglobin concentration was more than twice as high in controls as in soccer players, it was still within the normal range in soccer players, who also had a normal mean hemoglobin concentration and no reticulocytosis. The authors wisely point out that the soccer players, as a group, were not iron deficient and needed no supplemental iron. As they note, unwisely giving supplements of oral iron to iron-replete, male athletes can increase the risk of developing hemochromatosis and can interefere with the absorption of other vital metals, especially zinc.—E.R. Eichner, M.D.

References

1. 1989 YEAR BOOK OF SPORTS MEDICINE, pp 288–289.
2. 1990 YEAR BOOK OF SPORTS MEDICINE, pp 104–106.

Effects of Maximal and Submaximal Exercise Under Normoxic and Hypoxic Conditions on Serum Erythropoietin Level

Schmidt W, Eckardt KU, Hilgendorf A, Strauch S, Bauer C (Medizinische Hochschule Hannover, Germany; Universität Zürich, Switzerland)
Int J Sports Med 12:457–461, 1991   4–19

Purpose.—Exercise stimulates the erythropoietic system, but the mechanisms responsible for this stimulation have not been identified. The effects of exercise intensity and duration, and the combination of hypoxia and exercise on serum immunoreactive erythropoietin (EPO) levels were investigated.

Study Design.—Ten healthy, untrained, nonsmoking men with a mean age of 28.7 years were recruited for the study. First, the men performed maximal exercise under normoxic condition, followed by submaximal exercise under normoxia for 60 minutes at 60% of the maximal performance obtained in the first test. Thereafter, 9 men performed maximal exercise under normobaric hypoxia for which the inspiratory oxygen pressure was lowered by mixing nitrogen with air in a closed spirometer system. Five of the men were then exposed to hypoxia for 90 minutes under resting conditions, and 4 performed submaximal exercise under normobaric hypoxia for 60 minutes at 60% of the maximal performance obtained under hypoxia in the previous test. Blood samples were obtained at predetermined intervals during and after all 4 test regimens.

Results.—As expected, maximal performance and oxygen uptake markedly decreased under hypoxia. Heart rate increased under resting hypoxic conditions, but it was not different at the end of maximal and submaximal exercise under normoxia and hypoxia. Erythropoietin levels remained unchanged up to 5 hours after maximal and submaximal exercise under normoxia. Serum EPO levels were increased after 3 hours of resting under hypoxic conditions. Serum EPO levels were also increased at 3 hours after submaximal exercise under hypoxia, and they remained elevated for the next 48 hours. However, maximal exercise under hypoxia did not affect serum EPO levels. There was a slight negative correlation between serum EPO levels and hematocrit values, representing oxygen transport capacity. Reticulocyte counts were increased after all hypoxic experiments and after maximal exercise under normoxia, but reticulocyte counts showed no correlation to serum EPO levels.

Conclusions.—Exercise has no immediate effect on the serum EPO concentration. Other factors known to be elevated by exercise (e.g., human growth hormone, testosterone, or thyroxin) or their combined effects may be stimulating the erythropoietic system during exercise. The higher serum EPO levels observed 1–2 days after submaximal exercise under hypoxia could be the result of hemodilution.

▶ This study does not support that of Schwandt et al. (Abstract 4–20), in that the serum erythropoietin concentration here was not significantly increased by vigorous exercise. After the subjects cycled maximally or submaximally while breathing room air, there was no increase in serum erythropoietin concentration within 5 hours, and the delayed increase, at 24 or 48 hours, was not statistically significant. The results were mixed during the hypoxemia experiments, but the general trend was for the expected rise in serum erythropoietin concentration from the hypoxemia with little further modulation as a result of the exercise. The authors speculate that the metabolic acidosis from the exercise here may have blunted any tendency for the kidney to release erythropoietin. Then, too, this study was of relatively brief cycling, whereas that of Schwandt et al. was of prolonged running; conceivably such differences can contribute to different patterns of erythropoietin response. We need more research on exercise and erythropoietin. See also Abstract 4–13.—E.R. Eichner, M.D.

Influence of Prolonged Physical Exercise on the Erythropoietin Concentration in Blood

Schwandt H-J, Heyduck B, Gunga H-C, Röcker L (Institut für Leistungsmedizin; Physiologisches Institut der Freien Universität Berlin, Berlin)
Eur J Appl Physiol 63:463–466, 1991   4–20

Purpose.—Endurance-trained athletes are known to have enhanced blood volume and red blood cell (RBC) mass values compared with sedentary individuals. The regulation of RBC mass is believed to be under the control of erythropoietin (EPO), the main regulator of erythropoiesis. The effect of marathon running on plasma EPO levels at various time intervals after the run was examined.

Study Design.—Sixteen well-trained male marathon runners, aged 23–40 years, each ran 2 special test marathons on 2 separate days. Blood samples were collected 30 minutes before a run, within 1 minute after finishing the run, and 3 and 31 hours later.

Results.—Plasma EPO levels were slightly increased immediately after the run, but they were markedly increased 31 hours after the run. Reticulocyte counts did not change significantly during the observation period. Red blood cell, hemoglobin, and packed cell volume values were all significantly increased immediately after the run. At 3 hours after the run, there were no significant differences in RBC and packed cell volume values, but hemoglobin levels had significantly decreased. At 31 hours after the run, RBC, hemoglobin, and packed cell volume values were all significantly decreased. Plasma volumes had decreased by 7.4% immediately after the run, returned to control values 3 hours later, and had increased by 10% 31 hours later.

Conclusion.—The long-lasting increase in the EPO concentration after a marathon run is responsible for the increased RBC mass found in trained distance runners.

▶ Limited studies on the blood of elite endurance athletes, even those training at sea level, suggest they have a slight expansion of red blood cell mass and a moderate expansion of plasma volume, thus keeping their hematocrit low. In other words, compared with inactive persons, elite endurance athletes seem to have more blood, but thin blood. This study, and the one by Schmidt et al. (Abstract 4–19), explore the mechanism by which the red blood cell mass may expand in such athletes. In these 15 well-trained distance runners, the mean serum erythropoietin concentration was slightly, but not significantly, increased immediately after a marathon, and notably increased (41% over baseline) 31 hours later. The authors speculate that, during vigorous running, diversion of blood from internal organs to working muscle causes renal hypoxia, which then spurs the release of erythropoietin. In time, with repeated strenuous workouts, this mechanism could conceivably increase the red blood cell mass.—E.R. Eichner, M.D.

Impact of Smoking, Physical Training and Weight Reduction on FVII, PAI-1 and Hemostatic Markers in Sedentary Men

Gris J-C, Schved J-F, Feugeas O, Aguilar-Martinez P, Arnaud A, Sanchez N, Sarlat C (Centre Hospitalier Gaston Doumergue, Nimes, France)
Thromb Haemost 64:516–520, 1990   4–21

Background.—Little is known about the effect of reducing cardiovascular disease risk factors on hemostatic factors. The consequences of simultaneous physical training associated with smoking cessation on plasma proconvertin (FVII) and plasminogen activator inhibitor (PAI-1) levels were studied.

Methods.—Thirty sedentary men, including smokers and nonsmokers, were studied. Variations of FVII, PAI-1, thrombin-antithrombin III complexes, fibrinopeptide A, D-Dimers, and β-thromboglobulin plasma levels were assessed in a 6-month program of physical training and smoking cessation.

Results.—After 3 months, sustained physical training was associated with a reduction in FVII and PAI-1 levels. In the next 3-month period, mild exercise maintained normal FVII and PAI-1 activities. Participants who stopped training had increased FVII and PAI-1 plasma levels. Smoking habits did not affect FVII. Quitting smoking appeared to slightly potentiate the reduction of PAI-1 levels associated with mild exercise. Being overweight, FVII and PAI-1 levels were correlated. Weight reduction from training was related to the changes in the factors. Physical exercise among smokers was associated with a significant rise in hemostatic markers. This variation disappeared after 3 months of training in participants who quit smoking and reappeared in those who smoked again after the 6-month training.

Conclusions.—In young sedentary men, both smokers and nonsmokers, simultaneous regular physical training and smoking cessation for 3 months was associated with a drop in FVII-c and PAI-1 plasma levels. After the second 3-month training period, these decreased values were preserved in men who continued running once a week, even in those who resumed smoking.

▶ Plasma fibrinogen concentration is now thought to be a risk factor for cardiovascular disease (CVD), and regular exercise may help fend off heart attack and stroke not only by releasing tissue plasminogen activator and thus activating fibrinolysis, but also by reducing resting fibrinogen concentration (1). Some researchers have proposed that high plasma levels of coagulation factor VII and of plasminogen activator inhibitor (PAI) may also be CVD risk factors. This study shows that physical training, running 5 km every other day for 3 months, can lower plasma levels of factor VII and PAI in previously sedentary young men, and may thereby help prevent CVD. Loss of weight during the program was related to the decrements in factor VII and PAI. Smoking cessation seemed to potentiate the exercise-induced decline in plasma levels of PAI. This study also examined several plasma markers of activation of hemostasis. The physical training program apparently did not activate hemostasis, as gauged by these markers, except in smokers (see also Abstract 4–23). This study adds to our knowledge about the CVD risks imposed by the "hematology of inactivity (2)."—E.R. Eichner, M.D.

References

1. 1991 YEAR BOOK OF SPORTS MEDICINE, pp 90–91.
2. Eichner ER: *Rheum Dis Clin NA* 16:815, 1990.

Sickle Cell Trait in Ivory Coast Athletic Champions, 1956–1989
Le Gallais D, Préfaut C, Dulat C, Macabies J, Lonsdorfer J (Centre National de Médecine du Sport, Abidjan, Ivory Coast; Hôpital Aiguelongue, Montpellier, France; Institut National de la Santé Publique, Abidjan, Ivory Coast; Laboratoire de Physiologie et d'Explorations Fonctionnelles Abidjan, Ivory Coast)
Int J Sports Med 12:509–510, 1991   4–22

Introduction.—The percentage of sickle cell trait carriers (SCTC) among team sports players equals that found among the general black population. Although SCTC athletes have even participated in races and won some medals during Olympic games, the physical possibilities of SCTC athletes have not been studied. An epidemiologic study was conducted of Ivory Coast athletic champions from 1956 to 1989 to examine the exact physical possibilities of SCTC athletes.

Findings.—Of 129 Ivory Coast champions or record holders studied, 13 were found to be SCTC (10.1%). There were 9 male and 4 female SCTC. The percentage of SCTC among the general Ivory Coast population is 12%. The difference is statistically not significant. Thirty-three titles and national records (7%) were won by the 13 SCTC, of which 32 (12.5%) were won in races of 400 m or less and only 1 (.004%) was won in races of 800 m or more. The highest performing SCTC won 8 titles and national records, whereas 13 of the 116 non-SCTC won between 9 and 30 titles and records.

Conclusions.—Sickle cell trait carriers are able to compete in and win short-distance races, but they succeed less well than non-SCTC in long-distance events. Furthermore, SCTC athletes win considerably fewer events during their lifetime than do non-SCTC athletes.

▶ This survey of 129 Ivory Coast champion runners from 1956 through 1989 shows that the percentage of carriers of sickle cell trait (10%) among such athletes is not different from the percentage of sickle cell trait carriers (12%) among the general population. The authors then go on to suggest that runners with sickle cell trait are better able to win at shorter distances than longer. This part of their analysis, however, is suspect because they did not show that the sickle-trait runners participated in the longer races. In fact, no cogent evidence yet exists to prove that sickle cell trait limits exercise performance. As a recent example, when volunteers with sickle cell trait cycled to exhaustion at a simulated altitude of 2,300 m, cardiopulmonary and gas exchange responses were not different from those of control subjects (1). Then again, it has been shown that strenuous exercise at moderate (1,270 m) or high (4,000 m) altitude can induce sickling of some red blood cells in the effluent blood of exercising limbs, according to another study of volunteers with sickle cell trait (2). So, as recently reviewed (3), based on anecdotal reports, it seems plausible that rare persons and/or athletes with sickle cell trait who charge recklessly into all-out exercise, especially when new at altitude, are at some risk of sickling, fulminant rhabdomyolysis, lactic acidosis, shock, collapse, acute renal failure, and death.—E.R. Eichner, M.D.

References

1. Weisman IM, et al: *Am J Med* 84:1033, 1988.
2. Martin TW, et al: *Am J Med* 87:48, 1989.
3. Eichner ER: *Your Patient and Fitness* 5:15, 1991.

Effects of Exercise and Ethanol Ingestion on Platelet Thromboxane Release in Healthy Men

Numminen H, Hillbom M, Vapaatalo H, Seppälä E, Laustiola K, Benthin G, Muuronen A, Kaste M (University of Helsinki; University of Oulu, Finland; University of Tampere, Finland; Wihuri Research Institute, Helsinki; University of Stockholm)
Metabolism 40:695–701, 1991   4–23

Background.—Cardiovascular and cerebrovascular accidents may result from even occasional bouts of heavy drinking and from acute heavy physical exercise. To determine whether platelet activation could be precipitated by these factors, their combined effects on platelet aggregation and associated thromboxane release were studied.

Methods.—Ten healthy male volunteers, aged 20 to 24 and in good physical condition, were studied. The subjects performed graded 30-minute bicycle exercise 3 times in each of 2 sessions. In 1 session each subject drank ethanol, 1.5 g/kg mixed with fruit juice, before exercise, and in the other they drank fruit juice alone. Blood and urine samples for analysis were taken before and after exercise.

Results.—Adenosine diphosphate (ADP)-induced platelet aggregation and aggregation-associated thromboxane release decreased with morning exercise after fasting. These measures increased after the men drank fruit juice and performed a second bout of exercise at noon. When the men drank ethanol, however, the latter changes were negligible. When the men performed the third session of exercise in the evening, aggregation and associated thromboxane release again decreased during the control session but increased during the ethanol session. Urinary, 2,3-di-nor-6-keto-PGF$_{1\alpha}$excretion was increased by exercise.

Conclusions.—Platelet thromboxane release stimulated by ADP appears to be affected by both physical exercise and ingestion of ethanol with fruit juice. Neither factor seems to precipitate transient platelet hyperactivity. Thromboxane release is probably influenced by changes in plasma arachidonic acid concentration.

▶ Whether exercise activates platelets has been hotly debated in recent years, and this debate intensified when researchers correlated the morning peak in heart attacks with a morning increase in platelet aggregability (1). In the capricious land of platelet research, however, the results of clinical studies on exercise and platelet activation have been mixed. In fact, platelet aggregability after exercise has been reported to be increased, decreased, or unchanged. Here, in a study on the effects of exercise with or without ethanol ingestion, we have mixed results during the course of a single day. After the morning exercise bout, platelet aggregability decreased. After the afternoon exercise bout, aggregability increased in the control session but changed little in the ethanol session. And after the evening exercise bout, aggregability decreased in the control session but increased in the ethanol session. The researchers, no doubt exasperated by these results, concluded that they could not observe any significant platelet activation after exercise irrespective of whether the subjects were intoxicated by ethanol or not. Back to the drawing board.—E.R. Eichner, M.D.

Reference

1. Tofler GH, et al: N Engl J Med 316:1514, 1987.

Response of Red Cell and Plasma Volume to Prolonged Training in Humans

Green HJ, Sutton JR, Coates G, Ali M, Jones S (University of Waterloo, Waterloo, Ontario; McMaster University, Hamilton, Ontario; St. Joseph's Hosp, Hamilton; Cumberland College of Health Sciences, Lidcombe, New South Wales, Australia)
J Appl Physiol 70:1810–1815, 1991   4–24

Background.—The lower hematocrits (Hct) found in endurance-trained athletes may occur because of disproportional increases in plasma volume (PV) relative to red blood cell (RBC) mass (RCM), a condition called sports or athletic pseudoanemia. The lower hematocrit may also be caused by an actual reduction in RCM, a true anemia called athletic or sports anemia. A study was done to characterize the time-dependent alterations in vascular volumes, PV, and RCM in response to a protracted period of heavy training.

TABLE 1.—Training-Induced Changes in TBV, PV, and RCM

	Week		
	0	*4*	*8*
TBV	5,315±139	5,879±246*	
PV	3,068±104	3,490±126*	3,362±113*
RCM	2,247±66	2,309±128	

Note: Values are mean ± SE in mL.
*Significantly different from week 0 (P < .05).
(Courtesy of Green HJ, Sutton JR, Coates G, et al: *J Appl Physiol* 70:1810–1815, 1991.)

Methods.—Seven healthy active but untrained males finished an 8-week cycle-training program. Training was performed on a 3-1-3 cycle for approximately 8 weeks in 2-hour sessions. Intensity was initially set at 62% of maximal oxygen uptake ($\dot{V}O_{2max}$).

Findings.—Over 8 weeks, $\dot{V}O_{2max}$ increased by 17.2%. Plasma volume and PV plus RCM, or total blood volume (TBV), increased through week 4 and then stabilized. During the initial 4 weeks, RCM did not change, and no change was apparent during the final 4 weeks of training when RCM was estimated from PV and hematocrit (Table 1). During the first 4 weeks, reductions were noted in Hct, hemoglobin (Hb), and RBC count, and increases were noted in mean cell volume (MCV) and mean cell Hb. From weeks 4 to 8, no further changes were noted in Hb, RBC count, and MCV, and both mean cell Hb and Hct returned to pretraining levels (Table 2). Serum ferritin was reduced during the training (Table 3).

TABLE 2.—Training-Induced Changes in Selected Hematologic Indices

	Week		
	0	*4*	*8*
Hct, %	0.438±0.01	0.418±0.01*	0.429±0.01†
Hb, g/dl	15.0±0.30	14.4±0.28*	14.4±0.32*
RBC, 10^9/l	4.90±0.10	4.59±0.08*	4.70±0.11*
MCV, fl	89.6±0.83	91.0±0.76*	91.2±0.83*
MCH, pg	30.7±0.34	31.4±0.35*	30.7±0.34†
MCHC, g/100 ml	34.3±0.18	34.5±0.15	33.7±0.14*†
RDW	12.3±0.14	12.6±0.16	12.3±0.13
Reticulocytes, %	1.16±0.21	1.71±0.27	1.26±0.31

Note: Values are mean ± SE. *Abbreviations:* MCH, mean corpuscular Hb; MCHC, mean corpuscular Hb concentration; RDW, RBC window width.
*Significantly different from week 0 (P < .05).
†Significantly different from week 4 (P < .05).
(Courtesy of Green HJ, Sutton JR, Coates G, et al: *J Appl Physiol* 70:1810–1815, 1991.)

TABLE 3.—Training-Induced Changes in Serum Ferritin, Serum
Bilirubin, and RBC Creatine Concentrations

	Week		
	0	4	8
Ferritin, $\mu g/l$	78.6±1.3	40.5±7.2*	33.8±6.7*
Bilirubin, $\mu mol/l$	7.5±2.0	12.8±5.1	10.0±2.9
Creatine, mmol/l RBC	0.41±0.02	0.41±0.03	0.42±0.04

Note: Values are mean ± SE.
*Significantly different from week 0 ($P < .05$).
(Courtesy of Green HJ, Sutton JR, Coates G, et al: J Appl Physiol 70:1810–1815, 1991.)

Conclusions.—The initial response to training in 7 untrained males was a hypervolemia resulting in a pseudoanemia that persisted with continued training. The increase in mean cell volume over the first 4 weeks was sustained during the last 4 weeks and may reflect preferential loss of older RBCs and replacement with younger erythrocytes.

▶ This is a mechanistic study of the serial development of "athlete's anemia" in 7 untrained men who undertook a program of vigorous aerobic cycling. It confirms earlier research in showing that the fall in hemoglobin concentration in athletes is mainly "dilutional." The plasma volume, measured directly, was increased by 14% at the 4-week point but not further by 8 weeks. The red blood cell mass, gauged directly at 4 weeks and indirectly at 8 weeks, did not change; conceivably, with longer and harder training, it may have increased. Two other interesting findings were the increase in red blood cell mean corpuscular volume, presumably because of exertional hemolysis, as in "runner's macrocytosis" (1); and the decrease in serum ferritin, presumably because of dilution as well as because of incorporation of iron into newly formed myoglobin and newly formed reticulocytes to replace the older red cells destroyed by exertional hemolysis.—E.R. Eichner, M.D.

Reference

1. Eichner ER: Am J Med 78:321, 1985.

Development of Runner's Anemia During a 20-Day Road Race: Effect of Iron Supplements
Dressendorfer RH, Keen CL, Wade CE, Claybaugh JR, Timmis GC (William Beaumont Hosp, Royal Oak, Mich; Univ of California, Davis; Letterman Army Inst of Research, Presidio of San Francisco; Tripler Army Med Ctr, Tripler, Hawaii)
Int J Sports Med 12:332–336, 1991   4–25

Background.—Intense training for long-distance running is associated with decreased hemoglobin (Hb) levels and low iron stores. The value of iron supplementation to prevent "runner's anemia" is still debated. The relationship between iron status and the early stage of decreased Hb levels in male runners was assessed.

Methods.—Fifteen healthy men, aged 25 to 47, ran twice their regular training distance in 20 days during a 500-km race. Nine men took iron-containing tablets providing an average of 36 mg of iron daily. The remaining 6 took no supplements. Hematologic variables were examined.

Results.—Only 1 runner had a low Hb level before the race. After 10 days and 285 km, 12 of the men had low Hb levels. Six of them were taking iron supplements. After a 2-day rest period there were 5, and after 5 more days of running, there were 7 with low Hb levels. Serum iron, ferritin, total iron-binding capacity, and percent transferrin saturation remained normal and showed no significant changes. Reticulocyte counts rose progressively to 8 times baseline values, regardless of whether iron supplements were taken.

Conclusions.—Runner's anemia developed in 73% of the runners independently of their iron status and intake. Reductions in Hb were accompanied by parallel drops in red blood cell count and hematocrit and a significant reticulocytosis. The drop in Hb levels in these runners was acute, partially reversible with rest, and not preventable by iron supplementation. It was probably therefore a result of functional hemodilution.

▶ This clinical research conducted with 15 runners of the 20-day, 500-km Great Hawaiian Road Race documents a fall in mean hemoglobin concentration, almost surely "dilutional pseudoanemia" (see also Abstracts 4–27 and 4–24), as well as mild exertional ("footstrike") hemolysis and reticulocytosis, in response, presumably, to both the mild intravascular hemolysis and the 80-mL phlebotomy over the course of the race. One would not expect, in iron-replete runners such as these, an iron supplement taken for 2–3 weeks to make any difference whatsoever. Sure enough, it didn't.—E.R. Eichner, M.D.

Haemolytic Effects of Exercise
Weight LM, Byrne MJ, Jacobs P (University of Cape Town, South Africa; Groote Schuur Hospital, Cape Town)
Clin Sci 81:147–152, 1991   4–26

Background.—Several studies have suggested that impact exercise results in an accelerated erythrocyte breakdown that may lead to a negative iron balance in trained runners. There is also evidence of iron deficiency, anemia, and intravascular hemolysis in athletes in nonimpact sports, suggesting that mechanisms other than footstrike are responsible for this phenomenon. Erythrocyte survival rates were determined in male and

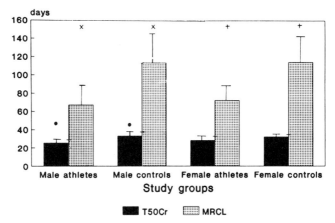

Fig 4–9.—T_{50}Cr (*solid boxes*) and MRCL (*stippled boxes*) in male and female athletes and sedentary controls. Values are mean + SD. Statistical significance: *dagger*, P < .01, male athletes vs. controls; *asterisk*, P < .01, female athletes vs. controls. (Courtesy of Weight LM, Byrne MJ, Jacobs P: *Clin Sci* 81:147–152, 1991.)

female distance runners by using radiolabeling techniques. Hematologic parameters were measured before and after marathon running to document erythrocyte destruction.

Methods.—Erythrocyte survival studies with ^{51}Cr were performed on 10 male and 10 female endurance-trained athletes. A control group was comprised of 5 men and 5 women who did not perform any regular exercise.

Findings.—The chromium half-disappearance time (T_{50}Cr) of the male but not the female athletes was significantly lower than that of the con-

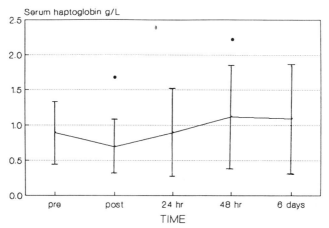

Fig 4–10.—Sequential changes in serum haptoglobin levels (mean ± SD) before and after prolonged strenuous exercise. Statistical significance: *dagger*, P < .05; *asterisk*, P < .01 compared with values before race. (Courtesy of Weight LM, Byrne MJ, Jacobs P: *Clin Sci* 81:147–152, 1991.)

trols. The mean erythrocyte lifespan (MRCL) of the male and female athletes was significantly shorter than that of the controls (Fig 4-9). The mean erythrocyte lifespan was not correlated with hemoglobin concentration, serum ferritin level, body mass, weekly training distance, number of years running, or daily protein intake. Mean cell volumes and reticulocyte counts were in the normal range both before and after completing a marathon race. After the race, plasma hemoglobin levels were elevated and serum haptoglobin levels were decreased (Fig 4-10).

Conclusions.—Significantly elevated plasma hemoglobin levels were found in runners at rest and after strenuous exercise, but there was no further increase after marathon running. The increase in erythrocyte turnover in athletes may precipitate an iron deficiency when dietary intake or absorption does not meet the accelerated erythropoietic demands.

▶ This cross-sectional comparison of distance runners with nonexercising controls tends to support the concept of "exertional hemolysis" by showing that chromium-labeled red blood cells disappear from the circulation faster in runners, both men and women, than they do in control subjects; as well as by showing that the serum haptoglobin concentration, a gauge of intravascular hemolysis, is reduced by running a marathon (see also Abstracts 4–24, 4–25, and 4–27). The conclusion, however, is too strong. The exertional hemolysis seen in endurance athletes is generally so mild that it causes no iron to leave the body. Rather, the iron released from hemolyzed red blood cells is recycled, and almost certainly reused promptly to make new red cells. Consequently, with very rare exceptions perhaps, exertional hemolysis is not likely to contribute to iron deficiency in athletes.—E.R. Eichner, M.D.

Athletes' Pseudoanaemia

Weight LM, Darge BL, Jacobs P (University of Cape Town; Groote Schuur Hospital, Cape Town, South Africa)
Eur J Appl Physiol 62:358–362, 1991   4–27

Background.—In endurance exercise, overall expansion of circulating blood volume occurs, but hemoglobin concentration and packed cell volume do not increase. As a result, endurance-trained athletes usually have a low-normal hemoglobin concentration. Standard radiolabeling techniques were used to further characterize this so-called sports anemia.

Methods.—The subjects were 24 distance runners who had been training for at least 2 years and ran between 50 and 120 km/week^{-1}. Half were men, mean age 34.3 years, and half were women, mean age 32.8 years. A comparison group of 5 men and 5 women who did not exercise regularly was also studied. Plasma volume, red cell volume, and total blood volume were measured with ^{125}I-labeled human serum albumin and ^{51}Cr-labeled erythrocytes.

The Plasma Volume, Red Cell Volume, and Total Blood Volume in Male and Female Distance Runners and Sedentary Controls

	Athletes				Controls			
	male (n = 12)		female (n = 12)		male (n = 5)		female (n = 5)	
	mean	SD	mean	SD	mean	SD	mean	SD
Haemoglobin (g·l⁻¹)	141.1	11.8	127.5	18.0	146.3	3.7	121.5	9.7
Packed cell volume	0.42	0.0	0.38	0.0	0.44	0.0	0.37	0.0
Plasma volume (ml·kg⁻¹)	52.8**	7.5	51.5	6.2	38.4**	7.6	43.6++	1.8
Red cell volume (g·kg⁻¹)	32.6**○○	3.6	25.9++○○	3.5	24.2**××	5.0	22.8+++××	2.5
Total blood volume (ml·kg⁻¹)	86.0**	10.1	77.7++	7.6	63.2**	12.3	67.2++	2.7

** $P < .01$ male athletes vs. male controls.
++ $P < .01$ female athletes vs. female controls.
∞ $P < .01$ male vs. female athletes.
×× $P < .01$ male vs. female controls.
(Courtesy of Weight LM, Darge BL, Jacobs P: *Eur J Appl Physiol* 62:358–362, 1991.)

Results.—In male athletes, the mean plasma volume was 37.5% higher than in controls; in females, mean plasma volume was 18.1% higher in athletes than in controls, which was a novel observation. Red cell volume was 34.7% higher in male athletes than in controls, but no such difference was seen between female athletes and controls (table). This finding may have resulted from an iron-limiting erythropoiesis; the red cell volume of the female athletes defined as clinically anemia was substantially lower than in the women without anemia. The expanded plasma volume of the female athletes resulted in part from the elevated plasma protein mass and concentration.

Conclusions.—Athlete's pseudoanemia, or decreased blood hemoglobin levels occurring in endurance-trained athletes, appears to be mainly a dilutional effect. Distance runners of both sexes have a disproportionately expanded plasma volume, but only the men have a concomitant increase in red cell volume. Plasma albumin concentrations are only slightly increased, whereas total globulin fraction is significantly increased.

▶ This cross-sectional comparison of 24 well-trained distance runners and 10 nonexercising controls supports earlier research suggesting that endurance athletes tend to have increases in both plasma volume and red blood cell mass (see also Abstract 4–20). Cross-sectional comparisons, of course, are strongly influenced by choice of subjects, but in this study the differences in both plasma volume and red cell mass were impressive. Among the men, the runners had a 38% greater mean plasma volume and a 35% greater mean red cell mass than did the controls. Among the women, the respective figures were 18% and 14%. The authors make less of the 14% expansion of red cell mass among the women runners, apparently assuming it would have been greater if the athletes had been more replete in iron. But it was statistically significant, so suffice it to say that male and female endurance athletes tend to have gains in both red cell mass and plasma volume, with the plasma volume "outgaining" the red cell mass, thus keeping the hematocrit on the low side. In short, the elite endurance athlete has more blood, but thin blood—blood that flows easily to working muscles. For an expert review on blood volume and its adaptation to endurance training, see Convertino's article (1).—E.R. Eichner, M.D.

Reference

1. Convertino VA, et al: *Med Sci Sports Exerc* 23:1338, 1991.

Biophasic Changes in Leukocytes Induced by Strenuous Exercise
Hansen JB, Wilsgard L, Osterud B (University of Tromso, Tromso, Norway)
Eur J Appl Physiol 62:157–161, 1991   4–28

Introduction.—Physical exercise for less than 1 hour at near-maximum intensity leads to immediate changes including evident lymphocytosis and an increase in the number of neutrophils. Delayed leukocytosis induced by exercise has also been reported. The dynamics of the delayed leukocytosis and how the duration of exercise influences the magnitude of leukocytosis was studied.

Methods.—Seven healthy male volunteers participated in short-, middle- and long-term runs at close to their maximum speed. Blood samples were taken before and immediately after exercise and at intervals over the next 10 hours.

Findings.—After exercise, there was a prompt mobilization of white cells, and lymphocytes in particular. The initial increase in lymphocytes was succeeded by a significant decrease to a level 32%–39% lower than preexercise levels (Fig 4–11). Plasma cortisol concentration peaked 30 minutes after exercise and declined below the control level in 4 hours. The initial increase in plasma cortisol concentration was closely correlated with subsequent lymphopenia. There appeared to be no correlation between the modest increase in the number of granulocytes after exercise and the comprehensive increase in polymorphonuclear (PMN) elastase concentration (Fig 4–12). A delayed granulocytosis of varying magnitude in all subjects reached a peak between 2 and 4 hours after exercise. The neutrophilic granulocytosis was not accompanied by a corresponding enhancement in PMN elastase concentration.

Conclusions.—In this study, neither the initial increase of plasma cortisol nor the subsequent decrease to a level lower than preexercise levels

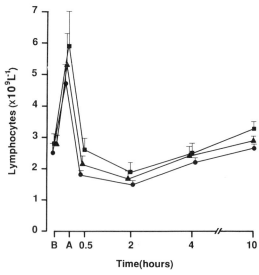

Fig 4–11.—The influence of strenuous physical exercise of short (*squares*), middle (*triangles*), and long (*circles*) duration on the number of circulating lymphocytes. Values are means and SEM. (Courtesy of Hansen JB, Wilsgård L, Osterud B: *Eur J Appl Physiol* 62:157–161, 1991.)

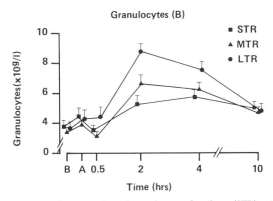

Fig 4–12.—Changes in circulating number of granulocytes after short- (*STR*), middle- (*MTR*), and long-term (*LTR*) runs close to maximal capacity. Values are means and SEM. *B* indicates measurement before exercise; A, after exercise. (Courtesy of Hansen JB, Wilsgård L, Osterud B: *Eur J Appl Physiol* 62:157–161, 1991.)

were essential for the magnitude of delayed leukocytosis. The magnitude of the leukocytosis was related to the duration of exercise.

Acute Phase Response in Exercise. II. Associations Between Vitamin E, Cytokines, and Muscle Proteolysis
Cannon JG, Meydani SN, Fielding RA, Fiatarone MA, Meydani M, Farhangmehr M, Orencole SF, Blumberg JB, Evans WJ (Tufts Univ, Boston)
Am J Physiol 29:R1235–R1240, 1991   4–29

Introduction.—Long-duration or damaging exercise may initiate reactions that resemble the host "acute phase response" to infection. Elements of the acute phase response have a common set of mediators, cytokines including interleukin 1β (IL-1β), tumor necrosis factor-α (TNF-α), and interleukin 6 (IL-6). The influence of damaging eccentric exercise on production and plasma concentrations of cytokines and their relationship to muscle protein breakdown was assessed.

Methods.—In a double-blind, placebo-controlled protocol, 10 male subjects were treated with vitamin E supplement and 11 males were treated with placebo for 48 days. Vitamin E or placebo supplementation was followed by an eccentric exercise session consisting of 3 15-minute periods of downhill running on a treadmill. Blood and urine samples were collected before, immediately after, and at intervals after exercise.

Findings.—Twenty-four hours after eccentric exercise, endotoxin-induced secretion of IL-1β in cells from the placebo subjects were augmented 154%, but there were no exercise-related changes in cells from the vitamin-E supplemented subjects. Secretion of TNF-α was increased in the placebo subjects, and the response was not inhibited in the vitamin-E supplemented subjects. In the placebo subjects, IL-6 secretion did

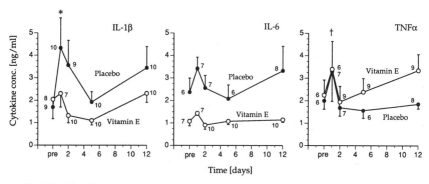

Fig 4–13.—Cytokine secretion by mononuclear cells isolated from morning blood samples. Cells were stimulated in vitro with 1 ng/mL lipopolysaccharide. Numbers next to each data point indicate sample size. *Significant increase ($P < .05$) over preexercise (placebo group only). †Significant increase ($P < .05$) over preexercise (both groups combined). (Courtesy of Cannon JG, Meydani SN, Fielding RA, et al: Am J Physiol 29:R1235–R1240, 1991.)

not change after exercise, but in the vitamin-E supplemented group, IL-6 secretion was significantly reduced throughout the 12-day observation period (Fig 4–13). Urinary 3-methylhistidine excretion correlated with mononuclear secretion of both IL-1β and prostaglandin E_2.

Conclusions.—An earlier study found a significant relationship between neutrophil function and muscle membrane permeability. Along with the present data, there is evidence that exercise initiates an acute phase response that may contribute to metabolic alterations after exercise. Dietary vitamin E significantly reduced IL-1β and IL-6 production.

▶ This study, part of ongoing research into the "acute phase response" to exercise, explored the influence of damaging, eccentric exercise on cytokine production and muscle proteolysis, and also gauged the influence of vitamin E supplementation. The exercise increased secretion of IL-1β and of TNF-α. Muscle proteolysis, as measured by urinary excretion of 3-methylhistidine, correlated with secretion of IL-1β, suggesting that cytokines triggered by exercise help regulate muscle proteolysis. The effects of supplementation with vitamin E were mixed and modest. That is, vitamin E affected secretion differently for each cytokine: interleukin-6 secretion was decreased overall; IL-1β secretion was reduced only after exercise, not at baseline; and secretion of TNF was not affected at all. We will be seeing more on the use of vitamin E and other "antioxidants" in attempts to reduce exercise-induced muscle damage in man.—E.R. Eichner, M.D.

The Effects of Moderate Exercise Training on Immune Response

Nehlsen-Cannarella SL, Nieman DC, Balk-Lamberton AJ, Markoff PA, Chritton DBW, Gusewitch G, Lee JW (Loma Linda Univ, Calif)
Med Sci Sports Exerc 23:64–70, 1991   4–30

Background.—Immunology of exercise is a research area of great interest, but there have been few prospective studies in humans. A randomized, controlled study was conducted to evaluate the relationship between moderate exercise and changes in immune system variables.

Serum Immunoglobulin Levels at Baseline, 6 Weeks, and 15 Weeks

Variable (g · l⁻¹)	Exercise Group			Nonexercise Group			Effect, Group × Time
	Base	6 wk	15 wk	Base	6 wk	15 wk	
IgG	9.59 (0.54)	11.84 (0.59)†	11.71 (0.56)†	11.21 (0.63)	11.70 (0.47)	11.30 (0.62)	0.008
IgA	1.62 (0.21)	2.04 (0.23)†	2.05 (0.23)†	1.87 (0.17)	2.08 (0.17)†	2.00 (0.15)†	0.001
IgM	1.43 (0.11)	1.71 (0.13)†	1.72 (0.13)†	1.69 (0.14)	1.83 (0.13)†	1.70 (0.14)	0.004

* Values are means, with SE in parentheses.

† $P < .05$ within research subjects' 6-week or 15-week values vs. baseline.

(Courtesy of Nehlsen-Cannarella SL, Nieman DC, Balk-Lamberton AJ, et al: *Med Sci Sports Exerc* 23:64–70, 1991.)

Methods.—The subjects were 36 sedentary, mildly obese, premeno-pausal women, who were randomized into exercise and nonexercise groups. The study was conducted during 15 weeks from January to May. The women in the exercise group performed moderate exercise in five 45-minute sessions per week, consisting of brisk walking and 60% of heart rate reserve. Subjects underwent body composition and treadmill testing and blood analysis at baseline, 6 weeks, and 15 weeks. Data were analyzed by repeated measures analysis of variance.

Results.—The 2 groups had a significantly different pattern of change in number of peripheral blood lymphocytes, T cells, B cells, and serum IgG, IgA, and IgM. No such differences were seen in spontaneous blas-togenesis or number of T helper/inducer or T cytotoxic/suppressor cells. After 6 weeks, women in the exercise group had significant de-creases in percentage and number of total lymphocytes and in number of T cells. At both 6 and 15 weeks, significant increases in all of the serum immunoglobulins were seen (table). In the nonexercising women, B cell number increased significantly at both 6 and 15 weeks, whereas no significant changes were seen in the exercising women.

Conclusions.—Moderate exercise training appears to be associated with a 20% increase in serum immunoglobulins and small changes in cir-culating numbers of immune system variables. These changes include significant decreases in circulating lymphocytes, especially T cells, and are apparent at 6 weeks, with some attenuation by 15 weeks. There is no improvement in lymphocyte function.

▶ The interaction of physical activity, immunity, and infection is a hot topic, and this is another report from researchers active in this field. In this study, 15 weeks of moderate exercise (i.e., regular, brisk walking) were associated with a mild decrease in the percentage and number of blood lymphocytes, especially T cells, and with a mild increase in levels of serum immunoglobu-lins. These changes were evident within 6 weeks, with some attenuation by 15 weeks. Why the lymphocyte count fell in the exercisers is not clear; total leukocyte count did not fall, and plasma volume was said not to change. Maybe the "lymphocytopenia" resulted from exercise-evoked changes in blood cortisol levels. The net 20% increase in serum levels of immunoglobu-lins in the exercisers is of dubious clinical import. Serum levels of immuno-globulin A and immunoglobulin M rose also in the nonexercisers, and group differences were not statistically significant at either 6 or 15 weeks. These researchers have also reported on infection rates before and after a mara-thon and on the effects of exercise training on natural killer cells and risk of upper respiratory tract infections (1). For a scholarly, insightful review on physical activity and the immune system, see reference 2.—E.R. Eichner, M.D.

References

1. 1991 YEAR BOOK OF SPORTS MEDICINE, pp 131–137.

2. Shephard RJ, et al: *Can J Sport Sci* 16:163, 1991.

Effect of Physical Exercise on In Vitro Production of Interleukin 1, Interleukin 6, Tumor Necrosis Factor-α, Interleukin 2 and Interferon-γ
Haahr PM, Pedersen BK, Fomsgaard A, Tvede N, Diamant M, Klarlund K, Halkjær-Kristensen J, Bendtzen K (Rigshospitalet, Copenhagen)
Int J Sports Med 12:223–227, 1991   4–31

Introduction.—Reported immunological changes during and after exercise range from a state of physical well-being with less susceptibility to infection to a stress stimulus that suppresses immunity. A study was done to examine the effect of physical exercise on production of interleukin-1α and 1β (IL-1α and IL-1β) by using ELISA and bioassay. The effect of exercise on the cytokines including interleukin-6 (IL-6), tumor necrosis factor-α (TNF-α), interleukin-2 (IL-2), and interferon-γ (IFN-γ) was also examined.

Methods.—Ten young, healthy volunteers underwent 60 minutes of bicycle exercise at 75% of maximal oxygen uptake ($\dot{V}O_{2max}$). Blood samples were collected before and during the last minutes of exercise and 2 and 24 hours after exercise.

Findings.—Levels of TNF-α, IL-2, and IFN-γ did not fluctuate in relation to exercise. Interleukin-2 and IFN-γ are mainly produced by CD4+ and CD16+ cells. Because the CD4+ subset decreases and the CD16+ subset increases during exercise, unchanged production of IL-2 and IFN-γ was expected. The production of IL-6 increased significantly, and production of IL-1α and IL-1β were enhanced (Figs 4–14 and 4–15). The

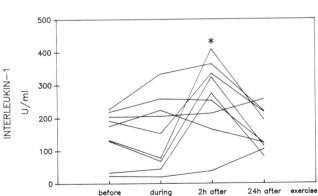

LPS–induced in vitro IL–1 synthesis following exercise

Fig 4–14.—Individual IL-1 in vitro production in 9 patients before, during, 2 hours after, and 24 hours after exercise. Friedman test: $P < .07$. Wilcoxon test: differences from the values before exercise are indicated. *Asterisk* indicates $P < .02$). (Courtesy of Haahr PM, Pedersen BK, Fomsgaard A, et al: *Int J Sports Med* 12:223–227, 1991.)

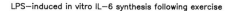

LPS—induced in vitro IL—6 synthesis following exercise

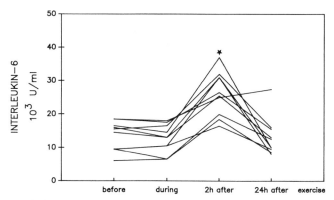

Fig 4–15.—Individual IL-6 in vitro production in 10 patients before, during, 2 hours after, and 24 hours after exercise. Friedman test: P < .01. Wilcoxon test: significant differences from the values before exercise are indicated. *Asterisk* indicates P < .01. (Courtesy of Haahr PM, Pedersen BK, Fomsgaard A, et al: *Int J Sports Med* 12:223-227, 1991.)

increased percentage and absolute number of blood monocytes 2 hours after exercise may explain the increased amounts of IL-1 and IL-6.

Conclusions.—The levels of cytokines predominantly produced by monocytes, IL-1, and IL-6, increased after exercise. Although produced mainly by monocytes, TNF-α levels did not increase with exercise. The production of IL-2 and INF-γ, predominantly performed by lymphocytes, was not changed by exercise.

▶ Research on physical activity, sports, and the diverse cytokines is still in its infancy, and results, as might be expected, are mixed. This study found that 1 hour of vigorous cycling increased the production of the monocyte cytokines, IL-1 and IL-6, but not of the monocyte cytokine, TNF-α, and not the lymphocyte cytokines, IL-2 and interferon-γ. In contrast, another recent study found that more prolonged exercise, 2.5 hours of running, increased plasma levels of TNF, as well as plasma levels of soluble IL-2 receptor (1). Similarly, an earlier study found that exercise increased plasma levels of interferon (2). We need more research to sort out the trends here, but obviously inflammatory and immunologic processes are involved in tissue injury and repair after vigorous exercise, especially eccentric exercise, as the working muscles are damaged ultrastructurally and are infiltrated by cytokine-rich leukocytes. See also Abstracts 4–29 and 4–30.—E.R. Eichner, M.D.

References

1. 1991 YEAR BOOK OF SPORTS MEDICINE, pp 128–129.
2. 1986 YEAR BOOK OF SPORTS MEDICINE, pp 165–167.

5 Cardiorespiratory Function, Other Medical Conditions

Effects of Exercise on Left Ventricular Diastolic Performance in Trained Athletes
Nixon JV, Wright AR, Porter TR, Roy V, Arrowood JA (Med College of Virginia; Virginia Commonwealth Univ, Richmond)
Am J Cardiol 68:945–949, 1991   5–1

Background.—Adaptive cardiac structural changes occur as a response to physical training. Dynamic exercise training may increase vagal tone, diminish resting heart rate, and increase cardiac stroke volume. The left ventricular (LV) wall mass increases to maintain normal wall stress. The effect of physiologic LV hypertrophy in trained athletes on M-mode and Doppler echocardiographic LV filling characteristics was examined during dynamic exercise.

Methods.—Six male and 4 female athletes were studied. Serial Doppler echocardiograms were obtained at rest, during supine graded bicycle exercise, and during recovery at heart rates of 80, 120, and 140 beats per minute. Results in the 10 trained athletes were compared with those in 10 age-matched controls.

Findings.—In the athletes at rest, there were significant increases in LV end-diastolic dimension and indexed LV wall mass. At heart rates of 140 beats per minute, there were differences between the athletes and controls in peak filling rates and in normalized peak lengthening rates. Doppler-derived variables of total time-velocity integral, early peak filling velocity, and its ratio to atrial filling velocity (E/A ratio) were different between athletes and controls. There were no significant differences in LV diastolic filling indexes at rest, but there was significant enhancement of these parameters in trained athletes at higher levels of dynamic exercise.

Conclusion.—Although LV diastolic filling in trained athletes is unchanged at rest, it is significantly enhanced during dynamic exercise in the presence of increased LV mass. Also, M-mode-derived peak filling and normalized peak lengthening rates, and Doppler-derived total time-velocity integral, early peak filling velocity, and E/A ratio were increased

189

in athletes. These parameters were found in the presence of significant increases in LV wall mass in the athletes.

▶ Resting echocardiographic measurements have shown significant LV wall mass differences as well as LV end diastolic dimensions between endurance athletes and controls (1). Within the athletic community there have been significant differences demonstrated between those performing endurance events and power events. In a more recent report studying over 900 subjects, upper limits for physiologic hypertrophy have been documented, enabling separation from a pathologic hypertrophic cardiomyopathy (2). Nevertheless, with increases in myocardial mass there has been concern that during exercise there would be an increased myocardial stiffness and impairment of diastolic filling at rest and even more so during exercise, although few studies have examined the diastolic function of trained athletes. The present study has extended our knowledge considerably and indicated the importance of making measurements at exercise and at rest because only significant differences were observed in the exercise state. Furthermore, the diastolic function of the trained athletes was enhanced, but particularly so during the active phase of diastole. There were several limitations to the study, not least of which was the failure to quantify the fitness of their subjects, although we may assume that being national collegiate athletes in division 1A basketball programs, they probably had well above average cardiorespiratory fitness as well as increased strength and power. A limitation pointed out by the authors was the likely difference in sympathetic activation of the 2 groups. Nevertheless I found this an important contribution to our understanding of exercise on cardiac function in athletes.—J.R. Sutton, M.D.

References

1. Maron BJ: *J Am Coll Cardiol* 7:190, 1986.
2. Pelliccia A, et al: *N Engl J Med* 324:295, 1991.
3. Hickson RC, et al: *Am J Physiol* 236:268, 1979.

Clinical and Electrophysiologic Characteristics of Exercise-Related Idiopathic Ventricular Tachycardia
Mont L, Seixas T, Brugada P, Brugada J, Simonis F, Rodríguez LM, Smeets JLRM, Wellens HJJ (University of Limburg, Maastricht, The Netherlands)
Am J Cardiol 68:897–900, 1991   5–2

Background.—It has been suggested that the idiopathic ventricular tachycardia (VT) that appears during or in relation to exercise is a catecholamine-sensitive arrhythmia that cannot be easily reproduced during programmed stimulation unless isoproterenol infusion is given. The clinical and electrophysiologic characteristics of patients who had exercise-related idiopathic VT were compared with those in patients who had VT not related to exercise.

Methods.—Among 53 patients with VT and no recognizable heart disease, 37 patients (group 1) had episodes of VT that were mainly related to exercise; 16 patients (group 2) had VT with no relation to exercise. Programmed electric stimulation was performed in all patients and 49 underwent a symptom-limited exercise test on a treadmill with use of the Bruce protocol.

Findings.—The 37 patients in group 1 with idiopathic VT related to exercise were younger and more often had dizziness during VT, compared to the 16 patients in group 2 with non–exercise-related VT. Four patients in group 1 needed cardioversion to terminate the arrhythmia, compared to 6 patients in group 2. Exercise-related VT was induced by programmed ventricular stimulation alone in about 50% of both groups. In group 1, VT was induced more easily by infusion of isoproterenol, and electrically induced VT was faster. Antiarrhythmic therapy was most effective with class III drugs and least effective with β-blocking agents. One patient with non–exercise-related VT died suddenly of unknown causes.

Conclusions.—Most patients with idiopathic VT had episodes related to exercise. Several distinctive clinical and ECG characteristics were observed in these patients, but no differences were observed in their response to antiarrhythmic drugs. The relationship of arrhythmia to exercise had no effect on long-term prognosis.

▶ The most feared arrhythmia during exercise is ventricular tachycardia (VT), and it has been suggested that this could be catecholamine related (1). By corollary, such arrhythmias (VT) should respond to β-blocking agents. A significant number of these patients do not have structural heart disease. In a group of 60 patients referred to their clinic, the authors studied 53 patients, 70% of whom had episodes of VT related to exercise and not surprisingly were more symptomatic during their episodes than those in whom the VT was not exercise related. Interestingly enough, with programmed stimulation the VT was equally reproducible in both groups, and the addition of isoproterenol was not significantly more effective in inducing the arrhythmia in the first group. In terms of therapy it was clear the class II drugs (i.e., β-blocking agents) were not particularly effective. Class I drugs (i.e., lidocaine, quinidine, procainamide, tocanide, disopyramide, etc.) were most effective, and most patients required 2 or more drugs in combination to be most effective. By and large, both groups had good long-term prognoses.—J.R. Sutton, M.D.

Reference

1. Mokotoff DM, et al: *Chest* 77:10, 1980.

Echocardiographic Assessment of Myocardial Performance After Prolonged Strenuous Exercise

Manier G, Wickers F, Lomenech AM, Cazorla G, Roudaut R (Université de Bordeaux II; Hôpital Pellegrin, Bordeaux, France; Régional d'Education Physique et Sportive, Talence, France; Hôpital Cardiologique du Haut-Leveque, Pessac, France)

Eur Heart J 12:1183–1188, 1991

5–3

Introduction.—Previous echocardiographic studies of left ventricular (LV) performance before and after a 24-hour race and a Hawaii Iron Man triathlon showed evidence of cardiac dysfunction. The rapid reversal of all changes suggested cardiac fatigue. This study was undertaken to assess myocardial performance in a group of nonelite middle-aged marathon runners.

Study Design.—Eleven nonelite competitive runners with a mean age of 37 years were studied before and during early recovery from the Aquitane championship marathon, a regional race. All runners had engaged in regular endurance training for several years. Each runner underwent 2 echocardiographic and 2 Doppler examinations performed by a cardiologist. Cavity dimensions, wall thickness, and fractional shortening were calculated from 2-dimensionally guided M mode echocardiograms. Dopper LV inflow tract recordings at the level of the mitral valve were analyzed for peak early and late velocities and their ratio. Seven runners wore a monitor to record the heart rate every 15 seconds throughout the race.

Results.—The runners ran the marathon at 87% of their maximal heart rate. At the end of the race, the LV diastolic dimension was slightly but significantly reduced. Fractional shortening did not vary, despite a decrease in systemic blood pressure and systolic wall stress. The LV filling pattern was unchanged. The ratio of early-to-late velocities remained constant. There was no significant relationship between the individual results and the time interval between the end of the race and the second examination.

Conclusion.—During the very early phase of recovery from a marathon race, there is a slight but consistent alteration of cardiac dimensions that is mainly caused by a change in loading conditions. This postexercise response will require further study to elucidate its significance.

▶ There has been much discussion in recent years regarding small and transient perturbations of cardiac function after participation in very prolonged and demanding athletic events. The present paper suggests that nonelite performers can complete a 42-km run for 3 hours or longer at an average 87% of their maximal heart rate with no evidence of change in myocardial performance, other than a constancy of end-systolic volume in the face of what is judged to be some reduction of after-loading. More sensitive tests might identify a minor decrease of myocardial contractility, but it is doubtful whether this has any clinical significance.—R.J. Shephard, M.D., Ph.D.

Prolonged Exercise Induces Left Ventricular Dysfunction in Healthy Subjects

Vanoverschelde J-LJ, Younis LT, Melin JA, Vanbutsele R, Leclercq B, Robert AR, Cosyns JR, Detry J-MR (University of Louvain Medical School, Brussels)
J Appl Physiol 70:1356–1363, 1991   5–4

Introduction.—Increases in heart rate and stroke volume during submaximal upright exercise result in increased cardiac output. A higher ejection fraction and a larger venous return both contribute to this increased stroke volume. During prolonged exercise, stroke volume and mean arterial pressure usually drop, and heart rate increases out of proportion to the work-rate. The effects of a moderately prolonged exercise on left ventricular systolic performance were studied in 23 healthy men, aged 18–61 years.

Methods.—The men exercised first on a treadmill, then completed a 20-km run on a later day. M-mode, 2-dimensional, and Doppler echocardiography and calibrated carotid pulse tracings were obtained at rest and less than 5 minutes after both brief and prolonged exercise. End-systolic stress-shortening relationships were determined to assess left ventricular systolic function.

Results.—Heart rate increased by 30% after both brief and prolonged exercise. The mean arterial pressure decreased from 99 to 92 mm Hg after prolonged exercise, but remained unchanged after brief exercise.

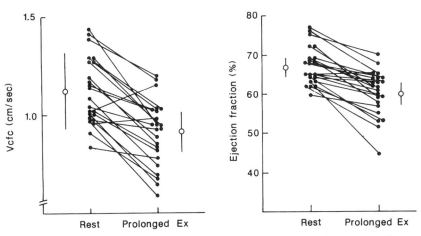

Fig 5–1.—Mean velocity of fiber shortening corrected for heart rate (V_{cfc}) (*left*) and ejection fraction (*right*) at rest and after prolonged exercise (Ex) in 23 normal individuals. (Courtesy of Vanoverschelde J-LJ, Younis LT, Melin JA, et al: *J Appl Physiol* 70:1356–1363, 1991.)

Left ventricular end-diastolic volume was reduced after prolonged exercise. Ejection fraction and rate-adjusted mean velocity of fiber shortening both decreased after prolonged exercise, despite a lower circumferential end-systolic wall stress. The relationship between ejection fraction and end-systolic wall stress was displaced downward at the end of the 20-km run (Fig 5-1).

Conclusion.—These data substantiate those of previous studies indicating that moderately prolonged exercise produces significant left ventricular dysfunction in healthy men. More studies are needed to determine the mechanisms underlying this impairment of the left ventricular systolic function and its physiologic significance.

▶ The increase of heart rate with continued exercise at a fixed intensity was traditionally attributed to cardiovascular drift, predominantly a consequence of a peripheral accumulation of the circulating blood volume in dilated veins and an increased tissue fluid space. Although such phenomena undoubtedly occur during exercise bouts of less than 30-minutes' duration, there are also an increasing number of reports suggesting that very prolonged events such as marathon, ultramarathon and iron-man competitions have a transient negative effect on myocardial contractility. Explanations that have been suggested include a depressant effect of free fatty acids (1), "stunning" after myocardial ischemia (although the lack of cardiac enzymes in the plasma does not support this suggestion), or a down-regulation of β-adrenoceptors in response to prolonged elevation of catecholamine levels (2). The present data were collected within 5 minutes of ceasing exercise, and it will be important to extend observations further into the recovery period to assess the long-term clinical consequences, if any.—R.J. Shephard, M.D., Ph.D.

References

1. Seals DR, et al: *Am J Cardiol* 61:875, 1988.
2. Ohman EM, et al: *J Cardiovasc Pharmacol* 10:728, 1987.

Measuring Physical Activity With a Single Question
Schechtman KB, Barzilai B, Rost K, Fisher EB Jr (Washington Univ, St Louis; Univ of Arkansas)
Am J Public Health 81:771–773, 1991   5–5

Background.—Physical inactivity, through its association with low high-density lipoprotein (HDL) cholesterol levels, obesity, and other physiologic parameters, has been linked with increased illness and death from a variety of causes. Measuring physical activity has therefore become a standard component of epidemiologic studies. Unfortunately, many of the measurement techniques described are complex, costly, and time-consuming. The usefulness of a single exercise question was assessed.

Methods.—Data on 1,004 subjects, mean age 36.6 years, were collected. Seventy-three percent of the participants were women. Of the 986 subjects providing baseline exercise information, 32% said they exercised regularly. Body mass index (BMI) and HDL cholesterol levels were also determined.

Results.—At baseline, after adjusting for age, subjects who said they exercised had a lower BMI, greater oxygen capacity, and higher HDL cholesterol levels than subjects who said they did not participate in regular exercise. After age adjustment, mean HDL cholesterol was not the same in men who said they did exercise at baseline and final assessment, who said they did not exercise at both times, or who said they did or did not exercise at baseline and gave the opposite answer at final assessment. There was an increase in HDL in those who said they did exercise at baseline and final assessment that was significantly different from the reduction in HDL cholesterol in those reporting they did not exercise at baseline and final assessment.

Conclusions.—In this study, a single self-reported measure of participation in regular exercise was significantly associated with BMI and oxygen capacity after adjusting for age in both women and men, and with HDL cholesterol in women. These findings support previous data suggesting that simple self-report methods can yield valuable data about participation in regular exercise.

▶ The assessment of physical activity is a very difficult matter, particularly in large-scale epidemiologic projects, where a small change of questionnaire wording has sometimes increased the apparent proportion of the population who are active from 9% to 78% in the same year! Some authors have argued that the precision of activity measurement can be improved by the use of a long and complex questionnaire, with verification of responses by a trained interviewer. But this is a very costly approach, and in some people an increase in the number and complexity of questions is counterproductive. Canadian investigators have thus argued for a long time that most of the measurable variance in exercise behavior can be assessed from responses to 1 or 2 simple questions (1,2). The present report substantiates this view. A single positive response increases aerobic power by 3.5 mL/kg.min in women and 6.5 mL/kg.min in men. This differential corresponds to much of the potential effect of training in a large population.—R.J. Shephard, M.D., Ph.D.

References

1. Shephard RJ, McClure RL: *Int Z Angew Physiol* 21:212, 1965.
2. Godin G, et al: *Can J Pub Health* 77:359, 1986.

Physical Activity and Ischaemic Heart Disease in Middle-Aged British Men

Shaper AG, Wannamethee G (Royal Free Hospital, London)
Br Heart J 66:384–394, 1991 5–6

Background.—Studies in middle-aged men suggest that exercise reduces risk of coronary events only if it is vigorous and sustained. It remains unknown whether low physical activity levels help in diminishing heart attack risk. Physicians have studied the relationship in a sample of middle-aged men selected to represent the socioeconomic distribution of men in the British population.

Methods.—The analysis included 7,735 men selected from 1 group general practice in each of 24 British towns. The men were participating in the British Regional Heart Study, a prospective, 8-year follow-up study. They were aged 40–59 years at their initial examination, which included a detailed history, several physical measurements, and blood sampling. Breathlessness, any preexisting ischemic heart disease, and physical activity level were also assessed. Subjects were assigned a physical activity score, which was validated against heart rate and lung function in men who had no apparent ischemic heart disease.

Results.—During 8 years, 488 subjects had at least 1 major heart attack. Men who participated in moderate and moderately vigorous activity had less than half as many heart attacks as inactive men. Heart attack rates were higher in vigorously active men than in the moderate or moderately vigorous activity groups. Among men who had symptomatic heart disease, risk was reduced with light and moderate activity and increased with more vigorous levels of activity. Case fatality decreased progressively, however. Vigorous activity, performed with any frequency, was associated with significantly lower heart attack rates; however, after exclusion of this group, there was still a strong inverse relationship between physical activity and heart attack risk in men without preexisting ischemic disease.

Conclusions.—In middle-aged men, overall physical activity level is an independent protective factor against ischemic heart disease. Vigorous sports activity has its own benefits, but it is not imperative to the protective effect. For middle-aged men who wish to begin a regimen of vigorous activity, a review of their cardiovascular state is recommended.

▶ There is growing evidence that whereas a moderate amount of exercise is good for you, an excessive amount can have less positive results. The present prospective trial supports this position; benefit plateaued over the 3 highest categories of physical activity, and the heart attack rate was actually a little higher in the most active group than in those who were undertaking a more moderate level of physical activity. This deterioration of prospects was most marked in those who had engaged in an excessive amount of physical activity, but was also seen in those who reported walking more than an hour per day, and in those who cycled for more than 30 minutes per day. In contrast with Morris and associates (1), the present authors also observed benefit when they deliberately excluded all patients who reported sports participation. The level of benefit observed in this study was of the order previously described, a twofold to threefold reduction in the risk of heart attacks being associated with moderate physical activity.—R.J. Shephard, M.D., Ph.D.

Reference

1. Morris JN, et al: *Br Heart J* 63:325, 1990.

The Upper Limit of Physiologic Cardiac Hypertrophy in Highly Trained Elite Athletes

Pelliccia A, Maron BJ, Spataro A, Proschan MA, Spirito P (Comitato Olimpico Nazionale Italiano, Rome; NIH, Bethesda, Md)
N Engl J Med 324:295–301, 1991   5–7

Introduction.—The athlete's heart is recognizable by increases in the diastolic dimension of the left ventricular cavity, in the thickness of the left ventricular mass, and in the calculated left ventricular mass. The thickness of the left ventricular wall may resemble cardiac disease such as hypertrophic cardiomyopathy. Differential diagnosis must distinguish between physiologic and pathologic hypertrophy.

Methods.—To study the upper limit of left ventricular wall hypertrophy, echocardiographic measurements were taken of left ventricular dimensions in 947 elite athletes.

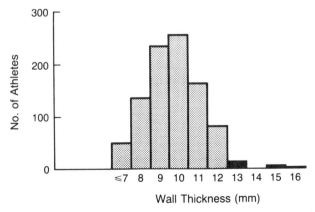

Fig 5–2.—Distribution of maximal left-ventricular-wall thicknesses in the 947 elite athletes. *Shaded bars* indicate wall thicknesses within the normal range; *solid bars,* within a range compatible with the diagnosis of hypertrophic cardiomyopathy (≥ 13 mm). (Courtesy of Pelliccia A, Maron BJ, Spataro A, et al: *N Engl J Med* 324:295–301, 1991.)

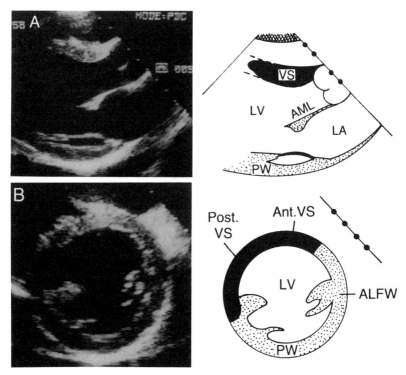

Fig 5–3.—Stop-frame 2-dimensional echocardiograms obtained during diastole and corresponding schematic drawings from a 21-year-old cyclist with a normally thick ventricular wall and a 25-year-old canoeist with a thickening of the left ventricular wall. In the cyclist, a parasternal long-axis view **(A)** shows normal anterior ventricular septal *(VS)* and posterior-wall *(PW)* thicknesses (11 mm and 10 mm) and an enlarged left ventricular *(LV)* cavity (61 mm) at end-diastole. A short-axis view **(B)** at the papillary muscle level shows normal thickness of all segments of the left ventricular wall. *(Continued.)*

Results.—Left ventricular wall thickness of 13 mm or greater is compatible with the diagnosis of hypertrophic cardiomyopathy. This thickness was found in 15 rowers or canoeists and 1 cyclist of 947 athletes (Fig 5–2). The group with a wall thickness of 13 mm or greater was only 7% of the 219 rowers, canoeists, and cyclists included in the group of 947 athletes. The athletes with walls 13 mm or greater also had enlarged left ventricular end-diastolic cavities. The upper limit for wall thickness increased by athletic training was 16 mm (Fig 5–3).

Conclusion.—A left ventricular wall thickness of 16 mm was the upper limit found in the athletes. An athlete with a wall thickness of more than 16 mm and a nondilated left ventricular cavity is likely to have primary pathologic hypertrophy such as hypertrophic cardiomyopathy.

▶ Sudden cardiac death in athletes is a particularly important problem. In those over the age of 35, it is invariably related to coronary artery disease. In younger athletes, however, various forms of congenital cardiac abnormali-

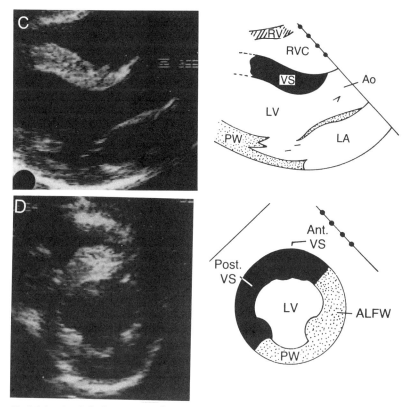

Fig 5–3 (cont).—C, In the canoeist, a long-axis view shows a thickening anterior ventricular septum (16 mm), exceeding the thickness of the posterior free wall, and moderate enlargement of the left ventricular cavity. A short-axis view **(D)** at the papillary muscle level on the same athlete shows localized thickening of the anterior septum, whereas the free wall and posterior septum *(Post. VS)* are normal. *ALFW* denotes anterolateral free wall; *AML,* anterior mitral leaflet; *Ant. VS,* anterior ventricular septum; *Ao,* Aorta; *LA,* left atrium; *RV,* right ventricle; and *RVC,* right ventricular cavity. (Courtesy of Pelliccia A, Maron BJ, Spataro A, et al: N *Engl J Med* 324:295–301, 1991.)

ties, including anomalous coronary arteries, Marfan syndrome, congenital valvular abnormalities, but most importantly, hypertophic cardiomyopathies, are generally the cause. The distinction between a pathologic cardiomyopathy and the cardiac hypertrophy associated with the so-called "athletes heart" is therefore of great importance. In the former there is a significant incidence of sudden death (1), whereas physiologic hypertrophy associated with the various forms of athletic training may well be cardioprotective. Until the advent of echocardiography, detailed studies of cardiac dimensions were not feasible. Since echocardiography has come into widespread use, there have been only scant studies with insufficient numbers of inappropriately chosen subjects to be able to make any global statements about the normal physiologic cardiac changes after training. However, the present study does have respectability of numbers in that they quantified the left ventricular dimensions of 947 elite athletes and only 1.7% had left ventricular wall thickness of greater than 13 mm, which would be compatible with a diagnosis of hypertrophic cardiac myopathy (15 of these were rowers and 1 was a cyclist). All of these, of course, had large left ventricular cavities that would immediately separate them from the patients with pathologic hypertrophic cardiomyopathies. We are therefore grateful for this relatively large survey so that we can extend the upper limits of normal, although as every echocardiographer knows, there are many other echocardiographic features that distinguish pathologic from physiologic cardiac hypertrophy.—J.R. Sutton, M.D.

Reference

1. Maron BJ, et al: *Circulation* 62:218, 1980.

Sports-Related and Non-Sports-Related Sudden Cardiac Death in Young Adults
Burke AP, Farb A, Virmani R, Goodin J, Smialek JE (Armed Forces Inst of Pathology, Washington, D.C.; Office of the Chief Medical Examiner, Baltimore)
Am Heart J 121:568–575, 1991   5–8

Background.—Many younger athletes who die during exercise have hypertrophic cardiomyopathy and anomalous coronary arteries, whereas most older than age 35 years have severe coronary atherosclerosis. To ascertain which conditions are preferentially seen in individuals who exercise, exercise and nonexercise-related sudden deaths were compared.

Methods.—All cases of natural, unexpected cardiac death in persons, aged 14–40 years, occurring in the state of Maryland during an 8-year period, were evaluated. Exercise-related sudden cardiac deaths were defined as those with symptoms occurring during or within 1 hour of en-

Exercise-Related Deaths: Distribution of Race/Sports			
Cause of death (n)	*Black*	*White*	*Sport*
Severe atherosclerosis (9)	1	9	Running (5) Other (4)
Hypertrophic cardiomyopathy (8)	6	2	Basketball (7) Swimming (1)
Anomalous coronary arteries (4)	2	2	Basketball (2) Baseball (1) Soccer (1)
Others (13)	6	7	Basketball (5) Running (4) Other (4)

(Courtesy of Burke AP, Farb A, Virmani R, et al: *Am Heart J* 121: 568–575, 1991.)

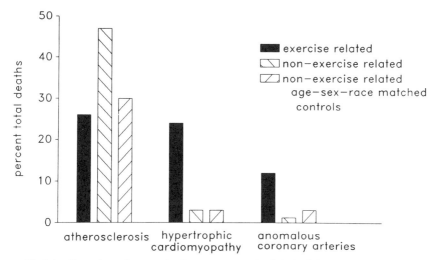

Fig 5–4.—Comparison of sports-related vs. non-sports-related deaths (atherosclerosis, hypertrophic cardiomyopathy, and anomalous coronary arteries. (Courtesy of Burke AP, Farb A, Virmani R, et al: *Am Heart J* 121:568-575, 1991.)

gaging in sports and with death occurring within 24 hours. Each such death was matched for age, sex, and race to 3 nonexercise-related deaths in random fashion.

Results.—Of 690 sudden cardiac deaths, 34 were sports-related, an incidence of 5%. Nine patients had severe atherosclerosis as the cause of death, 8 had hypertrophic cardiomyopathy with asymmetry, and 6 died of unknown causes; 2 of the latter patients had tunnel arteries (table). Other causes of death included coronary artery anomalies, idiopathic concentric left ventricular hypertrophy, myocarditis, right ventricular dysplasia, and Kawasaki disease. Compared to controls, exercise-related death was more likely to result from hypertrophic cardiomyopathy (Fig 5-4). The incidence of severe atherosclerosis was no different between the 2 groups. Mean age of subjects with hypertrophic cardiomyopathy was 24 years compared to 32 years for those with severe atherosclerosis.

Conclusions.—In younger persons with hypertrophic cardiomyopathy, exercise may result in sudden cardiac death. Of all exercise-related sudden cardiac deaths, the younger victims are usually black persons and have hypertrophic cardiomyopathy, and the older ones are usually white persons and have severe atherosclerosis. This information may be useful in counseling athletes and setting up preventive screening programs.

▶ To better understand the true causes of sports-related sudden cardiac death in young adults, this clinicopathologic study examined sudden deaths, both exercise-related and nonexercise-related, in a defined population of persons 14–40 years old. The autopsy findings from each athlete who died suddenly during sports play were compared with those from 3 persons who died suddenly when not exercising. Five percent of all deaths were sports-related. The breakdown of the sports involved jibes with the notion that basketball is the sport most commonly associated with sudden death; of the 34 sports-related deaths, 14 occurred during basketball (1). Running was the second most common sport on the "death list," tied to 9 deaths. One must emphasize, however, that this retrospective study lacks "denominator data"; that is, the number of athletes in the underlying population and the sports they played. Given these limits, hypertrophic cardiomyopathy (HCM) seemed especially likely to cause death during exercise as opposed to when not exercising. Of the 8 athletes who died from HCM during sports play, however, none had a family history of premature sudden death or a history of dyspnea, syncope, or angina. In other words, sudden death during exercise seemed to be the first manifestation of HCM. This suggests that symptom-based screening programs of all potential athletes would not be cost-effective, yet implies that directed screening of selected "competitive athletes" would be wise, if we can agree on how to define such athletes and how best to screen them. Intriguingly, in this study, blacks who died during sports play had a greater incidence of HCM than did whites and were younger. The sharp debate over the clinical import of tunnel coronary arteries was not settled here. For more on HCM and sudden death in athletes, see reference 1.—E.R. Eichner, M.D.

References

1. 1991 Year Book of Sports Medicine, pp 278–279.
2. 1990 Year Book of Sports Medicine, pp 215–216.

Hypertrophic Cardiomyopathy and Its Inherent Danger in Athletics
Smith AN, Bell GW (US Military Academy at West Point, NY; Univ of Illinois, Urbana/Champaign)
Athletic Training JNATA 26:319–323, 1991   5–9

Introduction.—Hypertrophic cardiomyopathy consists of a hypertrophied, nondilated left ventricle and interventricular septum without other cardiac or systemic disease that could produce the ventricular hypertrophy. This disease can result in sudden, unexpected death. The inherent danger of this disease in athletes was reviewed.

Discussion.—Hypertrophic cardiomyopathy is characterized by asymmetrical hypertrophy of bizarre cellular arrangement of muscle fiber of the cardiac wall. It uusually involves the left ventricle and interventricular septum. Cardiac hypertrophy, often found in endurance athletes, is an adaptive change that coincides with other skeletal muscle hypertrophy. The first sign of hypertrophic cardiomyopathy is often sudden death. Recognizing the disease is therefore important to athletic trainers and physicians. Many patients are asymptomatic. Trainers and physicians must make a concerted effort to identify athletes with risk factors, such as exertional syncope, chest pain, or dyspnea. Detailed personal and

---

Checklist for Athletic Trainers Pertaining to the Detection of Hypertrophic Cardiomyopathy and Other Cardiovascular Disease

- Record and inform the team physician of all episodes of dyspnea, syncope, and chest pain in athletes.

- With the assistance of the team physician, perform a preparticipation physical examination, including height, weight, vital signs, inspection, and palpation and auscultation of the heart.

- Implement a family history questionnaire to be completed by the athlete and/or the parent prior to participation. Ask questions pertaining to:
  - a personal or a family member having episodes of syncope, dyspnea, or chest pain,
  - the sudden death of a family member, especially at a young age,
  - a personal/family history of premature atherosclerosis or seizures.

- Know the physical characteristics associated with various cardiovascular abnormalities.
  - elongated appendages (incuding toes and fingers)
  - unsteady or irregular gait
  - abnormal joint flexibility
  - pes planus feet
  - dislocation of the optic lens
  - club-shaped fingernails

- Always seek a physician's assistance when questions arise about the physical well-being of a particular athlete.

(Courtesy of Smith AN, Bell GW: *Athlete Training* JNATA 26:319-323, 1991.)

---

family histories and physical examinations can aid in diagnosis (table). Echocardiography and ECG are often used for further diagnosis and monitoring. There are no specific or consistent physical or diagnostic tests related to the disease.

Conclusion.—Although sudden death from hypertrophic cardiomyopathy is rare in athletes, it is a great concern of athletic trainers and physicians. Risk factors and warning signs must not be taken lightly. Athletic participation is contraindicated until special testing has been performed to rule out this disease.

▶ Athletic trainers and all of those involved with preparticipation physical examinations must be aware of those athletes with the risk factors of "exertional syncope, chest pain, or dyspnea." The examination questionnaire should include family medical history and personal medical history. The examination itself should include "measuring vital signs and inspection and auscultation of the heart" by a qualified person.

Athletes identified with hypertrophic cardiomyopathy should be referred to a cardiologist and should not be allowed to participate in athletic activity. Athletes should also be offered counseling to help them adjust to a change in lifestyle.—F.J. George, A.T.C., P.T.

Sudden Death in Athletes: Risk Factors and Screening
Maron BJ (Natl Heart, Lung, and Blood Inst, Bethesda, Md)
J Musculoskel Med 8:63–78, 1991   5–10

Introduction.—The recent sudden deaths of well-known competitive athletes have led to much interest in what causes these deaths and how to prevent them. Although such deaths are uncommon, they produce a sense of alarm in a public that is becoming increasingly interested in sports.

Causes.—Hypertrophic cardiomyopathy is a common cause of sudden death in athletes younger than age 35 years. Coronary artery anomalies and Marfan's syndrome are other causes of sudden death in this age group. Those who lack evidence of organic cardiovascular disease at autopsy most likely die of primary arrhythmia. Most older athletes die of coronary heart disease. Mitral valve prolapse and hypertrophic cardiomyopathy also can cause sudden death in athletes older than age 35 years.

Screening.—It is feasible to screen young athletes on a small scale by using a personal and family history, physical examination, ECG, and echocardiogram. Larger scale efforts that make use of the history, examination, and ECG have failed to yield a substantial number of cases of cardiomyopathy, Marfan's syndrome, or other disorders disposing to sudden cardiac death. The cost of echocardiography has impeded its routine use in the primary screening of large populations.

Participation.—Clinicians must make some judgments about participation in athletics on an individual basis. Athletes often ignore symptoms or deny their significance. Hopefully, education in the potential lethality of underlying cardiovascular disease will lessen this tendency.

▶ As pointed out by the author, the published recommendation of the Sixteenth Bethesda Conference on cardiovascular abnormalities in the athlete held by the American College of Cardiology in the National Institutes of

Health in 1984 represent the most ambitious attempt at formalized guidelines for determining eligibility of athletes for competition on the basis of cardiovascular disease (1). It should be noted, however, that the guidelines recommended by this conference were essentially empiric recommendations. The ultimate decision to resume sports is the responsibility of the athlete and his or her parents after carefully discussing the possible risks, including death, with his or her physician.—J.S. Torg, M.D.

Reference

1. Mitchell JE, et al: *J Am Coll Cardiol* 6:1189, 1985.

Spontaneous Pneumopericardium: A Link With Weight Lifting?
Casamassima AC, Sternberg T, Weiss FH (New York Med College; Charleston Naval Hosp, Charleston, NC; Albert Einstein Med Ctr, Philadelphia)
Physician and Sportsmedicine 19:107–110, 1991   5–11

Introduction.—Spontaneous pneumopericardium (pneumopericardium occurring without associated pathologic findings or well known antecedents) is rare but was found in an adolescent weight lifter.

Case Report.—Male, 16, had throbbing, pressure-like substernal pain that worsened with deep inspiration or with bending forward but moderated when he lay prone. Symptoms began within 24 hours of his last weight-lifting session. A chest radiograph demonstrated pneumopericardium and pneumomediastinum. The patient was treated with generic ibuprofen. Ten days after presentation, physical examination and chest radiographs were normal.

Discussion.—The pathogenesis of weight-lifting–associated pneumopericardium probably involves performance of the Valsalva maneuver, which has also been cited as the cause of "weight lifter's blackout." The symptoms of pneumopericardium include syncope, upper abdominal pain, and shock. Physical findings include Hamman's sign, a short grade 2/6 systolic murmur, pulsus paradoxus, hyperresonance over the precordium, diminished intensity of heart sounds, hypotension with tamponade, jugular venous distension, tachycardia, and subcutaneous emphysema. The characteristic radiographic sign is a radiolucent band outlining the heart and defining the pericardial membrane. Most patients recover spontaneously.

Conclusion.—The American Academy of Pediatrics recommends that children and adolescents avoid weight lifting until they reach the Tanner stage 5 level of developmental maturity. Weight-lifting–associated pneumopericardium should be suspected in any adolescent with an acute on-set of chest pain.

▶ A diagnosis to consider when a young weight-training athlete has chest pain and dyspnea. This pain was substernal, continuous, present even at rest, worse with deep inspiration or when bending forward, and better when lying prone. The Hamman's sign, a holosystolic sound like "crackling cellophane," was a strong clue to air in the mediastinum, and the x-ray was diagnostic for pneumopericardium. Similar symptoms have been described in a patient with acute asthma and after being punched in the chest. At least 1 other case has been reported in a young weight lifter, a 14-year-old boy who had 2 episodes of pneumopericardium a year apart, both times after lifting weights. Presumably, the problem is repeated Valsalva maneuvers (i.e., forced expiration against a closed glottis) from lifting excessive weight. Fortunately, spontaneous resolution usually occurs within a few days.—E.R. Eichner, M.D.

Usefulness of Weightlifting Training in Improving Strength and Maximal Power Output in Coronary Artery Disease
McCartney N, McKelvie RS, Haslam DRS, Jones NL (McMaster University, Hamilton, Ontario)
Am J Cardiol 67:939–945, 1991   5–12

Background.—Traditionally, cardiac exercise rehabilitation programs have omitted systematic strength training, probably because of the abrupt rise in heart rate and arterial pressure that accompanies even moderate isometric contractions of small muscle groups. However, acceptable circulatory responses to weight carrying and weight-lifting have been reported in selected patients with coronary artery disease (CAD). The usefulness of weight-lifting in improving strength and maximal power output was investigated in 18 male patients with CAD.

Methods.—Ten men underwent 20 sessions of combined weight-lifting and aerobic training in a 10-week period and 8 others had aerobic training only. Indexes of strength and aerobic power were determined.

Results.—The 2 groups had similar initial test performances. After aerobic training, the maximal load that could be lifted once in a single-arm curl increased by 13%, single-leg press imprived by 4%, and single-knee extension exercises rose by 5%. The corresponding gains with combined weight-lifting and aerobic training were 43%, 21%, and 24%, respectively. The initial 1-repetition maximum could be lifted an average of 4 times after aerobic training and 14 times after combined training. Maximal progressive incremental cycle ergometer power output rose by 2% and 15% in the aerobic group and the combined training group, respectively. Cycling time at 80% of initial maximal power before attaining a Borg rating of perceived exertion of 7, or very severe, rose by 11% in the aerobic group and by 109% in the weight-trained group (Fig 5–5).

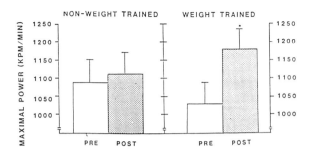

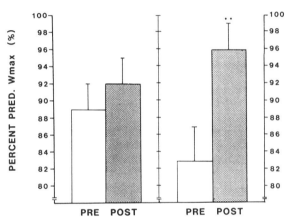

Fig 5–5.—Maximal power output in progressive incremental cycle ergometry exercise expressed as absolute (*upper panel*) and as percentage predicted (*Wmax*) for a healthy control population (*lower panel*), before (*open bars*) and after (*filled bars*) 10 weeks of either aerobic or combined training. *P < .05; **P < .01. (Courtesy of McCartney N, McKelvie RS, Haslam DRS, et al: *Am J Cardiol* 67:939-945, 1991.)

Conclusions.—Dynamic weight-lifting combined with aerobic endurance training is a more effective way to increase muscle strength and maximal power output in conditioned patients with CAD than is aerobic endurance training alone. There was also a marked reduction in perceived leg exertion during heavy submaximal exercise, which may result in improved function in many strenuous activities of daily living.

▶ For a long time, those training "postcoronary" patients were very careful to avoid all forms of resisted exercise. The fear of this type of activity probably dates back to the classical observations of Lind and McNicol (1), who showed a rapid rise of heart rate, systolic and diastolic pressures during isometric contractions at relatively small fractions of maximal voluntary force. It was reasoned that if such a rise of heart rate and pressures occurred in a cardiac patient, there would be a dramatic increase in double product, with a resultant increase in the risk of a cardiac catastrophe. Moreover, it was ar-

gued that a muscle strengthening regimen would detract from aerobic training, leaving the patient with a bulky body to be transported by an untrained
heart. One unfortunate consequence of exclusive aerobic programs such as
fast walking and slow jogging was that muscle strength was lost from the
upper part of the body. Thus, if occupational demands or some emergency
required a strong arm contraction, the postcoronary patient had to make this
effort with weakened muscles, and there was a greater rise of cardiac work-
rate than would have occurred if the patient had also undertaken some muscle building exercises.

More recently, it has been appreciated that the hypertensive response to
isometric efforts offer a "worse-case" scenario, and that moderately resisted
dynamic exercise (for example, repeated contractions at 40% of the 1-repe-
tition maximum) can be undertaken with no greater increase of systemic
blood pressure than would be seen with a bout of cycle ergometer exercise
(2, 3). Moreover, in many instances, such as the cases reported here by
McCartney and associates, aerobic effort is also limited by muscle weakness,
and the gains of aerobic power are thus greater if the regimen that is
adopted strengthens the main muscles of the body as well as focusing on
aerobic conditioning.—R.J. Shephard, M.D., Ph.D.

References

1. Lind S, McNicol GW: *Can Med Assoc J* 96:706, 1967.
2. Vander LB, et al: *Ann Sports Med* 2:165, 1986.
3. Haslam DRS, et al: *J Cardiopulm Rehabil* 8:213, 1988.

Resistance Training in Cardiac Rehabilitation
Franklin BA, Bonzheim K, Gordon S, Timmis GC (William Beaumont Hosp,
Royal Oak, Mich)
J Cardiopulmonary Rehabil 11:99–107, 1991   5–13

Background.—Traditionally, cardiac exercise programs have stressed
dynamic lower extremity exercise. More recent research, however, suggests that complementary resistance training has beneficial effects on
strength, cardiovascular endurance, hypertension, hyperlipidemia, and
psychosocial well-being.

Discussion.—Many cardiac patients lack the physical strength to perform the common tasks of daily living, and many others lack the confidence to attempt activities requiring even low levels of muscular exertion. Mild to moderate resistance training can be an effective way for
such patients to improve strength and cardiovascular endurance, modifying coronary risk factors and enhancing their quality of life. The safety of
resistance exercise can be attributed to the fact that heart rate and blood
pressure responses are not aggravated beyond clinically acceptable levels.
Proper preliminary screening, appropriate prescriptive guidelines, and
careful supervision play important roles in such a program. Resistance

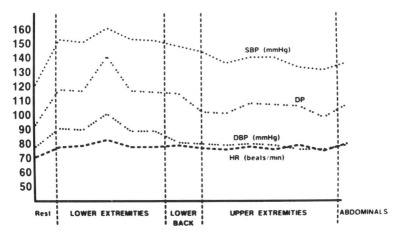

Fig 5–6.—Cardiovascular response at rest and during peak Nautilus exercise. *Abbreviations: SBP,* systolic blood pressure (mm Hg); *DP,* double product (beats/min $\times$ mm Hg $\times$ 10^{-2}; *DBP,* diastolic blood pressure (mm Hg); *HR,* heart rate (beats/min). (From Franklin BA, Bonzheim K, Gordon S, et al: *J Cardiopulmonary Rehabil* 11:99-107, 1991. Courtesy of Vander LB, Franklin BA, Wrisley D, et al: *Ann Sports Med* 2:165-169, 1986.)

training also provides a way to maintain interest and increase diversity so that long-term compliance with the exercise program may be improved. Resistance training should serve as a supplement to the patient's aerobic exercise prescription, not as a replacement for it (Fig 5–6).

▶ This review covers much of the discussion that has led to acceptance of strength training as an important component of cardiac rehabilitation. It cautions against overenthusiastic endorsement of heavily resisted exercise based on recovery blood pressure measurements by sphygmomanometer cuff. Intra-arterial measurements show that pressures fall rapidly immediately after exercise. Nevertheless, intra-arterial measurements during exercise support the use of resisted contractions to 40% of the 1-repetition maximal voluntary force. Franklin and associates suggest limiting such therapy to patients who have an ejection fraction > 45%, who can reach stage III of the Bruce protocol, have a blood pressure < 160/90 mm Hg, and are free of ST depression, angina, and uncontrolled arrhythmias. The one claim for the program that may need re-evaluation is the normalization of lipid profile (see Abstract 3–10).—R.J. Shephard, M.D., Ph.D.

Sensitivity of Exercise Electrocardiography for Acute Cardiac Events During Moderate and Strenuous Physical Activity: The Lipid Research Clinics Coronary Primary Prevention Trial

Siscovick DS, Ekelund LG, Johnson JL, Truong Y, Adler A (Harborview Med Ctr, Seattle; Univ of Washington, Seattle; Univ of North Carolina, Chapel Hill)
Arch Intern Med 151:325–330, 1991   5–14

Clinically Silent ST Segment Changes and Activity-Related
Acute Cardiac Events

Ischemic ST-Segment Changes	CHD During Activity†	No CHD
Entry Electrocardiogram		
Present	11	238
Absent	51	2907
Follow-up Electrocardiogram		
Present	12	434
Absent	39	2408
Any Electrocardiogram		
Present	23	672
Absent	39	2488

† Nonfatal myocardial infarction or CHD death.
(Courtesy of Siscovick DS, Ekelund LG, Johnson JL, et al: *Arch Intern Med* 151:325–330, 1991.)

Introduction.—The role of exercise electrocardiography for screening apparently healthy men before they begin a vigorous exercise program is controversial. Data from the Lipid Research Clinics Coronary Primary Prevention Trial were analyzed to determine whether an exercise electrocardiogram can predict acute cardiac events during moderate or strenuous physical activity.

Study Design.—Data from 3,617 apparently healthy but hypercholesterolemic men, aged 35 to 59, were studied. Subjects underwent submaximal exercise tests at entry and at annual follow-up visits in years 2 through 7. A positive test result was defined as an ST segment depression or elevation of at least 1 mm or 10 μV-sec. A record review was performed to assess the circumstances that surrounded each nonfatal myocardial infarction and coronary heart disease (CHD) death. The average follow-up period was 7.4 years.

Findings.—Sixty-two men had an acute cardiac event during moderate or intense acttivity. The cumulative incidence of activity-related acute cardiac events was 2%. The risk increased 2.6-fold in the presence of clinically silent, exercise-induced, ST segment changes at entry, even after adjusting for 11 other potential risk factors. Eleven patients had clinically silent, exercise-induced ischemic ST segment changes on the entry exercise electrocardiogram (table). A positive test result on entry had a sensitivity of 18% and a specificity of 92% for predicting acute cardiac events during activity. These rates remained unchanged when the length of follow-up was restricted to 1 year after testing. For a new positive test result at a follow-up visit, the sensitivity was 24% and the specificity was 85%. For any positive result during the study, the sensitivity was 37% and the specificity was 79%.

Conclusion.—The presence of a clinically silent, exercise-induced, ischemic ST segment change on the submaximal exercise test is associated with an increased risk of activity-related acute cardiac events. The test is not sensitive, however, when used to predict the occurrence of acute cardiac events during physical activity among asymptomatic, hyper-cholesterolemic men. The usefulness of the submaximal exercise test to assess the safety of physical activity among asymptomatic, middle aged men at risk for CHD is likely to be limited.

▶ The last 2 decades have seen vigorous debate about the necessity of an exercise stress test as a prelude to exercise prescription, with Canadian physicians tending to take a more liberal approach than their counterparts in the United States. The population involved in the Lipid Research Clinics trial seems just the group for whom stress-testing has been most strongly advocated—a high-risk population in the age range 35 to 59 years. The sample tested was of substantial size (3,617 subjects), and the follow-up was quite extensive (an average of 7 years). As anticipated, the risk of an exercise-related cardiac event was a little higher in those with silent ischemia during a stress test that was carried to 90% of the age-related maximal heart rate. The difference in risk, however, was not large enough to be able to offer much useful advice to the patient on the result of the stress test.

There were a total of 457 acute cardiac events in all over the 7-year period, 62 (or less than 14%) developing during moderate or vigorous activity. No details are given about events that occurred when the patients were not exercising, but earlier reports from the same trial suggest that clinically silent ischemia induced a similar increase of relative risk under resting and exercise conditions.

There remains one further note of caution. The patients were participating in a trial of cholestyramine rather than of exercise therapy, and the prediction of exercise-induced misadventure might have been clearer if patients had a stronger motivation to exercise vigorously. Whereas a stress ECG is not required if a person is only going to make a small increase in habitual physical activity, it may be wise to obtain such information if a patient is contemplating a dramatic change of lifestyle such as a return to serious competition.—R.J. Shephard, M.D., Ph.D.

Logistic Discriminant Analysis Improves Diagnostic Accuracy of Exercise Testing for Coronary Artery Disease in Women
Robert AR, Melin JA, Detry J-MR (University of Louvain Medical School, Brussels)
Circulation 83:1202–1209, 1991   5–15

Introduction.—The exercise ECG in women has a limited accuracy in detecting coronary artery disease. New diagnostic techniques based on computer and multivariate analysis have improved the diagnostic value of exercise testing in men.

Methods.—To determine whether the diagnostic value of exercise testing for women can also be enhanced using multivariate analysis of exer-

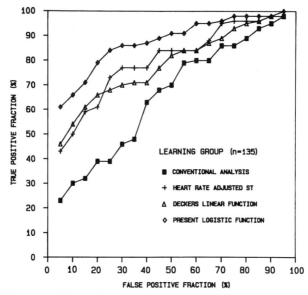

Fig 5-7.—Plot of sensitivities at fixed specificity for the prediction of coronary artery disease for conventional ST depression, heart rate-adjusted ST, discriminant function according to Deckers, and logistic function of the present study in the learning group of 135 catheterized female patients. (Courtesy of Robert AR, Melin JA, Detry J-MR: *Circulation* 83:1202-1209, 1991.)

cise data, 135 infarct-free women underwent cycle-ergometer exercise testing and coronary angiography in 1978-1984; 41% of the sample had significant coronary artery disease. Maximal exercise variables in the first group were analyzed in a stepwise logistic model. The variables selected for use in the diagnostic model were work-rate, heart rate, and $ST_{60}X$. This model was then tested in a second group of 115 catheterized women, 47% of whom had significant coronary artery disease, and 76 volunteers. The model was finally compared with conventional analysis of the exercise ECG, ST changes adjusted for heart rate, and a previously described analysis.

Results.—The current model had a better sensitivity in both groups than did the conventional analysis and the previously described analysis. The current model had a sensitivity of 66% and 70% for the 2 groups, respectively. No specificity was lost, those values being 85% and 93%, respectively. Receiver-operator characteristic curves also showed better accuracy with the current model (Fig 5-7).

Conclusion.—Logistic analysis of exercise variables improves the diagnostic accuracy of exercise testing for women. Sensitivity is significantly improved, with no loss of specificity.

▶ As others have shown previously, the diagnostic accuracy of an exercise stress test can be improved if other information is added to that derived from

ST segmental depression alone. In the present case, the variables proposed are peak work-rate and peak heart rate. The first is related to peak oxygen intake, and is thus the surrogate of stroke volume. The peak heart rate is related to a combination of age and symptom-limitation of effort; given the substantial age-spread of subjects in the present sample (31–59 years) and the marked influence of age on the extent of coronary vascular narrowing, it is surprising that the authors did not try inserting age as a variable into their diagnostic equation. Although the proposed discriminant function has a greater accuracy than a simple reading of ST depression, there is still a long way to go before the exercise stress test has much value for general population screening. For instance, if our goal is to identify 90% of patients with significant coronary narrowing, we will still have about 50% false positive results, so that the tossing of a coin would be just as effective a diagnostic procedure!—R.J. Shephard, M.D., Ph.D.

Usefulness of Severity of Myocardial Ischemia on Exercise Testing in Predicting the Severity of Myocardial Ischemia During Daily Activities

Benhorin J, Moriel M, Gavish A, Medina A, Banai S, Shapira M, Stern S, Tzivoni D (Bikur Cholim Hospital; Hebrew University Hadassah Medical School, Jerusalem)

Am J Cardiol 68:176–180, 1991   5–16

Introduction.—Patients with negative or mildly positive exercise testing responses rarely display spontaneous ischemic episodes during ambulatory ECG monitoring. However, the interrelations between ischemic indexes during exercise testing and ambulatory ECG monitoring among patients with ischemic changes on both tests has not been systematically studied.

Methods.—To determine the relation between myocardial ischemic indices on exercise testing and on ambulatory Holter recording, 60 patients with stable coronary artery disease who had an ischemic response to both testing procedures were studied. All patients performed a Bruce protocol exercise test and underwent 24-hour Holter recording within 2 weeks. No antianginal medications were given.

Results.—The mean exercise duration was 7.4 minutes; the mean heart rate at 1 mm ST depression was 118 beats per minutes; and the mean maximal ST depression during exercise was 2.2 mm. During Holter recording, the average number of ischemic episodes was 4.7 per patient, and the mean duration of daily ischemia was 62 minutes. The mean maximal ST depression was 3.2 mm, and the average heart rate at 1 mm ST depression was 93 beats per minute. Overall, the ischemic indices on both testing procedures was very weakly correlated. Heart rate at 1 mm ST depression was the only exercise variable to be correlated significantly with all Holter variables. However, it correlated very weakly with most Holter covariates, having a stronger correlation only with average heart rate at 1 mm ST depression during Holter monitoring.

Conclusion.—Ischemic indices on exercise testing are not accurate predictors of ischemic indexes on ambulatory Holter monitoring in this patient population. Much of the variability in Holter ischemic indices depends on factors other than those represented by exercise testing indices. Holter recording in the ambulatory setting may provide clinically relevant data in addition to those obtained by exercise testing in certain patient subgroups.

▶ One of the hopes of those undertaking exercise stress tests is that the intensity of exercise at which ST depression is observed in the laboratory will offer useful guidance in setting a safe exercise prescription. However, for this to occur, the increase of blood pressure observed at a given heart rate during treadmill or cycle ergometer exercise would need to match that developed during other forms of physical activity. Unfortunately, exercise is performed in various postures, under varying ambient conditions; small muscles are used as well as large, and there are varying elements of competition and excitement. For these reasons, the correlation between laboratory and "real-life" ECG findings is very weak. Even the closest correlation (the heart rate associated with an ST depression of 1 mm) has a correlation coefficient of only .51; this means that the laboratory test predicts only a quarter of the variance in ST segmental behavior observed while wearing the Holter monitor. If the laboratory test is to provide any guide to the safety of prescribed exercise, then the pattern of the prescribed exercise must match that of the laboratory test rather closely.—R.J. Shephard, M.D., Ph.D.

Exercise-Related Cardiac Arrest in Cardiac Rehabilitation: The Johannesburg Experience
Digenio AG, Sim JGM, Dowdeswell RJ, Morris R (Johannesburg City Health Department; National Institute for Virology, Johannesburg; University of Witwatersrand, Johannesburg)
S Afr Med J 79:188–191, 1991   5–17

Introduction.—Although physical activity is an important part of the rehabilitation of patients with coronary artery disease, exercise also carries the risk of myocardial infarction and cardiac arrest in some patients. The safety of a cardiac rehabilitation program was evaluated and possible factors that could identify patients at risk of sudden death were investigated.

Methods.—In 1982–1988, 1,574 patients were admitted to the study unit. The male/female ratio was 8:1. After undergoing a complete medical history, cardiovascular examination, and a resting ECG, the patients were required to exercise at their prescribed intensity 3 times a week for 30–50 minutes, first at the unit and then at home. They were reevaluated at 6 and 18 months after admission.

Results.—Of the 4 men in whom cardiac arrest resulted from ventricular fibrillation, 3 died despite immediate cardiopulmonary resuscitation and DC defibrillation. All collapsed suddenly during normal exercise. The mean age of the 4 patients was 60.5 years. All were exsmokers and all were thought to have been at low risk for sudden death on admission to the cardiac rehabilitation program. The incidence of cardiac arrest at the study unit (1/120,000) patient hours is similar to that of programs in the United States in 1980–1984.

Conclusion.—Although the usual high risk factors for sudden death were not present in these 4 patients, certain common factors were present: a combination of interior infarction with occluded dominant right coronary artery, good collateralization, and asymptomatic ischemia.

▶ The rate of cardiac incidents reported here is a little higher than the 1 in 300,000 patient hours seen in modern programs in Canada and the United States (1), although given the relatively small number of both patients (1,574) and critical incidents (4), not too much statistical importance should be attached to this difference. It would be helpful to those engaged in cardiac rehabilitation if a reliable indicator could be found that would identify those at risk of death during exercise, but experience in Toronto and elsewhere has proven that this goal is elusive. The one apparently useful pointer noted here (clinically silent exercise-induced ST depression in 3 of 4 patients) has already had considerable discussion (2). Although there is a statistical doubling of the risk of a further cardiac catastrophe in the patient with ST depression, the difference in prognosis is unfortunately not large enough to be helpful in advising the individual patient.—R.J. Shephard, M.D., Ph.D.

References

1. Van Camp SP, Peterson RA: *JAMA* 256:1160, 1986.
2. Shephard RJ: *Sports Med* 1:75, 1984.

Exercise Capability Failure: Is Cardiac Output Important After All?
Cowley AJ, Fullwood LJ, Muller AF, Stainer K, Skene AM, Hampton JR (University Hospital, Queen's Medical Centre, Nottingham, England)
Lancet 337:771–773, 1991   5–18

Background.—The lack of correlation between measures of cardiac function and maximum exercise capability may be partly the result of the inappropriateness of the exercise test. The relationship between a noninvasive measure of cardiac output and different forms of exercise tests was studied in 39 patients with moderately severe chronic heart failure.

Methods and Results.—Several methods were used to assess the patients' exercise ability, which was then compared with measures of cardiac output. Cardiac index and exercise tolerance measured on a treadmill were poorly correlated. However, exercise tolerance determined by

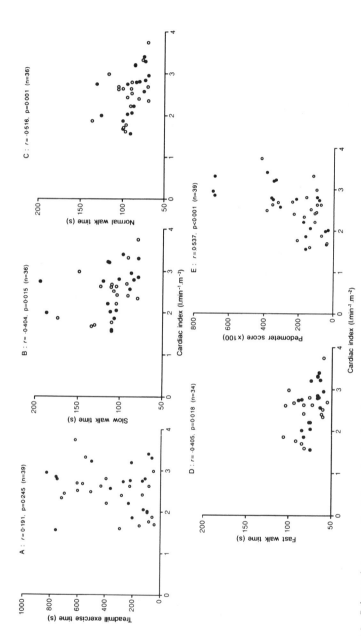

Fig 5–8.—Relations between cardiac index and various exercise tests in patients taking diuretics only (*filled circles*) and in patients taking diuretics and angiotensin-converting enzyme inhibitors (*open circles*). (Courtesy of Cowley AJ, Fullwood LJ, Muller AF, et al: *Lancet* 337:771–773, 1991.)

a series of self-paced corridor walk tests was moderately correlated with cardiac index. Customary activity assessed by step counting was better correlated with cardiac index (Fig 5–8).

Conclusions.—The type of exercise used to assess severity of heart failure appears to be extremely important. Tests that better represent a patient's normal activities may correlate best with direct measures of cardiac performance. Cardiac output may be a factor that determines patients' exercise capability when they choose their own walking speed but not when they are subjected to formal treadmill tests in the laboratory.

▶ I have always been a little puzzled why patients who are in moderately compensated congestive cardiac failure show so little correlation between measures of aerobic performance such as the maximal oxygen intake and measures of cardiac function such as the determinations of ejection fraction at rest and during standard exercise tests (1). One factor is undoubtedly that many of the clinical measurements of cardiac performance are done with the patient lying supine or semisupine; adoption of this posture inevitably has a large effect on venous return and thus both the resting stroke volume and the increment in stroke volume during exercise. A second concern is the use of ejection fraction, rather than a more direct measure of cardiac performance such as stroke volume or cardiac output. The present study obviated this problem by making observations on cardiac output, using the carbon dioxide rebreathing procedure at seated rest and during the first stage of treadmill walking. The third factor is the limited precision of treadmill testing when dealing with a patient who has a low peak oxygen intake; often, the treadmill exercise is halted by the onset of dyspnea rather than by the performance of the cardiac pump. Cowley and associates suggest this may be why they found a correlation coefficient of .52 between the resting cardiac index and the pace of walking, but the coefficient between treadmill endurance time and resting cardiac output was only .19. For technical reasons, they were only able to measure the exercise cardiac output at light work-rates, and even then in only a few of their subjects. But the findings do suggest that the best laboratory evaluation of exercise tolerance would be linked in some way to a determination of cardiac stroke volume in vigorous but submaximal exercise.—R.J. Shephard, M.D., Ph.D.

Reference

1. Franciosa JA, et al: *Am J Cardiol* 47:33, 1981.

Psychophysical Power Functions of Exercise Limiting Symptoms in Coronary Heart Disease
Sylvén C, Borg G, Holmgren A, Åström H (Huddinge University Hospital, Sweden; Stockholm University; Karolinska Hospital, Stockholm)
Med Sci Sports Exerc 23:1050–1054, 1991   5–19

Introduction.—Exercise stress tests are used objectively to measure physical capacity and its relation to perceptual modalities such as perceived general exertion, leg exertion, breathlessness, and chest pain. The purpose of the present study was to characterize the stimulus-response relations between exercise load and chest pain, leg exertion, and breathlessness and to assess the interrelation of these symptoms in patients with severe coronary heart disease (CHD) and in healthy controls of similar age.

Study design.—Thirty men with angiographically confirmed multivessel disease and 10 healthy volunteers underwent symptom-limited exercise testing on a cycle ergometer with stepwise increments of 10 W every minute. Chest pain, leg exertion, and breathlessness were rated every minute with the use of a 10-level category-ratio scale (CR-10), and psychophysical power functions were computed.

Results.—All patients with CHD had symptom-limited exercise capacity, 20 because of chest pain and 10 because of leg exertion or breathlessness. Both patient groups interrupted the exercise test at lower workrates and at lower symptom intensities than did healthy controls. Exercise capacity did not differ between those who terminated for chest pain and those who terminated for leg exertion or breathlessness. Patients and controls had similar psychophysical power functions for leg exertion. The growth of breathlessness was slower in patients who terminated for leg exertion or breathlessness than it was in patients who terminated for chest pain. The intensity of chest pain increased more rapidly than did leg exertion or breathlessness in patients who terminated for chest pain (Fig 5–9).

CR-10

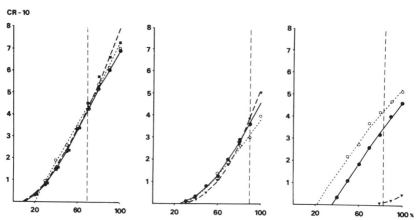

Fig 5–9.—Psychophysical power functions (indexed medians) of general perceived exertion (*squares*), leg exertion (*open circles*), breathlessness (*filled circles*), and pain (*triangles*) according to CR-10 scale (y-axis) and relative to exercise load in percent of symptom limited load (x-axis). General perceived exertion was evaluated only in patient groups. Vertical lines indicate 100 W. *Left,* 10 healthy controls; *center,* 20 patients who ended exercise test because of chest pain; *right,* 10 patients who ended test because of leg exertion or breathlessness, or both (Courtesy of Sylvén C, Borg G, Holmgren A, et al: *Med Sci Sports Exerc* 23:1050–1054, 1991.)

Conclusion.—Patients with CHD interrupt exercise stress testing at lower ratings of leg exertion and breathlessness than do healthy volunteers. The psychophysical power functions do not grow more rapidly for these sensory modalities in patients with CHD than they do in healthy volunteers.

▶ In theory, there seem a number of reasons why symptoms should grow more rapidly in the patient with severe cardiac disease than in a healthy person. Backward failure of the heart may cause a rising pulmonary capillary pressure, decreasing pulmonary compliance and enhancing breathlessness. Forward failure may impair the blood flow to the active muscles, increasing the accumulation of anaerobic metabolites at any given rate of working, and myocardial ischemia may cause anginal pain, exacerbating overall discomfort.

In practice, the present authors found lower ratings of general exertion, leg exertion, and breathlessness in the cardiac patients than in their controls, but this may reflect difficulties in comparing the data sets. Graphs are here plotted (as is usually the case) relative to the percentage of peak aerobic effort; however, such a basis of comparison becomes fallible if the peak work-rate is very low because of either poor general condition or the onset of chest pain.—R.J. Shephard, M.D., Ph.D.

Tracking of Elevated Blood Pressure Values in Adolescent Athletes at 1-Year Follow-Up
Tanji JL (Univ of California, Davis Med Ctr, Sacramento)
Am J Dis Child 145:665–667, 1991   5–20

Background.—Although borderline hypertension may exist for many years, the diagnosis is often not made until the third or fourth decade. This is partly because young people, particularly adolescents, do not often seek medical attention. Results of preparticipation physical examinations for high school sports were used to determine whether elevated blood pressures at this examination correlated with elevated blood pressures at 1-year follow-up.

Methods.—Examinations were done on 467 adolescents, 359 boys and 108 girls, mean age 16.2 years. Approximately 62% of the sample was white. Screening history and physical examination were done according to a published format. When significant elevations in blood pressure were found, follow-up checks were made within 3 months. Four hundred thirty-six subjects were reexamined after 1 year.

Results.—Significant elevations of blood pressure were found in 12.2% of patients. Of those patients, 79.6% had persistently elevated blood pressures at follow-up. There was a positive association between family history of hypertension and elevated blood pressure in 80.7% of cases, compared with 5.6% of controls. Mean body weight was 94.5 kg in the hypertensive group, compared with 75.2 kg in normotensive subjects. The hypertensive patients were also more likely to do heavy resistance training (71.9%) than the normotensive subjects (15.8%).

Conclusions.—Elevated blood pressure in adolescents can be detected by routine preparticipation examinations for high school sports. Stratification of blood pressures may begin before adulthood. A continued follow-up of this cohort in a prospective, longitudinal study to determine when the diagnosis of hypertension is made.

▶ This worthwhile project examined the prevalance of elevated blood pressure readings during preparticipation physical examinations of 467 adolescents who came out for high school sports. Nearly 1 in 8 had an elevated pressure (i.e., 142 mm Hg systolic or greater and 92 mm Hg diastolic or greater). Higher blood pressures were associated with a family history of hypertension, with heavier body weight, and with heavy resistance weight training. This latter association was unexplained, but the author specified that he used appropriate cuff sizes for arm sizes, and speculated about a possible link between high blood pressure and the illicit use of anabolic steroids among some weight lifters. At a 1-year follow-up, 80% of those with an initially high blood pressure continued to have a high blood pressure. As suggested by this study, team physicians can help in the early diagnosis of hypertension in young people.—E.R. Eichner, M.D.

Effects of Endurance Training on Baroreflex Sensitivity and Blood Pressure in Borderline Hypertension
Somers VK, Conway J, Johnston J, Sleight P (John Radcliffe Hospital, Oxford, England)
Lancet 337:1363–1368, 1991   5–21

Background.—Physical training is a potential nonpharmacologic strategy for controlling mild and borderline hypertension. However, its effect on blood pressure is still debated. The impact of endurance training on waking and sleeping blood pressure and baroreflex sensitivity in borderline hypertensive persons was studied.

Methods.—Eight patients were evaluated before and after a 6-month endurance training program. When it was clear that blood pressures were lower after training, another 8 patients were studied. This latter group was assessed at the end of the training and after 4 months' abstention from exercise. Baroflex sensitivity, blood pressure, R-R interval, and blood pressure and R-R variability were measured. Ambulatory blood pressures were measured in 7 trained and 6 detrained subjects, and sleep blood pressures were measured in 3 trained and 3 detrained subjects.

Results.—Increased fitness was associated with a decrease in resting arterial blood pressure of 9.7 mm Hg systolic and 6.8 mm Hg diastolic. It was associated with an ambulatory blood pressure drop of 4.8 mm Hg

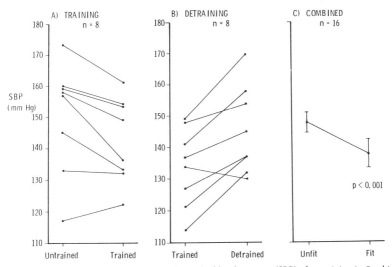

Fig 5–10.—Changes in resting intra-arterial systolic blood pressure (SBP) after training in 8 subjects (*left*), after detraining in 8 subjects (*middle*), and in combined changes with fitness for group of 16 (*right*). (Courtesy of Somers VK, Conway J, Johnston J, et al: *Lancet* 337:1363–1368, 1991.)

and 7.5 mm Hg, respectively. Baroreflex sensitivity was 14 ms/mm Hg in the detrained and 17.5 ms/mm Hg in the trained subjects. Despite longer sleep R-R intervals, sleep blood pressures were not lower in the trained group (Figs 5–10 and 5–11).

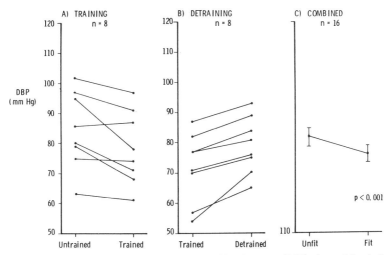

Fig 5–11.—Changes in resting intra-arterial diastolic blood pressure (DBP) after training in 8 subjects (*left*), after detraining in 8 subjects (*middle*), and in combined changes with fitness for group of 16 (*right*). (Courtesy of Somers VK, Conway J, Johnston J, et al: *Lancet* 337:1363–1368, 1991.)

Conclusions.—Endurance training lowers daytime blood pressure during both rest and activity. It also increases baroreflex sensitivity and R-R interval variability. Despite prolonged R-R interval during sleep, endurance training does not reduce sleep blood pressure.

▶ It is interesting that Somers and associates began their experiments from the viewpoint that the potential effect of training on blood pressure is controversial. In an exhaustive review of the topic, Tipton (1) wrote "it is no longer good scholarship or grantsmanship to state that exercise training will result in increases, decreases or no change in resting arterial blood pressure." Plainly, it takes some time for knowledge to percolate from the exercise scientists to the rarefied atmosphere of the *Lancet.* It is even more remarkable that the views of the present authors (and presumably the editors of the *Lancet*) were changed as the result of studies on 8 subjects. The decrease in waking blood pressure with training is of the order seen in substantial meta analyses. One nice feature of the experiment conducted on a further 8 patients was that blood pressures were measured after both training and detraining. Other useful features of the report are the demonstration of a decrease in baroreflex sensitivity, the recording of ambulatory pressures, and the comments regarding the absence of a change in pressures recorded during sleep. The last finding was explained on the basis that the sleeping blood pressure was already at a "floor" level, and thus could not be further reduced by training. This seems probable because initial ambulatory diastolic values dropped from 91 mm Hg to only 66 mm Hg during the night.—R.J. Shephard, M.D., Ph.D.

Reference

1. Tipton CM: *Exerc Sport Sci Rev* 19:447, 1991.

Changes of Blood Pressure and Lipid Pattern During a Physical Training Course in Hypertensive Subjects
Filipovský J, Šimon J, Chrástek J, Rosolová H, Haman P, Petříková V (Charles University, Plzeň; Czechoslovakia; Research Institute of Balneology, Mariánské Lázně, Czechoslovakia; University Hospital, Plzeň)
Cardiology 78:31–38, 1991   5–22

Objective.—Physical activity is an important component of nonpharmacologic management of hypertension. A study was conducted to determine the influence of an intensive physical training program in patients with hypertension and predominantly low leisure-time physical activity.

Methods.—Changes in several cardiovascular and biochemical parameters were monitored during a 5-week physical training course in 77 hypertensive patients with a predominantly sedentary way of life. Blood pressure (BP) exceeded 160/95 mm Hg in all patients. Antihypertensive

Changes in BP, Serum Lipids, Uricemia, and BMI

	I (n = 77)	II (n = 77)	III (n = 70)	Paired t tests		
				II vs. I (n = 77)	III vs. I (n = 70)	III vs. II (n = 70)
Systolic BP, mm Hg	156.8 ± 20.1	142.5 ± 19.9	161.6 ± 18.1	< 0.001	< 0.05	< 0.001
Diastolic BP, mm Hg	97.8 ± 10.5	89.2 ± 11.4	101.8 ± 11.5	< 0.001	< 0.01	< 0.001
TC, mmol/l	5.79 ± 0.82	4.68 ± 0.83	5.90 ± 1.11	< 0.001	NS	< 0.001
TG, mmol/l	2.07 ± 1.23	1.35 ± 0.56	1.61 ± 0.86	< 0.001	< 0.001	< 0.05
HDL-C, mmol/l	1.49 ± 0.49	1.35 ± 0.33	1.27 ± 0.22	< 0.001	< 0.001	< 0.05
HDL-C/TC ratio	0.262 ± 0.009	0.295 ± 0.005	0.220 ± 0.002	< 0.001	< 0.001	< 0.001
LDL-C, mmol/l	3.89 ± 0.89	3.06 ± 0.77	4.31 ± 1.01	< 0.001	< 0.001	< 0.001
Uric acid, µmol/l	345.6 ± 84.4	311.5 ± 73.9	313.5 ± 89.9	< 0.01	< 0.01	NS
BMI, kg/m^2	29.0 ± 3.5	27.4 ± 3.2	28.0 ± 1.0	< 0.001	< 0.001	< 0.001

Note: values are mean ±SD. *I* indicates values at admission; *II* values at the end of the intervention; *III*, values at follow-up.
(Courtesy of Filipovský J, Šimon J, Chrástek J, et al: *Cardiology* 78:31–38, 1991.)

medications were withdrawn from all but 25 patients. A low-cholesterol diet was recommended. Follow-up examinations were also performed an average of 15 months after the intervention.

Results.—At the end of the intervention, both systolic and diastolic BP were reduced significantly in 58 patients (75.3%) regardless of age, sex, duration of hypertension, previous BP levels, and antihypertensive drug therapy (table). There was a strong negative correlation between initial uricemia and the reduction in diastolic BP. The reduction in BP correlated positively with an increase in maximum oxygen uptake per kilogram during the intervention. In addition, serum levels of total cholesterol (TC), triglycerides (TG), high-density lipoprotein cholesterol (HDL-C), and uric acid as well as body mass index (BMI) were significantly reduced, and the HDL-C/TC ratio significantly increased after the intervention. These favorable changes were of short duration, disappearing 3 to 7 months after the intervention, except for BMI and TG and uric acid levels.

Conclusion.—A 5-week intensive physical training program provides a favorable but short-lived effect on BP and lipid patterns in the majority of hypertensive patients.

▶ A variety of authors have now demonstrated that exercise training induces a therapeutically useful reduction of blood pressure in hypertensive patients as well as in normotensive patients. For a very thorough review of this topic, please see reference (1). However, mechanisms remain uncertain. At first inspection, the relationship here reported between maximal oxygen intake and the decrease of diastolic pressure seems interesting. However, the correlation is quite weak (r=.29). The gain of maximal oxygen intake itself seems a little suspect, because the maximal work capacity increased only from 147 to 151 W, and the training period was rather short for much training to have occurred (despite what seems to have been a substantial weekly energy expenditure, in the European spa tradition). Further studies are needed, using a control group, and with training continued for longer than 5 weeks.—R.J. Shephard, M.D., Ph.D.

Reference

1. Tipton CM: *Exerc Sport Sci Rev* 19:447, 1991.

Abnormal Blood Pressure Response to Exercise in Borderline Hypertension: A Two-Year Follow-Up Study

Guerrera G, Melina D, Colivicchi F, Santoliquido A, Guerrera G, Folli G (Università Cattolica del Sacro Cuore, Rome)
Am J Hypertens 4:271–273, 1991   5–23

Background.—Borderline hypertension (BH) affects at least 10% of adults in Western cultures. Exercise blood pressure (BP) is considered a better indicator of the total BP burden during ordinary daily activities than resting BP. The prevalence of an abnormal BP response to exercise was assessed in a cohort of subjects with BH.

Data From the Initial Maximal Exercise Testing		
	Group 1 **(13 Subjects)**	**Group 2** **(15 Subjects)**
Maximal exertion SBP (mm Hg)	205 ± 9.67	222 ± 5.38*
Maximal exertion DBP (mm Hg)	92 ± 3.62	110 ± 4.47*
Maximal exertion HR (beats/min)	180 ± 6.20	180 ± 4.08†
Maximal workload (W)	181 ± 17.41	187 ± 15.45†
5th min recovery SBP (mm Hg)	145 ± 4.98	163 ± 5.35*
5th min recovery DBP (mm Hg)	87 ± 2.70	98 ± 2.20*
5th min recovery HR (beats/min)	95 ± 2.85	96 ± 3.84†

Abbreviations: SBP, systolic blood pressure; *DBP,* diastolic blood pressure; *HR,* heart rate.
* P < .001.
† No significant differences between the 2 study groups.
Group 1, normal blood pressure response to exercise; Group 2, abnormal blood pressure response to exercise.
(Courtesy of Guerrera G, Melina D, Colivicchi F, et al: *Am J Hypertens* 4:271-273, 1991.)

Methods.—Twenty-eight men underwent maximal exercise testing and were followed up for 2 years. All had BH according to the criteria of the World Health Organization.

Findings.—Fifteen men, or 53.6%, had abnormal BP behavior during exercise. Hypertension developed in 63% of those with an abnormal BP response to exercise and in only 15% of those with normal BP behavior. Maximal exercise testing had a sensitivity of 83.3% in predicting established hypertension development over 2 years. Its specificity, accuracy, positive predictive value, and negative predictive value were 68.8%, 75%, 66.7%, and 84.6%, respectively (table).

Conclusions.—These findings suggest that maximal exercise testing may be a useful clinical tool for identifying BH patients likely to develop established hypertension in the next few years. Because such testing requires special equipment and qualified personnel, further research is needed to define the cost-effectiveness of such an approach to BH management.

▶ Whereas the measurement of resting blood pressure is a well-established component of an office clinical examination, problems arise because a substantial proportion of patients fall in the "grey" area, where there is a suspicion of hypertension. The situation is further complicated, because many such individuals show a normal blood pressure if observations are repeated by a nurse or paramedical professional in a less threatening situation such as a fitness clinic or their own homes (1,2). Nevertheless, the fact that such individuals react adversely to a doctor's office may be a significant observation in itself. The present report suggests that a substantial proportion of such subjects have the further warning sign of an abnormal blood pressure response to exercise, with progression to established hypertension over the next two years. Although Guerrera et al. go on to calculate the sensitivity and specificity of such responses, the sample size (28 maximal tests and a 2-year follow-up) is not really adequate for their purpose. The findings have sufficient interest that further observations are warranted on larger samples.—R.J. Shephard, M.D., Ph.D.

References

1. Shephard RJ, et al: *Can J Public Health* 72:37, 1981.
2. Young MA, et al: *BMJ* 286:1235, 1983.

Blood Pressure Response to Exercise in Normotensives and Hypertensives
Franz I-W (Klinik Wehrawald der BfA, Berlin)
Can J Sport Sci 16:296–301, 1991   5–24

Introduction.—Systemic blood pressure (BP) is a highly variable parameter that can fluctuate markedly with the time of day and the momentary physical and emotional state of the individual. Because resting BP does not reflect the excessive increments of BP that occur in response to stress and exercise, one cannot determine from the resting BP whether complications of hypertension are related to the severity of physical stress-linked BP elevations.

Discussion.—Individuals with hypertension have lower cardiac outputs and stroke volumes, higher heart rates, and a markedly higher peripheral resistance than do normotensive persons at the same intensity of exercise. Patients with hypertension raise their BP excessively, even at very low levels of exertion. Even persons with mildly elevated resting BPs may experience alarming increases in BP when stressed by exercise, thus markedly increasing their myocardial oxygen demand during exercise. Because oxygen demand is determined not only by pressure load but also by the degree of ventricular hypertrophy, the following recommendations are made with regard to prescribing physical training for individuals with hypertension: Endurance training offers persons with hypertension a means of lowering exercise heart rate, reducing systolic BP and myocardial oxygen consumption, and improving physical work capacity. Recommendations for physical training should never be based on resting BP. All individuals with hypertension should undergo ergometric testing before embarking on an exercise program to avoid possible risks associated with the training. If ergometric testing shows a marked rise in BP at low levels of exertion, appropriate antihypertensive medications should be prescribed before initiating training. Antihypertensive drug efficacy should be assessed by pretraining ergometry.

▶ An excessive rise of blood pressure during exercise frequently serves as a warning that a person with a somewhat marginal resting blood pressure is at risk of developing hypertension. In established hypertension, the rise can be quite alarming. The author cites an example of 20 patients with an average resting pressure of 163/103 mm Hg who developed pressures averaging 240/126 after climbing only 4 flights of stairs. Such pressures can precipitate severe myocardial ischemia, particularly as the oxygen demand of the heart in such individuals is often augmented by cardiac hypertrophy.

In keeping with a number of reports from elsewhere, a training regimen reduced the adverse exercise response. However, it is also worth noting the recent criticism that, whereas exercise training reduces resting and exercise pressures, it does not seem to change the underlying anomaly and thus the basal or sleeping pressures.—R.J. Shephard, M.D., Ph.D.

Failure of Exercise to Reduce Blood Pressure in Patients With Mild Hypertension: Results of a Randomized Controlled Trial
Blumenthal JA, Siegel WC, Appelbaum M (Duke Univ, Durham, NC; New England Deaconess Hosp, Boston; Vanderbilt Univ, Nashville)
JAMA 266:2098–2104, 1991   5–25

Background.—Hypertension affects 18% of white adults and 35% of black adults in the United States. Antihypertensive therapy to minimize end-organ damage may include drug therapy and nonpharmacologic therapies (e.g., exercise and diet). The evidence suggests that exercise may be beneficial for patients with elevated blood pressure, but only 4 small, randomized, controlled trials of exercise have been conducted. The effects of aerobic training and strength training on blood pressure were assessed.

Methods.—In a randomized, controlled trial 99 male and female volunteers with untreated mild hypertension were assigned to a 4-month program of either aerobic exercise training or strength and flexibility training, or to a waiting-list control group. The groups were advised to make no changes in their diet or exercise behavior. Systolic and diastolic blood pressures were measured 4 times with a random zero sphygmomanometer on 3 separate days in a clinic setting.

Findings.—Small but statistically significant reductions in blood pressure occurred in all 3 groups, with no clear advantage for the subjects assigned to aerobic exercise. A differential decline of 5 mm Hg had been expected between the aerobic exercise and control groups. However, mean blood pressure differences in the 2 groups were only -1 mm Hg for systolic blood pressure and -1.2 at $\alpha = .05$ for diastolic blood pressure.

Conclusions.—Moderate aerobic exercise without dietary changes in nonobese patients with mild hypertension offers little benefit. A prescription of moderate levels of aerobic exercise should not be considered a replacement for pharmacologic therapy of hypertension. This was the first study to measure blood pressure in the clinic, in the laboratory during both exercise and mental stress testing, and in the usual environment with ambulatory monitoring.

▶ One recent review (1) concluded that the beneficial effect of exercise had now been clearly established, both for normotensive and for mildly hypertensive subjects. The present article does not cite this review, nor does it mention a meta analysis by Hagberg (2), which reached essentially similar conclusions to those of Tipton.

The present study was of 16 weeks' duration, and the gain in aerobic power was appreciable (from 31.8 to 36.9 mL/kg.min in the group receiving aerobic training). The negative results thus cannot be dismissed as being the result of an insufficient level of training. The authors were insistent on subjects maintaining a constant diet, and there was no change of body mass over the 16-week period. Given the close interaction between body mass and hypertension, it may be that some of the other studies where positive results have been reported induced a small decrease of body mass, and this was responsible for the decrease of blood pressures. The present authors conclude from their experiments that exercise should not be recommended as the primary treatment for mild hypertension. However, by insisting that weight be maintained at an above optimal level (82 kg, body mass index

27.2 kg/m², they were imposing an artificial constraint on their subjects. In the more reasonable situation where people were allowed to regress to an optimal body mass, benefit might well be obtained from an exercise regimen without recourse to drastic pharmacologic interventions.—R.J. Shephard, M.D., Ph.D.

References

1. Tipton CM: *Exerc Sport Sci Rev* 9:447, 1991.
2. Hagberg JM: in Bouchard C, et al (eds): *Exercise, Fitness and Health*. Champaign, Ill: Human Kinetics Publ, 1990.

Lone Atrial Fibrillation: It Needn't Slow Down an Active Patient
Cantwell JD, Lammert S, Kessler C (Georgia Baptist Med Ctr, Atlanta; Medical College of Georgia, Augusta)
Physician Sportsmed 19:71–82, 1991   5–26

Introduction.—Atrial fibrillation (AF) in the absence of rheumatic valvular disease is a common cardiac rhythm disturbance. However, it is not entirely benign because of an increased risk of stroke. Epidemiologic studies reported that more than 1 million Americans experience lone AF, and that 75,000 strokes per year are associated with it. The case reports of 8 apparently normal, physically active men who had AF were reviewed.

Patients.—Seven patients were regular endurance exercisers and 1 was a professional athlete. Triggers for AF included exercise and the consumption of coffee, caffeinated soft drinks, alcohol, ice-cold water, and ice cream. All patients had normal findings on physical examination, which included a thorough cardiac examination. None of the patients had clinical hyperthyroidism. Most patients were able to prevent recurrence by avoiding the triggers. However, 1 patient with persistent paroxysmal AF eventually suffered a right temporoparietal brain infarction, followed 20 months later by a more severe stroke that resulted in loss of speech and right-sided hemiparesis. He had been treated prophylactically over a 5-year period with a variety of anti-arrhythmic agents that failed to prevent frequent recurrences of AF.

Conclusion.—Atrial fibrillation is not a contraindication for vigorous athletic activity. In most cases, avoidance of precipitating factors will be sufficient. All patients with episodes of AF are advised to take 1 buffered aspirin tablet daily unless contraindicated. Anti-arrhythmic agents are indicated when AF persists.

▶ This is an informative and practical clinical article on how to deal with lone AF in athletic patients. Emphasis is on the common precipitating and contributing factors, including not only thyroid problems and exercise or emotion itself, but also cold drinks, ice cream, and common drugs like alcohol and caffeine. Reviewed within are the key studies on the risk of stroke among patients with AF. The studies suggest that, for chronic AF in a general medical population, warfarin may be slightly more effective than aspirin in preventing stroke. No study, however, is definitive on the relative merits of warfarin versus aspirin, and guidelines are even more uncertain for athletes with intermittent AF, who probably are at very low risk of stroke. Certainly, especially among athletes, warfarin would seem to carry a higher risk of bleeding than aspirin. The largest study, the Stroke Prevention in Atrial Fibrillation study, is still ongoing, and early results, as recently reviewed (1), do not allow a direct comparison of aspirin with warfarin, because there have been too few events among the patients in these 2 groups. Pritchett says that AF patients under 60 years old with no other clinical heart disease and no risk factors such as hypertension need no anticoagulation. Yet the advice here of 1 buffered aspirin a day unless contraindicated seems practical and prudent. Also included are other common sense guidelines on management.—E.R. Eichner, M.D.

Reference

1. Pritchett ELC: N Engl J Med 326:1264, 1992.

Maximum Intensity Exercise Training in Patients With Chronic Obstructive Pulmonary Disease

Punzal PA, Ries AL, Kaplan RM, Prewitt LM (Univ of California, San Diego)

Chest 100:618–623, 1991   5–27

Background.—For patients with chronic obstructive pulmonary disease (COPD), pulmonary rehabilitation, including exercise, can alleviate symptoms and improve function. However, there is controversy about the selection of appropriate exercise intensity targets for these patients. A randomized clinical trial was conducted to assess the value of and to create guidelines for high-intensity, symptom-limited endurance exercise training for these patients.

Methods.—The study sample was comprised of 52 patients with COPD who were taking part in a pulmonary rehabilitation program. Patients' mean age was 61.6 years. All patients were in stable condition, with moderate to severe disease and reduced exercise tolerance with ventilatory limitation. Patients first performed an incremental maximum treadmill exercise test, from which they were assigned a target work load of 95% of their baseline maximum treadmill work load. Training consisted of daily walking at this target level for 8 weeks. Training was supervised twice weekly for the first 4 weeks and once weekly for the last 4 weeks. Patients were followed up by pulmonary function testing and repeat maximum and endurance exercise testing.

Results.—At baseline, mean maximum treadmill work load was 4.7 metabolic equivalents. Patients were exercising at 85% of baseline maximum at 1 week, 84% at 4 weeks, and 86% at 8 weeks. After training, maximum work load had increased to 6.2 metabolic equivalents, maximum oxygen consumption per minute increased from 1.25 to 1.37 L/ minute, and endurance exercise time increased from 12.1 to 22 minutes. The 34 patients who did not reach anaerobic threshold reached 100% of their target work load compared with 85% for the 18 patients who did reach anaerobic threshold. However, these 2 groups had similar improvements in exercise performance and reduction of symptoms.

Conclusions.—For patients with moderate to severe COPD, exercise training can be at symptom-limited intensity levels that represent higher percentages of maximum than are normally recommended. Many patients, especially those with more severe disease and ventilatory limitations, can approach or even exceed their maximum level before training.

▶ The term $\dot{V}o_{2max}$ is widely used in the clinical literature, but it would probably be preferable to talk about peak oxygen intake when the treadmill performance of subjects such as the present sample is limited by a combination of anxiety and unpleasant symptoms rather than by a plateauing of cardiac function. It is difficult to envisage a true maximal oxygen intake when subjects have not even reached their anaerobic threshold! The study nevertheless points to the practical gains that can be realized when patients with chronic obstructive pulmonary disease are encouraged to exercise regularly at a level very close to this subjective limit.—R.J. Shephard, M.D., Ph.D.

Body Composition and Exercise Performance in Patients With Chronic Obstructive Pulmonary Disease
Schols AMWJ, Mostert R, Soeters PB, Wouters EFM (University of Limburg, Maastricht, The Netherlands; Asthma Centre, "Hornerheide," Horn, The Netherlands)
Thorax 46:695–699, 1991   5–28

Background.—Respiratory factors may impair the exercise capacity of patients with chronic obstructive pulmonary disease. Also, a compromised nutritional state may contribute to reduced exercise performance. Whether a compromised nutritional state limits exercise performance was investigated in patients with chronic obstructive pulmonary disease.

Patients.—Fifty-four patients with chronic obstructive pulmonary disease had severe airflow obstruction and an arterial oxygen tension of greater than 7.3 kPa. All patients were taking maintenance treatment, including theophylline, β_2 agonists, and inhaled or oral corticosteroids. The fat-free mass was assessed by skinfold measurements at 4 sites and by bioelectric impedance. Exercise performance was assessed from a walking test with the distance covered being measured after 2, 6, and 12 minutes.

Moving?

I'd like to receive my *Year Book of Sports Medicine* without interruption.

Please note the following change of address, effective: _____

Name: _____

New Address: _____

_____

City: _____ State: _____ Zip: _____

Old Address: _____

_____

City: _____ State: _____ Zip: _____

Reservation Card

Yes, I would like my own copy of the *Year Book of Sports Medicine*. Please begin my subscription with the current edition according to the terms described below.* I understand that I will have 30 days to examine each annual edition. If satisfied, I will pay just $59.95 plus sales tax, postage and handling (price subject to change without notice).

Name: _____

Address: _____

City: _____ State: _____ Zip: _____

Method of Payment

❑ Visa   ❑ Mastercard   ❑ AmEx   ❑ Bill me   ❑ Check (in US dollars, payable to Mosby-Year Book, Inc.)

Card number _____ Exp date _____

Signature _____

LS-0907

Your Year Book Service Guarantee:

When you subscribe to the *Year Book*, we'll send you an advance notice of future volumes about two months before they publish. This automatic notice system is designed to take up as little of your time as possible. If you do not want the *Year Book*, the advance notice makes it quick and easy for you to let us know your decision; and you will always have at least 20 days to decide. If we don't hear from you, we'll send you the new volume as soon as it's available. And, of course, the *Year Book* is yours to examine free of charge for 30 days (postage, handling and applicable sales tax are added to each shipment).

BUSINESS REPLY MAIL

FIRST CLASS MAIL   PERMIT No. 762   CHICAGO, IL

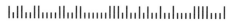

POSTAGE WILL BE PAID BY ADDRESSEE

Chris Hughes
Mosby-Year Book, Inc.
200 N. LaSalle Street
Suite 2600
Chicago, IL 60601-9981

‖‖₁‖‖₁₁₁‖‖₁‖‖₁₁₁₁‖‖‖₁‖₁‖₁₁‖₁‖₁₁₁‖‖‖₁₁₁‖

BUSINESS REPLY MAIL

FIRST CLASS MAIL   PERMIT No. 762   CHICAGO, IL

POSTAGE WILL BE PAID BY ADDRESSEE

Chris Hughes
Mosby-Year Book, Inc.
200 N. LaSalle Street
Suite 2600
Chicago, IL 60601-9981

‖‖₁‖‖₁₁₁‖‖₁‖‖₁₁₁₁‖‖‖₁‖₁‖₁₁‖₁‖₁₁₁‖‖‖₁₁₁‖

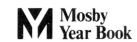

Mosby
Year Book

Dedicated to publishing excellence.

Findings.—The measures of body composition by bioelectric impedance and other measures had a high correlation, and the 2 measures of fat-free mass had good correlation. In 12 minutes of walking the mean distance covered was 845 m. There was good correlation between the distance walked and fat-free mass and total body mass in the whole group. Distance walked and fat-free mass also showed good correlation in a subgroup of 23 lean patients. On stepwise regression analysis, fat-free mass estimated by bioelectric impedance, maximal inspiratory mouth pressure, and arterial oxygen tension accounted for 60% of the variation in the distance covered in 12 minutes of walking.

Conclusion.—Although there was good correlation between body mass and the distance walked, the correlation between fat-free mass and walking distance was better. Fat-free mass, or muscle mass, is an important determinant of exercise performance in patients with severe chronic obstructive pulmonary disease, independent of the degree of airflow obstruction.

▶ Exercise training is often quite helpful to the patient with chronic obstructive pulmonary disease (COPD), but investigators have been puzzled as to why this should be so. There seems no inherent reason to expect any reversal of the pulmonary destruction in response to an exercise program, and tests of pulmonary function are generally unchanged at the end of a period of training. Small gains of performance may result from improvements in the mechanical efficiency of both walking and breathing, but as Mertens and associates first pointed out, much of the benefit from an exercise program can be attributed to a strengthening of the skeletal muscles (1). As these contract at a small fraction of their maximal voluntary force, there is a lesser accumulation of lactate, and ventilatory demand is reduced. This breaks the vicious cycle of dyspnea, anxiety, increasing inactivity, muscle weakening, and a further increment of dyspnea. The present paper demonstrates the importance of muscle mass to performance rather nicely, using the bioimpedance technique. However, for those who do not have access to such equipment, it is worth noting that gains of total body mass also reflect muscle strengthening, albeit a little less accurately. The practical lesson is that the patient with COPD should be encouraged to undertake regular resisted exercises to strengthen the main muscles of the body.—R.J. Shephard, M.D., Ph.D.

Reference

1. Mertens DJ: *Respiration* 35:96, 1978.

Psychological and Respiratory Physiological Effects of a Physical Exercise Programme on Boys With Severe Asthma

Engström I, Fällström K, Karlberg E, Sten G, Bjure J (Gothenburg University, Sweden)

Acta Paediatr Scand 80:1058–1065, 1991   5–29

Background.—Physical exercise programs for children with asthma are an important adjunct to pharmacologic treatment and environmental control. Pulmonary function has improved only marginally in several studies, but the programs have produced improved physical fitness and psychological gains. The immediate and long-term effects of a physical exercise program on pulmonary function and personality structure were evaluated in 10 boys with severe perennial asthma.

Methods.—Ten boys aged 9–12 years with severe perennial asthma participated in an 8-month program of gymnastics and swimming. Pulmonary function and psychological tests were performed before training, immediately after, and 1 year after the end of the exercise program. Indicators for pulmonary function were static lung volume, flow-volume variables, and histamine tolerance. Personality development was evaluated by ego structure, body image, social development, and concentration capacity.

Findings.—Before the study, the group had high functional residual capacity and residual volume, low forced expiratory volume in 1 second, forced expiratory flow when 50% and 25% of the forced vital capacity remains to be expelled (MEF50 and MEF 25), and low histamine tolerance. During training, the MEF50 and MEF25 increased slightly. Before training, all boys had at least one emotional indicator in the Human Figure Drawings test and 5 boys had signs of emotional instability. All the boys showed marked improvement in all psychological variables, and the positive effects remained during the year after the program.

Conclusions.—Although the improvements in clinical and pulmonary function changes were modest, there was a marked and lasting improvement in personality development. The feeling of safety and confidence inspired by the program allowed the boys to cope with asthmatic symptoms with less anxiety. This process of developing a positive and realistic body consciousness is important for future well-being.

▶ This study shows that, for children with asthma, an exercise program can benefit the psyche as well as the soma. These boys experienced a "catch-up" in personality development, gained more security and self-confidence, tended to need less emergency treatment in the hospital, and developed good relationships with peers with asthma. Benefits continued beyond the study year, and most of the boys undertook other physical activities, on their own, in the poststudy year.—E.R. Eichner, M.D.

Differentiation Between the Intensity of Breathlessness and the Distress it Evokes in Normal Subjects During Exercise

Wilson RC, Jones PW (St George's Hospital Medical School, London)
Clin Sci 80:65–70, 1991
5–30

Background.—The sensation of breathlessness has been compared to that of pain. Estimations of perceived breathlessness involve the individual's perception of the sensation and their reaction to it. People can reliably use subjective scaling to measure the intensity of their breathless-

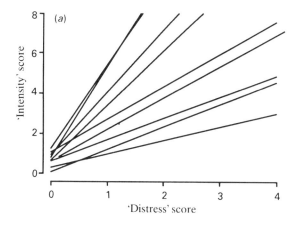

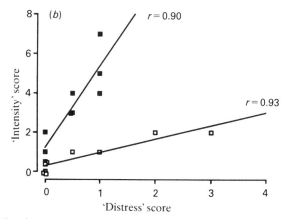

Fig 5–12.—The relationship between intensity score and distress score. **A,** individual data for 9 subjects. One subject who did not register any distress is not illustrated. In the 9 subjects there was a significant correlation between intensity score and distress score. The individual data points for each regression have been removed for clarity. **B,** data from the 2 subjects displaying the extremes of slopes of the relationship. Coincident points have been slightly displaced for clarity. (Courtesy of Wilson RC, Jones PW: *Clin Sci* 80:65–70, 1991.)

ness. This study examined whether normal subjects could differentiate between the intensity of breathlessness and the amount of distress it evoked by a suitable wording of instructions.

Methods.—Ten subjects performed 2 identical incremental cycle-ergometer exercise tests on separate occasions. During exercise, they were asked to quantify either intensity or distress, using modified Borg scales.

Results.—There was a significant correlation between intensity and minute ventilation in all cases. Eight of the 10 subjects also showed a significant correlation between distress and minute ventilation. One person had no correlation, and 1 reported no distress. Mean distress was lower than mean intensity. A significant correlation between intensity and distress was found within individuals. Among subjects, there was a wide scatter in the slope of this relationship. Maximum intensity and distress were uncorrelated. Different elements of the breathlessness sensation were identified and measured selectively, depending on the wording of instructions (Fig 5–12).

Conclusions.—Different aspects of the experience of breathlessness can be identified and measured selectively. Like pain, breathlessness is a multidimensional sensation. The precise wording of the instructions given to patients is therefore important. A universally accepted working definition of breathlessness is desirable for comparing study results.

▶ Psychologists have long recognized that a very small change in test instructions can dramatically modify the responses obtained from subjetcs. In the present experiment, a Borg 1–10 scale of breathlessness was modified by adding the descriptor "distress" (e.g., "very, very slight distress"). In different subjects, the response after the change of wording ranged from approximately unchanged to 6 units of breathlessness equals 1 unit of distress, with a typical 2:1 or 3:1 response ratio. Both scales also showed considerable interindividual variation in the relationship of ventilation to breathlessness, even among normal individuals. Departure from the anticipated relationship of ventilation to breathlessness was particularly large in patients with "disproportionate breathlessness" (1). Probably, variables increasing the breathlessness of such patients include not only a small vital capacity, but also an increased sensitivity of pulmonary receptors as the lungs become congested. This seriously limits the use of either the respiratory rate of perceived exhaustion or the "talk test" in the regulation of exercise prescription for the cardiac patient.—R.J. Shephard, M.D., Ph.D.

Reference

1. Burns BH, Howell JBL: *QJ Med* 38:277, 1969.

Respiratory Muscle Deoxygenation During Exercise in Patients With Heart Failure Demonstrated With Near-Infrared Spectroscopy
Mancini DM, Ferraro N, Nazzaro D, Chance B, Wilson JR (Univ of Pennsylva-

nia, Philadelphia)
J Am Coll Cardiol 18:492–498, 1991

Background.—Respiratory muscle underperfusion may be partly responsible for exertional dyspnea in patients with heart failure. Near-infrared spectroscopy, a new method, allows noninvasive evaluation of skeletal muscle oxygenation by monitoring changes in near-infrared light absorption. This technique was used to compare serratus anterior muscle oxygenation during maximal cycle ergometer exercise in patients with heart failure and in healthy persons.

Methods.—Ten patients with a mean ejection fracture of 16% were compared with 7 age-matched healthy control subjects. Measures were obtained for oxygen consumption, minute ventilation, and arterial saturation. Muscle deoxygenation was detected by changes in difference in spectral absorption between 760 and 800 nm wavebands, expressed in arbitrary units.

Results.—Normal subjects had minimal change in this difference in absorption during exercise, whereas patients with heart failure had progressive changes throughout exercise consistent with respiratory muscle deoxygenation. Compared with healthy subjects, patients with heart failure had significantly greater minute ventilation and respiratory rate but similar tidal volume at comparable work loads. At peak exercise, however, normal subjects had significantly greater minute ventilation and tidal volume, with a similar respiratory rate. There was no significant arterial desaturation in either group during exercise (Fig 5–13).

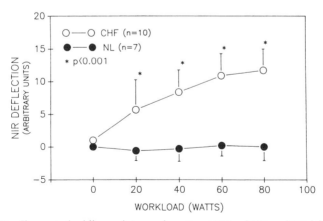

Fig 5–13.—Changes in the difference between absorption at 760 and 800 nm (NIR deflection) during exercise in heart failure and normal subjects. *Abbreviations:* CHF, congestive heart failure; NIR, near-infrared spectroscopy. *P < .001, normal subjects vs. patients with heart failure. (Courtesy of Mancini DM, Ferraro N, Nazzaro D, et al: *J Am Coll Cardiol* 18:492–498, 1991.)

Conclusions.—This study shows that respiratory muscle deoxygenation occurs in patients with heart failure during exercise. Deoxygenation may contribute to the exertional dyspnea noted in these patients.

▶ Some authors have maintained that pulmonary congestion is the main cause of exertional dyspnea in patients with heart failure. However, it is difficult to reconcile this explanation with persistence of the symptom after vagal blockade (1). An alternative possibility is that a poor cardiac output, an increase of respiratory work-rate, and possibly an increase of systemic vasoconstriction lead to ischemia of the respiratory muscles. Support for the hypothesis of respiratory muscle ischemia has already been obtained in animal experiments (2). The new technology of near infrared spectroscopy has now allowed similar observations to be made in patients with congestive heart failure. Although such experiments show that respiratory muscle ischemia occurs, further data are needed to establish a causal relationship between ischemia and the sensation of exertional dyspnea. If such a link is established, it may prove possible to increase the perfusion of the respiratory muscles by the use of drugs such as aminophylline or amrinone.—R.J. Shephard, M.D., Ph.D.

References

1. Killian K, Jones N: *Clin Chest Med* 9:237, 1988.
2. Aubier M, et al: *J Appl Physiol* 51:499, 1981.

An Infection Control Policy for the Athletic Training Setting
Webster DL, Kaiser DA (Central Michigan Univ, Mt Pleasant)
Athletic Training JNATA 26:70–74, 1991   5–32

Background.—Like other health-care providers, athletic trainers should be concerned about blood-borne infectious agents, notably the HIV and the hepatitis B virus. An infection control program will establish and implement policies and procedures relating to the control of infectious disease hazards where health-care workers may be exposed to body fluids.

Setting.—An infection control policy for Central Michigan University Sports Medicine has been established based on the following assumptions: athletic trainers are health-care workers, athletic training facilities are health-care facilities, and the duties performed by the athletic training staff may place a staff member at risk of exposure to infectious pathogens. The adoption of this policy includes the identification of exposure tasks and contaminated materials, the adoption of universal precautions, the collection of biohazardous wastes within the athletic environment, the disposal of biohazardous wastes in accordance with state regulations, the control of the environment, and the education and training of staff and student athletic trainers (Figs 5–14 and 5–15).

I. Exposure Category

Category II. Tasks that involve no exposure to blood, body fluids, or tissues, but employment may require performing unplanned Category I tasks.

The normal work routine involves no exposure to blood, body fluids, or tissues, but exposure or potential exposure may be required as a condition of employment. Appropriate protective measures should be readily available to every employee engaged in Category II tasks.

II. Identification of Risk Tasks

A. Injury/Illness Management:
CPR
Mouth to mouth resuscitation
Management of open wounds
Management of compound fractures/dislocations
Blister care

B. Environmental Management:
Soiled laundry/linen
Cleaning surfaces
Disposing of biohazardous bags/Sharp's box

III. Occupational Exposure to Blood-Borne Infectious Agents (Universal Precautions)

These precautions represent prudent practices that apply to preventing transmission of the AIDS virus (human immunodeficiency virus - HIV), Hepatitis B Virus (HBV), and other blood-borne infections, and should be used routinely.

1. When the possibility of exposure to blood or other fluids exists, appropriate barrier precautions to prevent skin and mucous membrane exposure should be followed. GLOVES should be worn for touching blood and body fluids, mucous membranes, or non-intact skin of all patients, and for handling items or surfaces soiled with blood or body fluids. Gloves should be changed after contact with each patient and disposed of in a proper waste container.

2. Hands and other skin surfaces should be washed immediately and thoroughly if contaminated with blood or other body fluids. Hands should be washed immediately after gloves are removed.

3. Sharp items should be considered as potentially infectious and handled with extraordinary care in order to prevent accidental injuries. After they are used, syringes, needles, scalpel

Fig 5–14 *(Continued)*

Fig 5–14   (cont).

blades, and other sharp items should be placed in a puncture-resistant container for disposal. The puncture-resistant container (Sharp's box) should be located as close as practical to the use area. Needles or blades should not be purposefully bent, broken, removed, or otherwise manipulated by hand.

4. Although saliva has not been implicated in HIV transmission, to minimize the potential for infection during emergency mouth-to-mouth resuscitation, mouthpieces, resuscitation bags, or other ventilation devices should be available for use.

5. Staff who have exudative lesions or weeping dermatitis should refrain from all direct patient care and from handling patient care equipment, until the condition resolves.

6. Pregnant staff should be especially careful to minimize the possible transmission of infectious pathogens to the fetus.

Fig 5–14.—Infection control, Central Michigan University. (Courtesy of Webster DL, Kaiser DA: *Athletic Training, JNATA* 26:70–74, 1991.)

I. COLLECTION OF BIOHAZARDOUS WASTE

Gloves, Gauze, Human Tissue, etc.

Each training room is to contain a covered waste container that is lined with a biohazardous trash bag. Materials that have become contaminated with blood, exudates, secretions, body fluid wastes, or other infectious agents are to be placed in these covered containers. Grossly soaked towels will be discarded in a biohazard bag.

Laundry

Towels that have been used and have moderate blood or body fluid contamination may be placed in the normal laundry bag. If there is any sign of blood or waste material on the laundry bag, gloves will be worn to take the laundry bag to the equipment room for laundering.

Sharps

A puncture-resistant container will be located in each training room. All scalpels and sharp objects contaminated with blood, exudates, body fluids, or other infectious agents will be discarded in the Sharp's box.

Tables, Counter Tops

All table and counter top surfaces will be cleaned with a 1:31 bleach to water solution.

II. DISPOSAL

The full-time athletic training staff is responsible for removing full biohazard bags from the covered waste containers, sealing bags securely, and transporting bags to a common collection site. Whenever the Sharp's containers are full, the container is removed and deposited at a common collection site.

Fig 5–15.—Environmental control, biohazardous waste, Central Michigan University. (Courtesy of Webster DL, Kaiser DA: *Athletic Training, JNATA* 26:70–74, 1991.)

Conclusion.—The transmission of blood-borne infectious agents remains a concern among health-care providers; and yet, the profession has been slow in implementing programs to prevent exposure to such pathogens. The infection control policy presented may serve as a model to encourage athletic trainers to address this concern.

▶ This paper is clear: "Athletic trainers are health-care workers. The duties performed by the athletic training staff may place a staff member at risk of exposure to infectious pathogens." As of January 1, 1992, the federal government made it compulsory for employers to provide free-of-charge immunization for any employees who may be exposed to blood-borne pathogens. I would urge all athletic trainers and student athletic trainers to take advantage of this policy and be immunized against hepatitis B virus. In addition, an infection control policy for your training room should be established and is now required by the same federal guidelines mentioned above. The authors state that these guidelines must address "the adoption of universal precautions; the identification of exposure tasks and contaminated materials; the collection of biohazardous wastes within the athletic environment; the disposal of biohazardous waste in accordance with state regulations; and the education and training of staff and student athletic trainers."

Many of us can receive help implementing these guidelines through our student health services or through an institutional designated officer, who is responsible for implementing these guidelines. The time has come for all of us to wear gloves when treating open wounds; to dispose of all contaminated materials properly; to never reuse needles, scalpels, or razors; and to use a 10% bleach solution to clean the training room. Be aware that some athletes we treat on a daily basis may be in the so called high-risk groups. Please refer to reference 1 for more information on this topic.—F.J. George, A.T.C., P.T.

Reference

1. 1990 Year Book of Sports Medicine, p 249.

The Role of the Athletic Trainer in the Detection and Prevention of Lyme Disease in Athletes
Pinger RR, Hahn DB, Sharp RL (Ball State Univ, Muncie, Ind)
Athletic Training JNATA 26:324–331, 1991   5–33

Introduction.—Lyme disease is of increasing concern in many areas of the country. Although athletes may be at particular risk for contracting Lyme disease, relatively few trainers are aware of the signs or potentially serious consequences of infection. The history of Lyme disease and the role of athletic trainers in its prevention and detection were reviewed.

Background.—Lyme disease was first reported in Lyme, Connecticut, in 1975. Within a decade it had become the most commonly reported tick-borne illness in the United States. The pathogen responsible for Lyme disease, *Borrelia burgdorferi*, is transmitted by members of the *Ixodidae* tick family. In most patients, the onset of the disease occurs during the summer months.

Stages of Lyme Disease.—The most obvious first sign, appearing in 60% to 80% of patients, is a rash known as erythema chronicum migrans (ECM). This rash expands from the site of the tick bite and may reach a diameter of more than 1 foot. The ECM is not painful, does not itch, and usually disappears in several weeks with or without treatment. Flu-like symptoms may also occur at this stage. If disseminated Lyme disease

---

Recommended Procedure for Removing Ticks

1. **Do not handle the tick with bare hands.** Use forceps or tweezers to remove the tick.
2. Grasp the tick as close to the skin surface as possible and pull upward with even, gentle pressure. **Do not twist or jerk** the tick as this may cause the mouthparts to break off and stay in the skin.
3. Do not squeeze, crush, or puncture the tick. Its fluids may contain infective agents.
4. After removing the tick, thoroughly disinfect the bite site and wash your hands with soap and water.
5. Safely dispose of the tick by placing it in a container of alcohol, flushing it down the toilet, or saving it for examination.
6. **Never** remove the tick by using fingernail polish, alcohol, or hot matches.

Note: Reproduced with modification from Needham GR: Evaluation of 5 popular methods for tick removal. *Pediatrics* 75:997-1007, 1985.
(Courtesy of Pinger RR, Hahn DB, Sharp RL: *Athletic Training JNATA* 26:324-331, 1991.)

---

develops, the infection spreads in the patient's blood or lymph and results in neurologic and/or cardiac problems. Intermittent attacks or arthritis occur at an average of 6 months after the onset of disease. The third stage of Lyme disease, late infection, is associated with a variety of cardiac, neurologic, and arthritic abnormalities. Infection during pregnancy may have serious consequences to the fetus.

Role of the Athletic Trainer.—Trainers should become familiar with the appearance of ECM. Athletes requiring careful attention are those whose sport takes them into grassy areas or woodlands, especially in states where Lyme disease is most prevalent. Joint pain with no obvious cause may reflect early or advanced Lyme disease. If a tick is found, new guidelines for tick removal (table) should be followed.

▶ This year we had 2 athletes report for their fall preseason physical examination who had sustained Lyme disease during the summer. This has become a significant problem in some areas of the country. Athletic trainers must be aware of the precautions to take with athletes who may be participating in tick-infested areas. The authors also state that most athletic training manuals indicate an improper method for tick removal from the skin. Please refer to Table 7 in the original article for the proper method to use. Athletic trainers must also recognize erythema chronicum migrans (ECM), a rash that occurs in the early stages for many Lyme disease patients. See Figure 7 in the original article.—F.J. George, A.T.C., P.T.

Cardiac Output and Oxygen Delivery During Exercise in Sickle Cell Anemia

Pianosi P, D'Souza SJA, Charge TD, Béland MJ, Esseltine DW, Coates AL
(McGill University-Montreal Children's Hospital Research Institute)
Am Rev Respir Dis 143:231–235, 1991   5–34

Introduction.—Intravascular sickling and vascular occlusion can result from desaturation in patients with sickle cell anemia (SCA). Exercise increases metabolic demands, which tends to increase oxygen extraction. This reduces saturation in the capillary bed and may predispose to sickling. An increase in cardiac output could minimize this.

Methods.—To assess the role of increased stroke volume (SV) in augmenting cardiac output ($\dot{Q}$) and to determine the role of enlarged arteriovenous O_2 content difference in maintaining oxygen (O_2) transport in children with SCA, 30 children with SCA and 16 healthy race-matched controls were studied. The 2 groups were of similar height and weight and performed incremental and steady-state exercise at 50% W_{max}. The indirect Fick method was used to measure cardiac output ($\dot{Q}$) during the steady state.

Results.—The slope of $\Delta HR/\Delta \dot{V}O_2$ during incremental exercise was greater in patients with SCA than in healthy controls, 4.01 vs. 2.8 beats per minute per mL/min/kg $\dot{V}O_2$. The $\dot{Q}$ for $\dot{V}O_2$ was abnormally high in the patients, especially in older patients with lower hemoglobin levels. Patients had higher HR and SV than controls. Multiple linear regression of $\dot{Q}$ percent predicted and SV percent predicted on hemoglobin and age demonstrated a positive correlation with age and a negative correlation with hemoglobin. The arteriovenous O_2 content difference was larger in controls because more hemoglobin was available. However, the

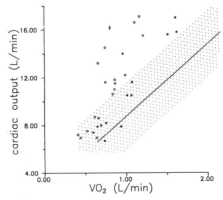

Fig 5–16.—Regression of $\dot{Q}$ (L/minute) vs. $\dot{V}O_2$ (L/minute STPD) for controls and patients with SCA. The *stippled area* is the 95% confidence interval for controls. The *solid circles* are patients with HbSC, and the *open circles* are those with HbSS. The slope of the regression was significantly greater in paitents than in controls. (Courtesy of Pianosi P, D'Souza SJA, Charge TD, et al: *Am Rev Respir Dis* 143:231–235, 1991.)

percentage of available O_2 extracted at 50% W_{max} was higher in the patients (Fig 5–16).

Conclusion.—Older children with SCA have greater cardiac output on exercise than normal to a degree inversely related to the severity of anemia. This results mainly from a progressive increase in stroke volume out of proportion to somatic growth.

▶ Patients with sickle cell anemia have an abnormal form of hemoglobin (hemoglobin-S). Substitution of a valine for a glutamate residue makes the hemoglobin molecule "sticky," and it tends to clump together in long chains. This is not a problem if the hemoglobin remains oxygenated, because a coiling of the hemoglobin molecule "hides" the sticky sector. However, deoxygenation causes the molecule to uncoil, allowing adhesion at a rate proportional to the tenth power of the concentration of deoxygenated hemoglobin. This change of molecular configuration accounts for the effects of vigorous exercise and increased stroke volume, as discussed in this article.

Because the venous oxygen saturation of the sickle cell patient is low, the primary reason for the large cardiac output in the affected children seems to be their anemia rather than any attempt to compensate for the sickling disease. However, it is interesting that the cardiac output is increased as much by a large stroke volume as by tachycardia. The contrast with, for example, a dietary anemia, probably reflects good overall nutrition. There may also be some ventricular hypertrophy in response to the afterloading of the heart and peripheral hypoxia induced by red cell clumping (1).—R.J. Shephard, M.D., Ph.D.

Reference

1. Vayo MM, et al: *Microvasc Res* 30:195, 1985.

Food-Dependent, Exercise-Induced Anaphylaxis: A Study on 11 Japanese Cases

Dohi M, Suko M, Sugiyama H, Yamashita N, Tadokoro K, Juji F, Okudaira H, Sano Y, Ito K, Miyamoto T (University of Tokyo, Do-ai Memorial Hospital, Tokyo)
J Allergy Clin Immunol 87:34–40, 1991   5–35

Background.—Exercise-induced anaphylaxis (EIAn), a distinct form of physical allergy, is characterized by symptoms such as collapse or upper respiratory tract obstruction associated with flushing or urticaria, a rise in plasma histamine, and pathologic findings of mast cell degranulation. A series of patients with food-dependent EIAn in Japan was reviewed.

Patients.—The patients were 7 women and 4 men, aged 18 to 43, known to have food-dependent EIAn.

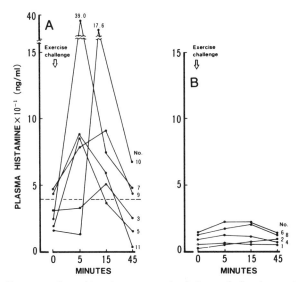

Fig 5–17.—Changes in plasma histamine concentration before and after the exercise challenge in patients with food-dependent EIAn. Plasma histamine concentration increased over the maximal value observed in controls (.4 ng/mL) in 6 of 11 patients (**A**) 5 to 15 minutes after challenge. Five patients (**B**) did not demonstrate any increase in plasma histamine concentration. (Courtesy of Dohi M, Suko M, Sugiyama H, et al: *J Allergy Clin Immunol* 87:34–40, 1991.)

Findings.—Seven patients had anaphylactic symptoms after eating certain foods, including shellfish, wheat, and grape, before exercising. The other 4 patients were predisposed to anaphylaxis by the act of eating. Their anaphylactic symptoms could be distinguished clearly from cholinergic urticaria by history. The 7 patients who had anaphylactic symptoms before the age of 20 were atopic or had atopic first-degree relatives. Six had elevated serum IgE levels, and 4 had IgE antibodies against the causative food allergens detected by skin prick or RAST. Patients who began to have symptoms after age 30 seemed to have a less atopic background. Levels of IgE were within the normal range in 3 of 4 of these patients. Three of these patients also developed symptoms after ingesting food made of wheat before exercise. All patients were sensitive to wheat according to the skin prick test. Six patients had a marked rise in plasma histamine levels after exercise challenge with treadmill alone. Food intake followed by exercise induced a further increase in 1 patient (Fig 5–17).

Conclusions.—Of 11 patients with food-dependent EIAn, exercise challenge alone caused a rise in plasma histamine concentrations in 6. Patients with EIAn may have increased histamine releasability from mast cells in response to exercise relative to normal individuals. Food intake may accelerate this process.

▶ Exercise-induced anaphylaxis is a very rare phenomenon, but can nevertheless be life-threatening. A number of these patients had eaten allergenic seafoods before exercising, but in 6 of 11 cases, plasma histamine was increased by an exercise challenge without food intake. This suggests that the mast cells of vulnerable patients release histamine over-readily even when such individuals are fasting.—R.J. Shephard, M.D., Ph.D.

Case Report: 30-Yr-Old Female With Exercise Induced Anaphylaxis
Briner WW Jr, Bruno PJ (Lutheran Gen Hosp, Park Ridge, Ill; Nicholas Inst of Sports Med and Athletic Trauma, New York)
Med Sci Sports Exerc 23:991–994, 1991   5–36

Introduction.—As the exercise boom continues, physicians can expect to see more cases of exercise-induced anaphylaxis (EIA). Identifying this specific condition and correct treatment are essential to avoid morbidity and mortality.

Case Report.—Woman, 30, experienced pruritic rash with exercise and 1 occurrence of lightheadedness. Side effects of treatment with hydroxyzine were poorly tolerated, and she was switched to inhaled cromolyn sodium with successful resolution of symptoms. An anaphylaxis epinephrine kit was also prescribed, and she was instructed to have it with her at all times when she was exercising.

Discussion.—If at all possible, exercise activity should not be limited or eliminated in patients with EIA. Correct diagnosis and proper drug therapy will alert the patient to the problem and hopefully eliminate the accompanying reactions.

▶ This case report includes a concise review of the 3 common types of exercise-induced physical allergy, or urticaria: cholinergic, anaphylactic, and variant. This young woman is classified as having the variant type, but in some ways—provocation of urticaria also by hot showers and lack of true collapse—the cholinergic type seems more likely here. The authors mention that exercise-induced anaphylaxis may well be a continuum rather than several distinct entities. They also describe how this condition interfered with the young woman's active life, and how inhaled cromolyn relieved her symptoms and allowed her to exercise freely. This, the authors say, is the second reported case of exercise-induced anaphylaxis to respond to inhaled cromolyn. For more on exercise allergies, see references (1-3).—E.R. Eichner, M.D.

References

1. 1986 YEAR BOOK OF SPORTS MEDICINE, p 105.
2. 1988 YEAR BOOK OF SPORTS MEDICINE, pp 168–169.
3. 1990 YEAR BOOK OF SPORTS MEDICINE, pp 233–234.

Effect of Cimetidine on Marathon-Associated Gastrointestinal Symptoms and Bleeding

Moses FM, Baska RS, Peura DA, Deuster PA (Walter Reed Army Med Ctr, Washington, DC; Uniformed Services Univ of the Health Sciences, Bethesda, Md)

Dig Dis Sci 36:1390–1394, 1991   5–37

Introduction.—Gastrointestinal bleeding occurs in 8% to 30% of marathon runners and in most ultramarathon runners. Hemorrhagic gastritis is the most frequent endoscopic abnormality seen in endurance athletes with gastrointestinal bleeding. The cause of these symptoms remains unknown, but acid-mediated ischemic damage has been proposed as a cause. A prospective, randomized, double-blind trial was undertaken to determine the impact of cimetidine on gastrointestinal symptoms and bleeding during a marathon.

Study Design.—Forty-two participants in the 1990 Marine Corps Marathon and New York City Marathon were randomly allocated to 800 mg of cimetidine by mouth 2 hours before the start of the race or to placebo. All participants were asked to complete a prerace questionnaire, return 3 double-window Hemoccult (HO) cards, and collect a single stool sample for Hemoquant (HQ) analysis during the week before the race. After the race, they were asked to complete a second questionnaire, return 3 more double-window HO cards, and send in another HQ sample. A runner was considered to be HO positive if any of the 3 cards showed a positive change.

Results.—Thirty participants (71%) returned both questionnaires, and all required stool HO and HQ specimens as requested. Two runners assigned to cimetidine forgot to take it and were included in the placebo group. Thus, there were 13 evaluable runners in the cimetidine group and 17 in the placebo group. Three runners with positive HO cards before the race were excluded from the analysis. After the race, 5 of 14 runners who were given placebo (36%) and 2 of 13 runners who took cimetidine (15%) had positive HO cards. Prerace HQ values were not significantly different from postrace HQ values, and all values were within the normal range. Although digestive symptoms during the race were common, there was no difference between the runners who took placebo and those who had taken cimetidine with respect to the frequency or severity of their symptoms.

Conclusions.—Cimetidine does not significantly affect endurance running-associated occult gastrointestinal bleeding as measured by HO or HQ results. Marathon-associated gastrointestinal bleeding and symptoms may be caused by lesions other than acid-mediated disease or hemorrhagic gastritis.

▶ It must be stressed that the GI bleeding that occurs in up to 30% of marathoners and 85% of ultramarathoners is generally occult and clinically trivial.

Surveys suggest that no more than 2% of recreational marathoners and triathletes, for example, have seen blood in their stool at least once during racing or training. The background of this topic has been covered in recent YEAR BOOKS (1-3). Another recent report documented occult GI bleeding in 5 of 15 women during a marathon (4). In general, GI bleeding in endurance athletes is infrequent, minor, and brief. Anecdotally, some of the more dramatic examples, in well known triathletes for example, have been linked to use of nonsteroidal anti-inflammatory drugs before and during the competition. The stomach and, less often, the colon, have been identified endoscopically as sites of GI bleeding in runners. In the stomach, hemorrhagic gastritis during a race may result from a blend of stress, drugs, and exercise-induced ischemia, perhaps compounded by gastric acid secretion. Recently, a prospective but nonrandomized and unblinded study showed that cimetidine lessened GI symptoms and reduced the frequency of GI bleeding in runners during a 100-mile race (3). In this follow-up study, however, whereas the postrace Hemoccult conversion rate was higher for placebo (36%) than cimetidine (15%), the difference was not statistically significant. Therefore, in this controlled study, cimetidine had no clear cut benefit on either GI symptoms or GI bleeding during a marathon.—E.R. Eichner, M.D.

References

1. 1988 YEAR BOOK OF SPORTS MEDICINE, pp 128–133.
2. 1990 YEAR BOOK OF SPORTS MEDICINE, pp 106–107.
3. 1991 YEAR BOOK OF SPORTS MEDICINE, pp 273–276.
4. Lampe JW, et al: *Int J Sports Med* 12:173, 1991.

Hematuria in a Young Recreational Runner
Elliot DL, Goldberg L, Eichner ER (Oregon Health Sciences Univ, Portland; Univ of Oklahoma, Oklahoma City)
Med Sci Sports Exerc 23:892–894, 1991   5–38

Background.—Although hematuria may occur after prolonged or intense exertion, other causes must be excluded before it is attributed to exercise. In a runner with gross hematuria, exercise precipitated hematuria from underlying genitourinary pathology.

Case Report.—Man, 27, was seen after a second episode of rust-colored urine after a 2-mile run. He ran 2 to 3 miles several times a week. He had undergone surgery for a twisted hydatid of the right testicle at age 8 years, and his father had a history of calcium oxalate nephrolithiasis. Physical examination was normal. He had a slightly elevated creatine kinase level of 249 U/L and 4 to 8 red blood cells/hpf on urinalysis. A filling defect in the right posterior bladder wall was seen on an intravenous pyelogram, and a 3-cm pedunculated tumor originating lateral to the right ureteral orifice was seen at cystoscopy. The lesion was resected transurethrally and proved to be a grade I to II superficial transitional cell bladder carcinoma. The patient returned to jogging 1 week later and has had no recurrence of hematuria or tumor over 2 years of follow-up.

Conclusions.—The diagnosis of exercise-induced hematuria should be one of exclusion. Other causes should be examined, particularly when the patient has features that increase the likelihood of an underlying abnormality. Factors pointing to a cause other than exercise include female sex, gross hematuria, exercise that is not prolonged or intense, and microscopic hematuria persisting for more than 48 hours.

▶ This graphic case report reminds us that not all hematuria in athletes is benign. Indeed, recreational and professional athletes alike are prone to diverse causes of hematuria, and proper diagnosis hinges on careful history, physical examination, and urinalysis, as well as on the wise use of screening tests and diagnostic maneuvers such as intravenous pyelography, ultrasound, CT, and/or cystoscopy (1). In runners, for example, hematuria can be benign (e.g., pseudonephritis) (2) or painful and gross, apparently owing to bladder trauma; the latter can plague male distance runners especially. Painless gross hematuria, however, as reported here, can be ominous, and calls for scrutiny. Four other cases of bladder cancer in patients seen for exercise-induced gross hematuria—3 in men between the ages of 22 and 41—were reported in 1988 (3). I know of a sixth case in a young professional football player. Running and/or aerobics, it seems, can "unmask" an otherwise covert, early, curable bladder cancer, thus serving as a life-saving "exercise stress test."
—E.R. Eichner, M.D.

References

1. 1991 YEAR BOOK OF SPORTS MEDICINE, p 278.
2. 1988 YEAR BOOK OF SPORTS MEDICINE, pp 126–128.
3. 1990 YEAR BOOK OF SPORTS MEDICINE, pp 245–246.

An Outbreak of Herpes Gladiatorum at a High-School Wrestling Camp

Belongia EA, Goodman JL, Holland EJ, Andres CW, Homann SR, Mahanti RL, Mizener MW, Erice A, Osterholm MT (Centers for Disease Control; Univ of Minnesota Hosp and Clin; Minnesota Dept of Health, Minneapolis)
N Engl J Med 325:906–910, 1991   5–39

Background.—Herpes simplex virus type 1 (HSV-1) can cause herpes gladiatorum, a cutaneous or ocular infection among athletes involved in contact sports. It is primarily transmitted by skin-to-skin contact. An outbreak of herpes gladiatorum during a 4-week intensive-training wrestling camp with 175 high-school wrestlers is investigated.

Methods.—Cases of infection were identified by review of medical records, interview and examination of the wrestlers, and culture of the skin lesions. Oropharyngeal swabs were obtained for HSV-1 culture and serum samples for serologic studies. Isolates of HSV-1 were compared by restriction-endonuclease analysis.

Findings.—Sixty wrestlers (34%) were diagnosed with HSV-1 infection. The lesions were on the head in 73% of the wrestlers, the extremities in 42%, and the trunk in 28% of the wrestlers. In 21 wrestlers, HSV-1 was isolated, and in 39 wrestlers, the infection was identifed by clinical criteria. Common constitutional symptoms included fever, chills, sore throat, and headache. Five wrestlers had conjunctivitis or blepharitis. The attack rate varied among the 3 wrestling practice groups. Four strains of HSV-1 were identified by restriction-endonuclease analysis, suggesting concurrent transmission of different strains within different groups.

Conclusion.—Herpes gladiatorum was transmitted primarily by direct skin-to-skin contact and not by saliva. Two strains of HSV-1 accounted for most of the cases within different practice groups. Routine skin examinations of the athletes and prompt exclusion of potentially infected wrestlers is one strategy to control herpes gladiatorum.

▶ This outbreak of herpes gladiatorum was unusual because of its size, the high attack rate in the heavyweight group, which was never explained, and the spreading of 4 distinct HSV-1 strains. Behavioral factors contributed to the spread. Several wrestlers continued to wrestle after the onset of skin lesions. Half of the afflicted wrestlers recalled having a prior abrasion or break in the skin at the site of the vesicular rash, possibly from mat burns. Skin-to-skin contact was the dominant mode of spread. Saliva was not a major source of transmission; nor was headgear, soap, or water bottles. Prior herpes labialis did not protect against herpes gladiatorum. Although many wrestlers had typical vesicular lesions, there was great variability in the appearance of the rash. Because the clinical appearance may be unreliable, all suspicious skin and eye lesions should be cultured for HSV-1. Wrestlers with open skin lesions should not compete until a physician certifies that the condition is not communicable. During the subsequent camp season, all the wrestlers were regularly examined by their trainers and encouraged to report all skin lesions promptly. No outbreak occurred.—E.R. Eichner, M.D.

Muscle Rehabilitation: Its Effect on Muscular and Functional Performance of Patients With Knee Osteoarthritis

Fisher NM, Pendergast DR, Gresham GE, Calkins E (State Univ of New York at Buffalo; Erie County Med Ctr, Buffalo; Batavia VA Ctr, Batavia, NY)
Arch Phys Med Rehabil 72:367–374, 1991   5–40

Introduction.—Osteoarthritis (OA) is a common cause of functional limitation and dependency, especially when the knees are involved, as often occurs in the elderly. Muscle rehabilitation improved function in a

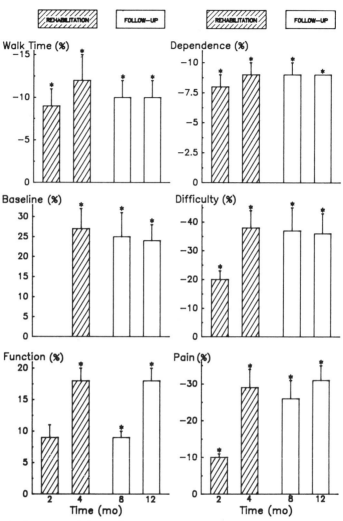

Fig 5–18.—Percentage of changes for various measures of functional performance presented for 2 and 4 months of rehabilitation and 4 and 8 months after rehabilitation (8 and 12, respectively). Values are presented as a percentage of prerehabilitation values. *Asterisks* indicate significant differences from prerehabilitation values (analysis of variance, $P < .05$). (Courtesy of Fisher NM, Pendergast DR, Gresham GE, et al: *Arch Phys Med Rehabil* 72:367–374, 1991.)

large proportion of elderly nursing home patients participating in a pilot study.

Methods.—Fifteen men with a mean age of 68 years who had OA of the knees undertook a 4-month, 3-times-weekly exercise program. The quadriceps muscle group was exercised at knee angles of 60, 90, and 135 degrees at hip angles of 90, 120, 150, and 180 degrees.

Results.—Initially muscle strength and endurance were 50% less in the patients with OA than in controls. Strength and endurance both increased 35% after rehabilitation, and speed increased 50%. Gain in strength was most marked at muscle lengths of 55 cm. The Jette Functional Status Index showed a 10% decrease in dependency after rehabilitation. Walking speed increased significantly. Muscle function and functional performance were unchanged from postrehabilitation levels 8 months after the program (Fig 5–18).

Conclusion.—A formal rehabilitative program can improve functional performance in elderly persons with OA more than traditional quadsetting. A combination of this program and aerobic exercises, either on land or in water, might be optimal.

▶ A loss of knee stability related to osteoarthritis is a common cause of disability in the elderly, and there have been frequent suggestions that function could be improved by a program to increase local muscle strength. The present study demonstrates such a response to a program that combined isometric with progressive isotonic exercise over the 4-month period. The Jette index includes assessments of ability to climb stairs, arise from a chair, stand, and walk, and there was a 30% decrease in the difficulty and pain encountered in such endeavors after conditioning. Probably in part because of initial dependency, the average body mass was 94 kg, and I was surprised to find no suggestion that this should be reduced. A decrease of obesity would in itself greatly reduce the load imposed on the deteriorating joints, and it should be an important tactic in the treatment of osteoarthritis.—R.J. Shephard, M.D., Ph.D.

Exercise Training Reduces Intraocular Pressure Among Subjects Suspected of Having Glaucoma
Passo MS, Goldberg L, Elliot DL, Van Buskirk EM (Oregon Health Sciences Univ; VA Med Ctr, Portland; Good Samaritan Hosp, Portland)
Arch Ophthalmol 109:1096–1098, 1991   5–41

Introduction.—Although studies in healthy, nonsedentary individuals have shown that exercise training lowers the intraocular pressure (IOP), no studies have evaluated the effect of exercise training on the IOP in previously sedentary individuals. The present prospective study was designed to determine whether regular aerobic exercise would lower the IOP in patients suspected of having glaucoma.

Patients.—The patients were 13 otherwise healthy sedentary adults aged 25–60 years who were being followed up for an elevated IOP of 22 mm Hg or greater in each eye on at least 2 separate occasions. All patients performed exercise testing to volitional exhaustion on a cycle ergometer before being enrolled in a supervised 12-week aerobic exercise conditioning program. Patients trained on a stationary exercycle for 40 minutes 4 times per week at a training level between 70% and 85% of maximum heart rate, as determined by their exercise test. After the 12 weeks of exercise conditioning, patients resumed their sedentary lifestyle. Measurements of IOP were obtained weekly until the IOP returned to the prestudy sedentary level.

Results.—Four patients did not complete the study, leaving 5 men and 4 women aged 29–57 years who did. At the end of the 12-week conditioning period, the mean IOP had decreased by 4.6 mm Hg (20%). However, 3 weeks after the cessation of exercise, the mean IOP had returned to its elevated preconditioning level.

Conclusion.—Regular aerobic exercise can lower an elevated IOP in sedentary patients suspected of having glaucoma. An aerobic exercise program may be an effective nonpharmacologic alternative or addition to medical therapy in these patients.

▶ When Ken Cooper first began preaching the gospel of aerobics, one of the promised rewards of the faithful that was viewed sceptically by many of his listeners was a reduction of intraocular pressure, although the findings of his group had already been documented in a respected professional journal (1). These observations have since had independent confirmation from a number of laboratories. The mechanism is still unclear—one suggestion has been a β-adrenergic antagonistic effect, or an alteration of the parasympathetic/sympathetic balance, because many of the front-line drugs used to treat glaucoma fall in this category. The 20% training-induced reduction of intraocular pressures observed in the present group of patients with high initial intraocular pressures is of the order associated with β-blockade, and the disappearance of benefit 2–3 weeks after withdrawal of treatment also shows a similar time course.

When making assessments, both of initial intraocular pressures and of the response to treatment, it is finally important to control the time of exercise sessions, because an acute bout of exercise lowered pressures by 29% before training and (perhaps because of the lower resting readings) by only 22% after training.—R.J. Shephard, M.D., Ph.D.

Reference

1. Lemper P, et al: *Am J Ophthalmol* 63:1673, 1967.

Physical Activity and Risk of Developing Colorectal Cancer Among College Alumni
Lee I-M, Paffenbarger RS Jr, Hsieh C-C (Harvard Univ, Boston; Stanford Univ, Calif)
J Natl Cancer Inst 83:1324–1329, 1991   5–42

Background.—Recent studies have provided evidence that increased physical activity protects men against colon cancer, but physical activity over the long term can be difficult to assess. In this prospective study

17,148 Harvard alumni aged 30 to 79 years, were followed up from 1965 through 1988. Levels of physical activity were assessed in 1962 or 1966 and again in 1977, occurrence of colon and rectal cancer was determined, and a relationship between the 2 was sought.

Methods.—Data on physical activity were drawn from self-reporting questionnaires that asked about the number of flights of stairs climbed, amount of walking, and kinds and duration of sports played in the past week and in the past year. From the answers estimates of energy expenditures per week were made, and alumni were categorized according to activity level as inactive or moderately or highly active. The relative risk of rectal or colon cancer at different levels of activity was calculated and then corrected for potential confounding by age and body mass index.

Results.—Two hundred twenty-five incidents of colon cancer and 44 cases of rectal cancer occurred in this population. The use of either the 1962 or 1966 activity assessment or the 1977 assessment showed decreases in risk rates of colon cancer with increasing activity, but these decreases were not significant. When activity assessments based on 1962/1966 and 1977 findings were used for analysis, it was found that moderate activity at both assessments was associated with a .52 relative risk of developing colon cancer and that a high level of physical activity was associated with a relative risk of .5, compared to inactive alumni. Alumni who had higher activity levels at the later assessment were at slightly but not significantly lower risk of having colon cancer than those who did not. Those who had decreased activity at the later assessment had no less risk of colon cancer than those who were less active at the earlier assessment. Increased activity did not seem to be protective against rectal cancer.

Conclusions.—In this population either higher levels of activity over long periods of time are necessary to protect against colon cancer, or this relationship can be seen only when 2 assessments are combined for the analysis. No evidence was found that increased physical activity was protective against rectal cancer.

▶ A great deal of useful information has emerged from a painstaking long-term analysis of the behavior of Harvard alumni in relation to their subsequent health experience. One area where the data have seemed somewhat at variance with other studies has been in terms of the influence of physical activity on the incidence of colon cancer. In the present report, 2 assessments of activity were made (1962–1966 and 1977). However, it was necessary to combine information from both studies to demonstrate the significant twofold protection against colonic cancer that has been reported by other investigators. It remains unclear whether use of the 2 data sets gives a better differentiation of activity habits or provides a measure of sustained involvement in physical activity. However, in support of the second possibility, many of the studies where the risk of colonic cancer was reduced involved occupational activity, something that is likely to continue for 20–30 years.—R.J. Shephard, M.D., Ph.D.

Effects of Spontaneous Physical Exercise on Experimental Cancer Anorexia and Cachexia
Daneryd PL-E, Hafström LR, Karlberg IH (Sahlgrens Hospital, University of Göteborg, Sweden)
Eur J Cancer 26:1083–1088, 1990   5–43

LTW 56 (PRE-EXERCISED)

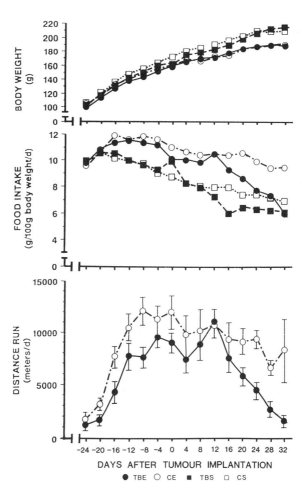

n = 10 in each group

Fig 5–19.—Body weight, food intake, and running distance in rats with 24 days of adaptation/training before tumor implantation. (Courtesy of Daneryd PL-E, Hafström LR, Karlberg IH: *Eur J Cancer* 26:1083–1088, 1990.)

Background.—Early experiments have shown that physical exercise has beneficial effects on tumor growth. Its effects on the tumor host, however, have not been assessed. A study was done to see whether spontaneous physical exercise delays the onset and reduces the extent of cancer anorexia and cachexia.

Methods.—Two transplantable experimental tumors were assessed in rats. Tumor-bearing Wistar Furth rats fed ad libitum and with free access to a running wheel were compared with nonexercised tumor-bearing rats and nonexercised non–tumor-bearing control rats.

Results.—The exercised rats had a delayed onset of anorexia compared with the control rats. Exercised tumor-bearing rats displayed normal behavior and were able to run the same daily distance as non-tumor-bearing control rats until the onset of cachexia. Exercised rats had a reduced carcass wet weight and lipid stores but an increased carcass dry weight. Despite a greater food intake, physical exercise resulted in a decreased final tumor weight without water content changes. Skeletal and cardiac muscle tissue did not differ in water content, but RNA/protein quotient was increased in the exercising tumor-bearing rats (Fig 5-19).

Conclusions.—Spontaneous physical exercise can apparently modify the deleterious changes induced by a malignancy on tumor host metabolism. A more detailed analysis of tumor host metabolism is needed before the clinical implications of these findings are established.

▶ Given that neoplasms lead to cachexia, and moderate exercise encourages protein retention in normal individuals, it is logical to test the possible benefit of physical activity as a palliative measure in those patients with tumors. The present experiment was conducted in rats rather than in humans, an important distinction (since the tumor is then experimental rather than spontaneous in origin). In view of the potential adverse effects of stress on immune function and thus tumor progression, the exercise was voluntary (use of a running wheel) rather than the commonly used techniques of enforced swimming or treadmill running in response to electric shocks). In the early stages of tumor growth, the exercise was indeed beneficial, increasing lean tissue mass. Perhaps more importantly, although the exercising rats had a larger food intake, the tumor grew more slowly than in the sedentary controls. But as the tumor became larger, a point was eventually reached where the rate of muscle wasting became greater than in sedentary controls. Presumably, at this stage, metabolism was unable to support the combined demands of exercise and tumor growth. There is a need to extend these findings to human volunteers, and to determine how long humans with cancer may usefully be encouraged to augment their physical activity.—R.J. Shephard, M.D., Ph.D.

Cardiac Output During Exercise in Paraplegic Subjects
Jehl JL, Gandmontagne M, Pastene G, Eyssette M, Flandrois R, Coudert J
(Faculté de Médecine, Clermont-Ferrand and Lyon; Hôpital Henry Gabrielle, Saint-Genis Laval, France)
Eur J Appl Physiol 62:256–260, 1991   5-44

Background.—Studies of exercise adaptation in paraplegics have focused mainly on gaseous exchanges during maximal arm exercise. Cardiac output using the CO_2 rebreathing method was examined during submaximal and maximal arm cranking exercises in paraplegics who had a high level of spinal cord injury.

Methods.—Six male paraplegics were compared with 8 able-bodied men not trained in arm exercise. The site of the paraplegics' spinal cord injury was superior or equal to T6, higher than sympathetic regulation of hepatosplanchnic and kidney circulation and higher than would permit the possibility of venous constriction below the cord injury. The paraplegics were active in daily life but did not participate in sports.

Findings.—Maximal O_2 consumption was lower in the paraplegics than in the able-bodied men. The 2 groups had similar maximal cardiac

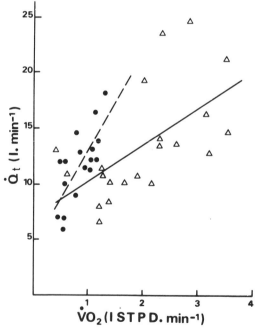

Fig 5–20.—Relationship between cardiac output (Q_t) and O_2 consumption ($\dot{V}O_2$) in 6 male paraplegics with high-level spinal cord injury (*circles*) and in 8 able-bodied men (*triangles*). (Courtesy of Jehl JL, Gandmontagne M, Pastene G, et al: *Eur J Appl Physiol* 62:256–260, 1991.)

output. The same result was obtained in the 2 groups for maximal heart rate and maximal stroke volume (Fig 5-20).

Conclusions.—Little difference was observed in maximal cardiac output between paraplegics and able-bodied men. However, the paraplegics' maximal oxygen consumption was half that of the able-bodied group. A major change in oxygen transport capacity to active muscle mass in paraplegics may result from alterations in vasomotor regulation below the level of the lesion.

▶ The majority of previous authors have used a similar technology (CO_2 rebreathing) to measure cardiac output in patients with spinal cord injuries. Typically, they have estimated a smaller than normal peak cardiac output, with stroke volume reduced by a peripheral pooling of blood in the inactive limbs (1,2). In contrast, the present report finds no difference of peak cardiac output between paraplegics and able-bodied individuals. But it makes 2 rather daring assumptions in reaching this conclusion. First, it is assumed that subjects can attain the necessary steady-state and carry out 15 seconds of rebreathing while performing maximal exercise, and second, it is assumed that there is no significant recirculation of blood during the 15-second interval. Both of these postulates are open to serious question, and this may be why the results are at variance with much previous work. It would be surprising if an abnormality of peripheral vasoregulation alone could account for the large difference of maximal oxygen intake between paraplegics and the able-bodied subjects in the face of a similar increment of cardiac output.—R.J. Shephard, M.D., Ph.D.

References

1. Hjeltnes N: *Scand J Rehabil Med* 9:107, 1977.
2. Davis GM, Shephard RJ: *Med Sci Sports Exerc* 20:463, 1988.

Epilepsy and Sports Participation
Gates JR (Univ of Minnesota, Minneapolis)
Phys Sportsmed 19:98–104, 1991   5–45

Background.—As diagnosis and treatment of epilepsy improve, affected patients are more than ever leading full, active lives. These patients often seek advice about physical activities, and recommended precautionary measures often go beyond what is reasonable and necessary. Issues related to exercise for epileptic patients are reviewed.

Discussion.—Regular physical activity should be encouraged for people with epilepsy. Such patients feel better and report better seizure control when they exercise regularly. Restrictions on activity for children with epilepsy should be minimized, although there is consensus that epilepsy patients should not participate in sports when a dangerous fall could result if a seizure occurred without warning. The increased ventilation during exercise is different from hyperventilation and will not cause seizures as hyperventilation does in some patients. Many patients are affected by epilepsy during their prime competitive sports years. In selecting a sport, the risks, the patient's frequency and timing of seizures, medication, and strength of the patient's preference should be considered. Sports such as rope or rock climbing, scuba diving, and bicycle riding should be avoided by patients who suffer frequent seizures. Contact sports appear to be allowable for those with no history of head injuries or significant structural lesions. Swimming is approved as long as there is close supervision. If seizures usually occur at a certain time of day, it is probably safe to engage in sports at other times.

Conclusions.—Patients should be warned that medications must be taken as prescribed, and that changes in weight may require adjustment of dose. Although children should be allowed to choose their activities, realistic limitations should be set if they show interest in a high-risk activity. Family, friends, and coaches should have basic knowledge of epilepsy and first aid.

▶ An eloquent and informative plea for wide access to sports and a full, active life for the 2% of our population with epilepsy, more than 4 million Americans. This paper outlines the salient clinical features of the 3 common types of epilepsy: generalized tonic-clonic seizures, or grand mal; absence attacks, or petit mal; and complex partial seizures, or psychomotor epilepsy. It provides commonsense guidelines for choosing activities and explains step-by-step what to do in the event of a seizure. There is a review of studies showing that many adults with active epilepsy, defined as at least 1 seizure a month, lead sedentary lives with limited social contact, and that physical training benefits them without meaningfully changing seizure rate or serum levels of antiepileptic drugs. The author reminds us that children with epilepsy have no higher rate of injury during daily activities than normal children, and that 75% of cases are diagnosed before the age of 20, so that many people are affected by epilepsy during their prime competitive sports years. Even swimming is generally safe, at least in the presence of an informed lifeguard. The article concludes that almost all patients with epilepsy can participate fully in sports.—E.R. Eichner, M.D.

The Preparticipation Exam: Special Concerns for the Special Olympics
Tanji JL (Univ of California, Sacramento)
Phys Sportsmed 19:61–68, 1991   5–46

Background.—Special Olympics athletes are many times more likely to have sports-significant impediments. To keep the participation of these athletes safe, physicians may sometimes have to disqualify an athlete from 1 event and recommend another. Pre-participation examinations tailored to the special needs of these athletes were evaluated.

Guidelines.—Annual examinations are necessary, because 39% of the athletes in the Special Olympics have sports-significant abnormalities. Because of the frequency of abnormalities among these athletes and because diagnoses are often associated with clusters of abnormal findings, a single-examiner method is best. Interpersonal communication is also enhanced when an examiner works one-on-one with an athlete. The physical examination includes assessment of height, weight, blood pressure, visual acuity, ear, nose, throat, eye, cardiorespiratory auscultation, and the abdomen, checking for hernia. Screening orthopedic assessment includes checking for scoliosis. If the patient's history is positive for injury, focused orthopedic examination is needed. Neurologic screening is also done. Findings that are of particular concern are loss of consciousness, sudden death in a relative younger than age 50 years, seizures, heat stroke or heat exhaustion, chronic medical problems and surgery, medication use, recreational or ergogenic drug use, fractures or dislocations, menstrual problems, asthma, and use of contact lenses, denture, or prosthetic devices. Athletes with Down syndrome must have 1 lateral cervical spine x-ray series in neutral, flexion, and extension positions to exclude atlantoaxial instability.

Conclusions.—Physicians can screen Special Olympics athletes most effectively by being alert to the clusters of findings associated with syndromes common to these athletes. A single-examiner approach to preparticipation assessment is recommended.

▶ A thoughtful and balanced approach to screening and encouraging Special Olympians. The most common disabilities are Down syndrome, cerebral palsy, seizure disorder, and developmental problems. Common findings include poor visual acuity, clonus, spasticity,, scoliosis, and heart murmur. Besides the cervical spine x-ray recommended for Down syndrome athletes, the examiner should look for metatarsus primus varus, pes planus, patellar instability, scoliosis, slipped capital femoral epiphysis, and various cardiac lesions, including ventricular septal defect. If an athlete must be disqualified from his or her chosen sport, it is important that the physician suggest an alternate, encourage the athlete, and stress a healthy lifestyle.—E.R. Eichner, M.D.

6 Injuries and Rehabilitation; Epidemiology and Prevention

A Three-Phase Analysis of the Prevention of Recreational Softball Injuries
Janda DH, Wojtys EM, Hankin FM, Benedict ME, Hensinger RN (St Joseph Mercy Hosp, Univ of Michigan, Ann Arbor; Huron Valley Hand Surgery, Ypsilanti, Mich)
Am J Sports Med 18:632–635, 1990   6–1

Introduction.—The prevention of recreational sports injuries — which are costly to society — is a major public health goal. It is impractical to make sliding illegal in baseball, a sport deeply steeped in tradition. As an alternative, the use of break-away bases was evaluated. As many as two thirds of injuries in recreational softball come from base sliding, most of them during rapid deceleration against a stationary base.

Observations.—In a prospective comparison study, 45 sliding injuries occurred in 627 softball games played with stationary bases, and only 2 occurred in 633 games played with break-away bases. Medical costs for the former injuries were nearly 80-fold greater. In a follow-up series of 1,035 games played with break-away bases, the 2 sliding injuries constituted 1 in more than 500 games. One of the players was injured when catching his cleat on the ground before reaching base.

Recommendation.—A significant number of serious softball injuries can be prevented by using break-away bases. These cost less than twice as much as standard stationary bases, and their use would avoid very substantial acute medical care costs.

▶ This paper represents an outstanding effort in the area of injury prevention for which the authors were awarded the American Orthopaedic Society for Sports Medicine 1989 excellence in research awarded in epidemiology. The break-away bases used in the study were manufactured by the Rogers Sports Corp. based in Elizabethtown, Penn. Apparently, each set of 3 bases costs $350.00, which is less than twice the cost the set of standard stationary bases. On the basis of the findings of this study, the Center for Disease

262 / Sports Medicine

Control estimated that 1.7 million injuries would be prevented at a savings of $2,000,000,000 per year nationally in medical care costs. Obviously, the next step is implementation.—J.S. Torg, M.D.

Profile of Sport/Leisure Injuries Treated at Emergency Rooms of Urban Hospitals
Pelletier RL, Anderson G, Stark RM (University of Ottawa; University of British Columbia; Ottawa General Hospital)
Can J Sport Sci 16:99–102, 1991   6–2

Objective.—An increase in the number of Ontario residents engaging in regular exercise has been accompanied by an increase in the number and severity of related injuries. Preliminary data were gathered on the number and nature of sport/leisure injuries in an urban Canadian population treated in hospital emergency rooms.

Findings.—During the 1-week survey period, 244 respondents, 4% of the total case load in 6 hospital emergency rooms, were treated for sport/leisure injuries. The injured persons were mostly males (73.4%) in the under-30 age group (86.3%) active at least once weekly (57.5%). The highest number (71.5%) of injuries was in noncontact sports such as touch football or soccer. Although almost two thirds of the injuries occurred during supervised activities, more than 55% of the injured persons received no treatment or first aid on site. Potentially serious injuries such as sprains, fractures, dislocations or separations, and concussions accounted for 52.9% of the injuries. Lack of first aid or proper on-site care could have serious consequences.

Conclusions.—The increasing number of injured athletes warrants increased community-oriented injury prevention and first-aid programs. These programs should be aimed at the most active individuals, those 30 years of age and younger, with special emphasis on the 11- to 20-year-olds.

▶ This study presents several problems. The occurrence of sports-related injuries is not presented on an injury rate basis, and severity criteria have not been included. Also, injuries that may have been treated by nonemergency physicians or, injuries in which no treatment at all was received have obviously been omitted. The authors also state that "there has been an overall increase in the number of Ontario residents who engage in regular exercise, coupled with an apparent increase in the number and severity of related injuries," the latter observation having been made by others. The observation that 4% of the total patient visits to emergency units is in keeping with a previous study by Watters et al. (1). It appears that between 4% and 7% of cases seen in emergency units are attributed to sports/leisure injuries.—J.S. Torg, M.D.

Reference

1. Watters D, et al: *Arch Emerg Med* 2:105, 1984.

Predictability of Sports Injuries: What Is the Epidemiological Evidence?
Meeuwisse WH (University of Calgary, Alta)
Sports Med 12:8–15, 1991   6–3

Introduction.—It is recognized that certain types of injury tend to occur in certain sports activities. Examples include the occurrence of otitis externa and shoulder disorders in swimmers and stress fractures in runners. Although there is a degree of overall predictability in sports injuries when rules, equipment, and playing conditions remain constant, it is much more difficult to predict injuries in individual athletes.

Prevention.—If risk factors are identifiable that predict injuries with some degree of certainty, athletes can take steps to prevent their occurrence. Removal of a risk factor is the most obvious approach. If several factors are involved, attempts can be made to modify them. A knowledge of the overall risk of injury will allow athletes to make a more informed decision about whether or not to participate.

Structural Measures as Predictors of Injury in Basketball Players
Shambaugh JP, Klein A, Herbert JH (NutriKinetics, Washington, DC)
Med Sci Sports Exerc 23:522–527, 1991   6–4

Introduction.—A wide range of factors have been studied in a search for predictors of sports injuries. To relate readily acquired structural measures to the occurrence of injury in basketball players, 45 players in a community center basketball league were studied.

Methods.—Measurements included bilateral weight, quadriceps girth, calf girth, the Q-angle of the knee, ankle dorsiflexion, forefoot and rearfoot valgus, and true and apparent leg lengths. Injuries that caused the player to miss a game were recorded during the 16-game season.

Results.—Injured players had average values for bilateral weight, quadriceps girth, Q-angle of the knee, rearfoot valgus, and leg length at least 1 SD greater than those for noninjured players. A logistic regression equation based on 3 of these variables (weight, Q-angle on both sides) correctly predicted the injury status of 91% of the players. When the equation was used prospectively to predict injuries in members of a college baseball team, the only player to miss a game from injury was identified as the most likely to be injured.

Conclusion.—Structural analysis can serve to predict the likelihood that basketball players will be injured. It should help in using manipulation, orthotics, and special training measures to reduce structural imbalances and therefore the risk of injury.

Etiologic Factors Associated With Patellofemoral Pain in Runners
Messier SP, Davis SE, Curl WW, Lowery RB, Pack RJ (Wake Forest Univ, Winston-Salem, NC)
Med Sci Sports Exerc 23:1008–1015, 1991   6–5

Introduction.—Overuse injuries and patellofemoral pain (PFP) are common in runners. Causative factors in PFP may be intrinsic or extrinsic, but research is needed to compare injured and noninjured runners under controlled conditions. Relationships among anthropometric, biomechanical, muscular strength and endurance, and training variables and runners afflicted with PFP were analyzed.

Methods.—The study sample was comprised of 20 uninjured and 16 injured runners both male and female aged 16 to 50 years. All had been running at least 4 days/week for at least 1 year. Diagnoses of PFP were made by an orthopedic surgeon. Subjects were analyzed by high-speed photography, force platform testing, and isokinetic dynamometry to evaluate rearfoot motion, ground reaction forces, and knee strength and endurance. The different categories of variables were compared by stepwise discriminant function analyses.

Results.—The injured and noninjured groups could be significantly discriminated by the Q angle. There were several significant discriminators in the muscular endurance data, with the injured group being weaker in knee extension endurance. Several significant discriminators were detected by kinetic analysis, but rearfoot movement was not a good discriminator. In addition, the injured patients ran significantly fewer miles per week than controls.

Conclusions.—A Q angle of more than 16 degrees appears to be a significant discriminator between runners with and without PFP. Several other muscular endurance and kinetic variables may also be important in the cause of PFP. Mileage and rearfoot movement do not appear to be important discriminators.

Patellofemoral Pain Caused by Overactivity: A Prospective Study of Risk Factors in Infantry Recruits
Milgrom C, Finestone A, Eldad A, Shlamkovitch N (Hadassah Hospital, Ein Kerem, Jerusalem; Israeli Defense Forces Medical Corps)
J Bone Joint Surg 73-A:1041–1043, 1991   6–6

Introduction.—There are a number of possible causes of patellofemoral pain. Repeated activities that generate high contact forces can result in overuse patellofemoral pain syndrome, a condition frequently observed in military trainees. This prospective study examined possible risk factors for the syndrome in a group of Israeli infantry recruits.

Methods.—The 390 male trainees underwent physical examinations before basic training. They were surveyed on their participation in sports before induction and asked to complete several physical fitness tests. Measurements were obtained on the medial tibial intercondylar distance in each of the trainees. Modified basketball shoes were randomly issued to 187 recruits and standard lightweight infantry boots to the remaining men. All were issued knee pads during the 14 weeks of training to protect the patellae from direct trauma.

Results.—Patellofemoral pain related to overactivity was diagnosed in 77 knees of 60 (15%) recruits. The time of onset of pain was distributed equally during the training period. The incidence of patellofemoral pain syndrome was not related to the type of footwear, but was significantly related to a greater than average medial tibial intercondylar distance and increased strength of the quadriceps. Recruits who could generate higher patellofemoral contact forces because of stronger extensor muscles of the knee had a higher rate of patellofemoral pain related to overactivity.

Conclusion.—This report appears to be the first prospective study of this condition. Findings support the idea that patellofemoral pain resulting from overactivity is caused by an overload of patellofemoral contact forces.

▶ Meeuwisse, in his article on "Predictability of Sports Injuries" (Abstract 6–3), clearly differentiates between the existence of risk factors for injury and epidemiologic evidence for predicting individual injury. He further points out that the next generation of injury prevention research should concern itself with "the factor in predicting injury." The articles by Shambaugh et al. (Abstract 6–4), Messier et al. (Abstract 6–5), and Milgrom et al. (Abstract 6–6) deal with this latter aspect.—J.S. Torg, M.D.

On the Importance of Planned Health Education; Prevention of Ski Injury as an Example
Kok G, Bouter LM (University of Limburg, The Netherlands)
Am J Sports Med 18:600–605, 1990   6–7

Introduction.—Together, health education specialists and sports injury specialists may be effective in preventing sports injuries. An educational strategy using the community approach for planning and evaluating health education was developed and applied to prevention of ski injury.

Planning.—The 10 questions to be addressed in planning and evaluating health education to prevent sports injuries are as follows:

1. How serious is the problem?
2. What behavior is involved?
3. What are the determinants of the behavior?

4. What options are there for change?
5. How can they be implemented?
6. Has the implementation been carried out as planned?
7. Has the intervention been received as planned?
8. Have the determinants of the behavior changed?
9. Has the behavior changed?
10. Has the problem been lessened?

Pitfalls.—The most common mistake is that of skipping steps, for example, jumping from problem to intervention without considering the planning steps. Other pitfalls include developing an intervention for a nonexistent problem, basing an intervention on a misconception, developing the wrong intervention, having an effective intervention but the wrong implementation, or being unjustifiably satisfied with the intervention. Behavior determinants must be taken into consideration, and intervention should be multisectoral. Pretesting is important in developing effective material aimed at changing behavior.

Conclusions.—The prevention of sports injuries can be achieved through cooperation and health education. Careful analysis must be made of the problem, behavior, determinants, intervention, implementation, and the relationship between these aspects.

▶ It is interesting that the authors conclude "until now, prevention of sports injuries has been dominated by sports injury specialists." Rather, it has been my observation that until now, prevention of sports injury has been virtually ignored by sports injury specialists. Furthermore, it is interesting to note that the authors also conclude "we believe that with respect to the prevention of most sports injuries, we still have not reached the stage where we know exactly what to advise people. Epidemiologic studies followed by research on the behavior determinants are necessary to fill in the gaps in our knowledge".
—J.S. Torg, M.D.

Promoting Bicycle Helmets to Children: A Campaign That Worked
Rogers LW, Bergman AB, Rivara FP (Harborview Injury Prevention and Research Ctr, Seattle)
J Musculoskel Med 8:64–77, 1991   6–8

Introduction.—Although bicycle helmets reduce the incidence of serious head and brain injuries, their use is unpopular, especially among children. A program was developed that was successful in inducing children to wear bicycle helmets.

Methods.—The campaign was based on a 2-step strategy, first to encourage parents to purchase helmets and then to encourage the children to wear them. The effort focused on children aged 5–9 years. Based on a consumer poll of third-graders and their parents, several themes evolved.

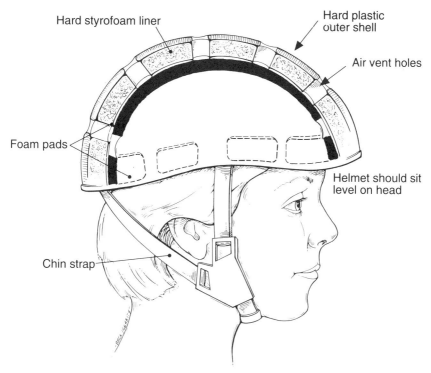

Hard styrofoam liner

Hard plastic outer shell

Air vent holes

Foam pads

Helmet should sit level on head

Chin strap

Fig 6–1.—Patient education guide. (Courtesy of Rogers LW, Bergman AB, Rivara FP: *J Musculoskel Med* 8:64–77, 1991.)

Parents needed education about the problem, low-cost helmets had to be available, children had to be encouraged to wear them, and public awareness had to be heightened. The program involved a coalition of 18 health, bicycling, helmet industry, and community-based organizations. Health care providers were encouraged to provide counseling and materials to patients and families (Fig 6–1). A coupon program for making helmets affordable, media coverage, and contributions from a variety of organizations and volunteers were important components. Incentive prizes were publicized and distributed by bicycle club volunteers. Cost was difficult to evaluate, but communities that had a strong coordinator had the greatest success. Helmet use among area children increased from 5% to 33%.

Conclusion.—Important components of such a program include active participation and involvement of physicians, sustained mass media support, and affordability of helmets.

▶ The importance of "educating parents and overcoming peer pressure" with regard to the use of bicycle helmets in children is clearly indicated in data from the National Electronic Injury Surveillance System (1). Specifically, bicycle injuries to children and adolescents result in over 400,000 emergency room visits and 500–600 deaths in the United States every year. As the authors have pointed out, although the bicycle is considered a toy, it is a major cause of serious head injury in children. One fourth of all significant brain injuries in children 14 years or younger are bicycle related. National Safety Council data indicate that children account for 70% of all bicycle-related injuries treated in hospital emergency rooms and for more than half of all bicycle-related deaths (2).—J.S. Torg, M.D.

References

1. The National Electronic Injury Surveillance System. MMWR 36:269–271, 1987.
2. National Safety Council: *Accident Facts*, 1982, pp 45–91.

Prevention of Cervical Spine Injuries in Football: A Model for Other Sports
Fine KM, Vegso JJ, Sennett B, Torg JS (Univ of Pennsylvania Sports Medicine Ctr, Philadelphia; Healthsouth, West Palm Beach, Fla)
Physician Sportsmed 19:54–64, 1991   6–9

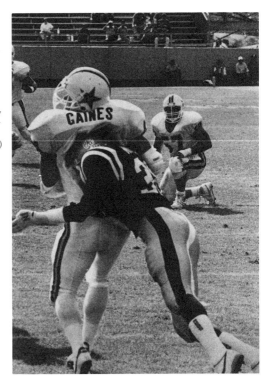

Fig 6–2.—A college defensive back (*dark jersey*) is shown ramming an opposing ball carrier with his head, resulting in severe axial loading of his cervical spine. The defensive player had fractures of C4, C5, and C6 and was rendered quardriplegic. The injury occurred October 28, 1989. (Courtesy of Fine KM, Vegso JJ, Sennett B, et al: *Physician Sportsmed* 19:54-64, 1991.)

Introduction.—Catastrophic injuries to the cervical spine and cord are not unknown in football and other collision sports, but often they are regarded as freak occurrences. Nevertheless, identifying mechanisms of injury can help implement effective preventive measures.

Mechanisms of Injury.—When the cervical spine is straightened with the neck flexed and force is directed along its longitudinal axis, angular deformation and buckling can occur, with failure of the intervertebral disks and/or the bony elements (Fig 6–2). Subluxation, facet dislocation, or fracture-dislocation may result. The critical role of axial loading in these injuries has been confirmed by studies of athletes in sports other than football, including rugby, diving, and ice hockey. Biomechanical studies also have shown the importance of axial loading in producing severe cervical spine injuries.

Conclusion.—The adoption of rules against "spearing" has dramatically reduced the number of serious cervical spine injuries occurring in college football. Cases of quadriplegia decreased from 34 in 1976 to 5 in 1984. Comparable steps might well decrease the occurrence of many types of injury in a wide range of sports.

▶ The data presented in this paper should be interpreted in light of more recent data published by Mueller and Shindler (1), which indicate an increase in the number of permanent cervical cord injuries among football players occurring in the 1988, 1989, and 1990 seasons. It appears that this apparent increase indicates a lack of both proper coaching techniques and enforcement of the rules by the officials. Certainly, this is a matter that those responsible for the conduct of the game should deal with.—J.S. Torg, M.D.

Reference

1. Mueller F, Shindler R: *Annual Survey in Football Injuries Research 1931–1991.* Mission, Kans, NCAA and NFCA, 1991.

Snowmobile Trauma: An Eleven-Year Experience
James EC, Lenz JO, Swenson WM, Cooley AM, Gomez YL, Antonenko DR (Univ of North Dakota, Grand Forks)
Am Surg 57:349–353, 1991   6–10

Background.—The first snowmobile was designed by a Canadian in 1923. Modern machines may weigh as much as 600 pounds and may be capable of speeds of up to 100 mph. The center of gravity of a snowmobile is low, but it is not a stable machine and can easily turn over on a slope or incline. Because registration is not necessary for snowmobiles used on private property, figures for registered snowmobiles in North Dakota dropped from 14,000 in 1982 to 6,415 in 1987. From 1977 through 1987, 88 patients were admitted to 1 hospital for snowmobiling injuries.

Findings.—Data collected included age, sex, method and degree of injury, use of safety attire, and risk factors. The 77 male and 11 female patients were treated for a total of 205 injuries, which required 760 hospital inpatient days. One hundred percent of injuries in 17 children younger than age 16 years involved extremities caught in the track of the snowmobile. There were 106 fractures in 71 patients; 18 patients had more than 1 fracture. Eleven patients had a loss of consciousness. There were 3 fatalities.

Conclusions.—The leading contributors to accidents in 88 patients seen over an 11-year period in 1 hospital were driver inexperience or carelessness, prior use of alcohol, excessive speed, and poor adherence to the manufacturer's recommendations. Education to promote the safe handling of snowmobiles, required safety courses and licensure of drivers, and mandatory protective footwear and helmets are all recommended.

▶ The authors call attention to the generally recognized fact that the snowmobile is a dangerous device. They effectively point out that children are too small to control the weight, speed, and power of a snowmobile. Also, although a relationship between substance abuse and injuries was not documented, alcohol was implicated in all 3 fatalities. It is worth taking note of their proposed regulations to improve safety:

1. Register all snowmobiles for tags at the time of purchase.

2. Require a course in safety for owners and all prospective drivers. The course should involve training in handling the snowmobile and familiarization with safety hazards before operation.

3. Strict prohibition of individuals under 16 years of age from operating snowmobiles.

4. Required licensure for snowmobile operation only after the successful completion of this safety course for individuals 16 years of age or older, regardless of whether the person has a valid automobile driver's license or age of the person.

5. Require safety-designed footwear for operation of snowmobiles.

6. Mandatory use of safety helmets for all drivers and passengers.

7. Yearly public awareness efforts through the media on safety requirements for the use of snowmobiles.—J.S. Torg, M.D.

Badminton Injuries
Krøner K, Schmidt SA, Nielsen AB, Yde J, Jakobsen BW, Møller-Madsen B, Jensen J (Univ Hosps of Aarhus, Denmark)
Br J Sports Med 24:169–172, 1990   6–11

Introduction.—Since badminton is such a popular sport in Denmark, with more than 170,000 club players, physical injuries should be a common occurrence from this physically demanding sport. The epidemiology and traumatology of badminton injuries during a 1-year period were assessed.

Methods.—A total of 4,303 patients with sports-related injuries were seen. A total of 217 badminton injuries in 208 patients were included. The age range was from 7 to 72 years, and badminton injuries were 4.1% of the registered sports injuries during the year.

Results.—Most players spent 2 hours a week playing badminton, and 44.8% had less than a 15-minute warm-up. Twenty percent had taken 30 minutes or more to warm up before playing. The over-30 age group spent significantly less time warming up than did the younger group. Only 10 players used prophylactic measures of any sort (e.g., taping, bandaging, or protective eyewear). Lower extremities were more often involved in injuries (82.9%) than were upper extremities (11.1%), and eyes were involved in 2.3% of the injuries. Most injuries (62%) were caused by falling or stumbling while playing. Most were minor and required treatment in the casualty department only (62.2%). Sprains and ligament ruptures were more frequent in younger players, and muscle injuries were more common in older players.

Conclusions.—Longer warm-up times, especially among older players, may decrease the risk of significant injury. Prophylactic interventions are recommended, such as protective eyewear, more intensive muscle exercises, taping, and stabilizing orthoses.

▶ The relative frequency of injury types reported by Kroner et al. differs from those of other authors. Specifically, Izen (1) and Mills (2) reported prominent badminton injuries to include lacerations, back and shoulder injuries, and fractures. In this study, these problems were infrequent. Also, Hensley and Paup (3) reported 7% eye injuries resulting from badminton compared to 2.3% reported by Kroner et al. Although the majority of injuries reported in this study were classified as "minor," it should be noted that a third of the injuries were severe enough to require hospitalization.—J.S. Torg, M.D.

References

1. Izen JA: Physical activity Sports, games and exercise; chronic injury, in Larson (ed); *Encyclopedia of Sport Sciences and Medicine.* New York: Macmillan, 1971.
2. Mills DMS: *Br J Sports Med* 11:51, 1977.
3. Hensley LD, Paup DC: *Br J Sports Med* 13:156, 1979.

Soccer Injuries Among Elite Female Players

Engström B, Johansson C, Törnkvist H (Huddinge University Hospital Huddinge, Sweden)
Am J Sports Med 19:372–375, 1991   6–12

Introduction.—Female soccer is becoming increasingly popular and now is played in 50 countries. In Sweden, soccer is the most popular female team sport. Injuries were reviewed over 1 year in 2 elite female soccer teams.

Results.—Of 41 players, 33 sustained a total of 78 injuries during the year of study. Nearly 90% of injuries were limited to the lower extremity. Traumatic injuries predominated at the start of the competitive season, whereas overuse injuries occurred mainly during preseason training and at the start and end of competition. Most injuries were minor, but there were 12 major injuries. The most common diagnosis was ankle sprain. Most traumatic injuries occurred during contact between 2 players. About 1 in 5 injuries were recurrences.

Conclusion.—Injury was very frequent in this survey of female soccer players in Sweden. Most injuries were minor, but there was a substantial number of major knee injuries. Changes in training probably would prevent many overuse injuries.

▶ This report of injuries occurring among a small but well documented study group raises 2 interesting points. First, the incidence of injury in this group, 12 per 1,000 hours, was twice that of the incidence of 5 per 1,000 hours reported for male elite soccer players (1). Also, in this group of 41 female players surveyed for 1 season, there were 7 knee ligament or meniscal tears. Thus, the authors have reported 1 "major knee injury" per 7 participants per year. —J.S. Torg, M.D.

Reference

1. Engström B, et al: *Am J Sports Med* 18:101, 1990.

Paragliding Injuries
Krüger-Franke M, Siebert CH, Pförringer W (Staatliche Orthopädische Klinik, Munich, Germany; Chirurgische Universitätsklinik Bonn, Germany)
Br J Sports Med 25:98–101, 1991   6–13

Introduction.—Paragliding is growing in popularity as a sport. Because serious injuries are associated with paragliding, the German Department of Transportation has issued guidelines regulating the sport. The types of injuries sustained during paragliding in Germany, Austria, and Switzerland were examined.

Methods.—There were 283 injuries in 218 paragliders documented in the study area from 1987 through 1989. Patients ranged in age from 15 to 59 years, with a mean age of 29.6 years; the majority (181) were men. A questionnaire was used to gather data on the patients, the type and site of injury, treatment, outcome, and the flight phase during which the injury occurred.

Results.—The majority (83%) of the 283 injuries occurred during planned or emergency landings. Twenty-eight injuries were sustained during take-off and 9 during flight. Fifty-nine patients suffered multiple injuries. Two deaths occurred, 1 following head trauma and 1 related to fracture-dislocation of the cervical spine. The lower extremities were affected in 41.3% of the cases. Only 13.4% of all cases involved the upper extremities. Almost 70% of the patients returned to paragliding.

Conclusion.—The landing phase of paragliding is particularly hazardous because of the likelihood of uneven terrain, unexpected obstacles, and forced landings in unfamiliar areas. Forces resulting from ground contact predispose to compression fractures of the thoracic and lumbar spine and calcaneus. Compression and rotation forces can lead to ankle injuries. Improvements in training and equipment may help to reduce the severity and rate of injuries.

▶ For the uninitiated, paragliding differs from both hang gliding and parachuting. Specifically, the paraglider is a single seat, nonmotorized advanced form of the parachute consisting of upper and lower sails. They are able to start from ground level without requiring a free-fall phase and are controlled by 2 steering lines attached to the chutes. It is interesting to note that of the injuries that resulted in paraplegia reported by the Arbeitsgemeinschaft Deutscher Querschnttszentren, a German organization of spinal trauma centers, for the period 1981–1989, 11 were the result of paragliding, 14 of hang gliding, and 12 of parachuting. Although the rate of injuries in general and those involving the spine in particular are not known, it certainly appears that this activity will keep the orthopedist busy.—J.S. Torg, M.D.

Snowboarding Injuries: An Analysis and Comparison With Alpine Skiing Injuries
Abu-Laban RB (Mineral Springs, Hosp, Banff, Alberta)
Can Med Assoc J 145:1097–1103, 1991   6–14

Background.—Snowboarding, in which small surfboards having fixed straps to anchor the feet are used, produces unique injuries. Most snowboards do not have quick-release binding systems such as those seen on alpine skis. The types of injuries and associated factors for snowboarders reported between 1988 and 1990 were assessed.

Methods.—All patients with injuries from snowboarding seen in the emergency department at the 20-bed Mineral Springs Hospital in Banff National Park from 1988 through 1990 were included in the study. Data on skiers injured in collisions with snowboarders also were obtained. When possible, patients completed a 23-item questionnaire that measured snowboard experience and accident history, fitness level, snow conditions, alcohol use, and other parameters.

Results.—A total of 115 injured snowboarders (87 males, 28 females) entered the emergency department during the study period. Of the 115, 73 (63%) completed the questionnaire; data for the other 42 were obtained from emergency records. The 115 snowboarders had a mean age of 20.3 years. Seven collisions with alpine skiers had occurred, with most of the skiers receiving only minor sprains or contusions. The 115 snowboarders had 132 injuries. Questionnaire results indicated that 83% of respondents had an excellent or above-average fitness level, 36% had no previous snowboard experience, 39% rated snow conditions as excellent, 59% reported light ski traffic on their hill, and 7% had ingested alcohol before the accident. The upper and lower body received equal amounts of injuries, but 75% of lower-body injuries affected the left or lead leg. Snowboarders had significantly different injuries compared with alpine skiers, with the former more likely to have spinal injuries, foot or ankle injuries, and distal radius fractures.

Implications.—These findings suggest that snowboarding is associated with a unique set of injuries, many of which can be prevented through athlete education and better equipment design.

▶ These 2 papers (Abstracts 6–14 and 6–15) describe the same snowboarding-associated injury patterns described by Pino and Colville (1). In view of the increasing numbers of snowboarders on the ski trails, it is most important that injury data be collected and analyzed. The more important question to be answered is, what impact do snowboarders and Alpine skiers have on one another. Specifically, has the presence of snowboards on downhill ski trails contributed to injuries to Alpine skiers? Abu-Laban did document 7 cases in which Alpine skiers collided with snowboarders. Although most of the skiers' injuries were mild, there was 1 fractured tibia in this small group. Also, Abu-Laban noted that his study had several design limitations. He pointed out that specific questions regarding speed, boot type, and injury mechanisms would have been in order, and he noted that some of his conclusions were speculative. He also recognized that data giving an accurate estimate of injury rates would be most desirable.—J.S. Torg, M.D.

Reference

1. Pino EC, Colville MR: *Am J Sports Med* 17:778, 1989.

Snowboarding: What Injuries to Expect in This Rapidly Growing Sport
McLennan JC, McLennan JG (Univ of Nevada, Reno; Northern Inyo Hosp, Bishop, Calif)
J Musculoskeletal Med 8:75–89, 1991   6–15

Introduction.—In the past 6 years the number of snowboarders has increased to more than 290,000 according to industry sources. The initial reluctance of ski areas to allow snowboarding has decreased in response to crossover participation by downhill skiers, fewer injuries than were anticipated initially, and reduced recreational demand in a recessionary economy.

Discussion.—In snowboarding the rider stands sideways, facing downhill, on a broad, wide ski. Turns are accomplished by weight changed in the hips and legs and by foot pressure. The newer boards are asymmetric in the nose and tail, thereby increasing control and stability. Soft-shell boots are less expensive than hard boots but do not protect as well against ankle injury. The hard boot is similar to a downhill ski boot, with a beveled toe and heel and binding clamps for the toe and heel. The snowboard stance is naturally triangulated, with the knees together and the feet apart. The components of riding (e.g., pressure control, edging, upper body positioning, and high-low positioning) are similar to those in skateboarding, watersurfing, and other sports. Injuries most commonly involve the soft tissues, with a slight predominance of upper extremity injury. More than half of all injuries have been muscle-ligament sprains and half of these were ankle injuries. In a 6-year period, the injury rate was 1.7/1,000 snowboard days, compared to 2-4 injuries per 1,000 downhill ski days.

Treatment of Injuries.—All injuries, except for the most minor, should be evaluated by a physician. Sprains, strains, contusions, and nondisplaced fractures should be treated with rest, elevation, immobilization, ice, and nonsteroidal anti-inflammatory agents followed by rehabilitation. The current trend in sports medicine for the treatment of displaced fractures or ligamentous injuries is delayed surgical intervention. The physician's role encompasses not only recognizing and handling or referring injuries but also patient education in preventing snowboarding accidents.

Common Cycling Injuries: Management and Prevention
Mellion MB (Sports Med Ctr, Omaha)
Sports Med 11:52-70, 1991   6-16

Purpose.—Traumatic and overuse injuries may well increase as more persons participate in athletic forms of bicycling. At present cycling injuries account for 500,000 visits per year to emergency rooms in the United States.

Types of Injury.—Over half of these accidents involve motor vehicles, and road surface and mechanical problems with the bicycle are also common causes of accidents. Head injuries account for most fatal accidents in cyclists. Abrasions, lacerations, and bruises are the most common injuries. Other traumatic injuries may involve contusions, sprains, and fractures, especially in the hand, wrist, lower arm, shoulder, ankle, and lower leg. Incorrect adjustment of the handlebar and seat may cause abdominal and genital injuries.

Treatment.—Management of overuse injuries may involve mechanical adjustment of the bicycle fit, seat, padding, pedals, and handlebars, as well as medical management. Neck and back pain may affect up to 60% of riders. Although helmets are effective and should always be used, victims of head injuries have rarely been wearing them.

Safety Measures.—Cyclists must take precautions against sun and heat injuries, especially dehydration and sunburn. Mirrors, eyewear, lights, and reflective clothing also protect the cyclist from the environment and make the cyclist visible to motor vehicles.

▶ An excellent review of the subject matter. The original article is recommended to the interested reader.—J.S. Torg, M.D.

Hazards of Horse-Riding as a Popular Sport
Silver JR, Parry JML (Stoke Mandeville Hospital, Aylesbury, England)
Br J Sports Med 25:105–110, 1991   6–17

Background.—Horseback riding is a popular sport in England, where there are estimated to be over 3 million riders. There has been a growing concern about the fact that the sport carries a high risk of morbidity and mortality. Many riding accidents result in serious head and spinal injuries. The extent to which riding accidents might be preventable was studied.

Methods.—A questionnaire was designed to cover the major factors thought to be responsible for accidents. Patients seen at the study institution were interviewed as soon as possible after the riding accident. Other patients with serious injuries were interviewed some years after the accident. Twenty cases were analyzed in greater detail for information about the horse, the rider, and the circumstances and outcome of the accident. Riders involved in minor accidents were compared with those sustaining serious spinal injuries.

Results.—The typical accident occurred on a summer afternoon in good weather and involved a relatively inexperienced rider on a mare from an unapproved riding establishment. Fractures were the most common injury. The horse was usually excitable and became uncontrollable. Although the equipment was not faulty, the setup was often incorrect. Ten of the 20 selected accidents were entirely preventable and 2 were possibly preventable.

Conclusion.—In this limited survey, spinal injuries were more serious than head injuries. Thus protective head gear will not eliminate all major injuries. Many accidents might be prevented, however, by the choice of a horse and a route suited to the rider's level of experience.

▶ The authors point out that the concept that "accidents are inevitable" and may be "viewed as an act of God" is to be questioned. Rather, they subscribe to the premise that equestrian accidents are caused by human errors and are thus preventable. Putting things in perspective, they point out serious injuries from motorcycles occur at a rate of 1/7,000 hours, whereas those from horse riding occur at 1/350 hours. Thus, on the basis of these data, it appears that horse riding is 20 times as dangerous as motorcycling. Also pointed out is the fact that "many impacts are not entirely directed to the head so the concentration only on the value of preventative head gear will not eliminate serious spine injuries".—J.S. Torg, M.D.

Do Asymptomatic Marathon Runners Have an Increased Prevalence of Meniscal Abnormalities? An MR Study of the Knee in 23 Volunteers

Shellock FG, Deutsch AL, Mink JH, Kerr R (Cedars-Sinai Med Ctr; Univ of California, Los Angeles)
AJR 157:1239–1241, 1991   6–18

Introduction.—The increased number of runners has led to a rise in injuries related to the sport. These injuries are caused basically by the forces generated in running. Magnetic resonance imaging was used to examine 23 asymptomatic marathon runners to determine the incidence of meniscal abnormalities in this population.

Methods.—The 15 women and 8 men had an average age of 40 years. All underwent MRI with a 1.5-T MR scanner and a transmit/receive extremity coil. The runners had trained for an average of 10 years at an average training distance of 41 miles per week. The MRI scans were reviewed by 3 musculoskeletal radiologists to determine whether the meniscus showed any signs of intrameniscal signals or morphological abnormalities.

Findings.—Of the 92 meniscal horns studied, 49 received a grade 0 signal, 29 a grade 1 signal, 12 a grade 2 signal, and 2 a grade 3 signal. The overall prevalence of meniscal tears was 9% in the asymptomatic runners. The prevalence of meniscal tears was 6% in the athletes younger than age 45 years and 14% in those 45 years or older. No associations were observed between the runner's age and signal abnormalities in the meniscus or between the meniscal signal abnormalities and the number of years of training.

Conclusions.—The prevalence of meniscal tears in the marathon-running population is not higher than that found in sedentary individuals. These runners appear to have the same amount of meniscal degeneration as is observed in nonrunner athletes. These findings may possibly relate to compensatory alterations that occur in the menisci as a result of prolonged physical training. The adaptations experienced by the marathon runners may actually preserve the integrity of the meniscus area in the older athlete, delaying normal degeneration of the meniscus.

▶ The sample is extremely small; however, what this paper has identified is the following: no symptoms, no pain, no findings.—J.S. Torg, M.D.

Postoperative Pulmonary Edema in Young, Athletic Adults
Holmes JR, Hensinger RN, Wojtys EW (Univ of Michigan, Ann Arbor)
Am J Sports Med 19:365–371, 1991   6–19

Background.—Laryngospasm after extubation may lead to pulmonary edema, which is life-threatening unless diagnosed and treated promptly. Only 7 such cases have been reported in adults; however, the situation may be much more common, as 7 cases were observed at 1 institution in a 2-year period.

Patients.—The patients were young, healthy, athletic men, with an average weight of 218 lb. Five patients competed on the collegiate and/or professional level. All of the men were undergoing relatively minor, uncomplicated operations—mostly orthopedic procedures—under general anesthesia. Immediately after extubation and mask anesthesia, clinical laryngospasm was noted, followed shortly by pulmonary edema. Clinical

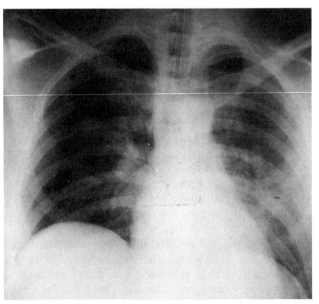

Fig 6–3.—Chest roentgenogram obtained within 1 hour of obstructive event, demonstrating diffuse pulmonary edema. (Courtesy of Holmes JR, Hensinger RN, Wojtys EW: *Am J Sports Med* 19:365–371, 1991.)

examination, arterial blood gas measurements or pulse oximetry, and chest radiography were done to confirm the diagnoses (Fig 6–3).

Outcome.—Four patients had to be reintubated. In all cases but 1, the edema resolved rapidly with prompt diagnosis and treatment with oxygen, diuretics, reintubation, and/or positive pressure ventilation. Pulmonary edema was not immediately recognized in the remaining patient, and it progressed to a florid state. The patient required emergency intubation 14 hours later, followed by mechanical ventilation for 3 days. The condition may have resulted from combined cardiogenic and neurogenic mechanisms, as well as hypoxia. In the present series, the most likely mechanism was excessive negative intrathoracic pressure generated by forced inspiration against a closed glottis.

Conclusions.—Young, healthy, athletic men may be at increased risk of postoperative pulmonary edema, probably because of their ability to generate extreme negative intrathoracic pressures. This knowledge could affect the choice of anesthesia, precautions on extubation, prolonged monitoring in the recovery phase, and rapid intervention in such patients.

▶ This experience on the part of the authors certainly presents a compelling argument for the routine use of regional and local anesthesia. In our institution, patients are encouraged to have epidural anesthesia for all major lower extremity procedures. All diagnostic and surgical arthroscopy procedures of the knee, ankle, and shoulder joints are routinely done under local anesthesia with intravenous sedation.—J.S. Torg, M.D.

7 Head, Neck, Back, Shoulder, and Arm

Head, Neck, and Back

Concussion in Sports: Guidelines for the Prevention of Catastrophic Outcome

Kelley JP, Nichols JS, Filley CM, Lillehei KO, Rubinstein D, Kleinschmidt-DeMasters BK (Univ of Colorado, Denver)
JAMA 266:2867–2869, 1991   7–1

Introduction.—Concussion, a traumatically induced alteration in mental status, is an extremely common injury in contact sports. Repeated concussions can lead to brain atrophy, neuropsychological deficits, or death. A high school football player died after repeated concussions without loss of consciousness.

Case Report.—Boy, 17 years, had a concussion without loss of consciousness in a football game and complained of headache for a week thereafter. The next week, he played again, wearing a professional-caliber padded-style helmet. He was struck on the side of the helmet by the helmet of a tackler, and was stunned, but his mental condition improved quickly and he re-entered the game. In the next play, his helmet made light contact with those of several tacklers. After rising from the pile of players, he fell, unconscious. He had minimal sponaneous movements of all limbs, rapid shallow breathing, no response to voice or shaking, little response to pain, and anisocoria. After an ambulance ride to a hospital, he arrived totally unresponsive with fixed and dilated pupils. He did not improve after hyperventilation and the administration of mannitol, furosemide, and dexamethasone, and he was transferred by air ambulance to a trauma center. There, CT showed a diffusely swollen brain and compression of the suprasellar and quadrigeminal cisterns, the fourth ventricle, and the cerebral sulci. The lateral ventricles were slightly enlarged, and an initial intracranial pressure of 35 mm Hg was recorded with an intraventricular catheter. No treatment was successful in controlling the intracranial pressure, which increased to 56 mm Hg after 4 hours. Cerebral angiography showed slow blood flow through the carotid and vertebral arteries and no intracranial blood flow. He was pronounced dead 15 hours after his final injury. At autopsy, massive swelling and vascular congestion of the brain, with no evidence of significant brain hemorrhages, anoxic damage, or diffuse axonal injury, and little edema were found.

Conclusion.—Vascular engorgement appears to have led to the severe brain swelling that caused the death of this patient. This phenomenon has been reported after severe traumatic brain injury and repeated mild head injuries over a short period of time. Catastrophic outcomes can follow repeated concussions. Even concussions that occur without loss of consciousness can lead to diffuse brain swelling after a second injury. Close observation and proper assessment using the Colorado guidelines may eliminate this preventable problem.

▶ The authors have reintroduced the concepts of "the second impact syndrome," "malignant cerebral edema," and "diffuse cerebral swelling" as a sequelae of minor head trauma. Emphasized is the fact that a life-threatening situation can result without loss of consciousness. Although the guidelines on the management of the concussion in sports represent nothing new, they should certainly be known and implemented by those caring for young athletes.—J.S. Torg, M.D.

The Prolonged Burner Syndrome
Speer KP, Bassett FH III (Duke Univ, Durham, NC)
Am J Sports Med 18:591–594, 1990   7–2

Background.—One of the most common injuries in tackle football occurs when a player makes contact with his head and shoulder and experiences intense burning pain, and in many cases, numbness about the shoulder. Pain may radiate into the arm or hand and often is followed by a heavy or dead feeling in the extremity. Recovery is prolonged in a small number of athletes.

Experience.—Nineteen university football players who reported a burner during the 1987 season were evaluated. Recovery was delayed in 6 of the athletes. Four of the players had weak deltoid, biceps, and/or spinatus muscles. Electrodiagnostic studies, done 4 weeks after injury, showed abnormalities in 3 of the 6 players, which in 2 instances suggested possible nerve injury. Positive findings correlated best with muscle weakness 72 hours after injury. Two of the 3 patients with electrodiagnostic abnormalities were clinically well at the time of study.

Discussion.—The C5 and C6 nerve segments are most often involved in the burner syndrome. Prolonged weakness may occur without significant axonal loss. The clinical findings should, in large part, guide the return to play. The use of better cushioned shock-absorbing shoulder pads and a custom rubber neck roll will help prevent reinjury. Neck-strengthening exercises also are important.

▶ This paper presents several interesting observations. Although there was no correlation between initial physical findings and the results of electrodiagnostic testing, evidence of muscular weakness at 72 hours after injury did correlate with positive electrodiagnostic findings. This study is also in keeping with the findings of Bergfeld et al., which demonstrated that of those players with brachial plexus injuries with an initial abnormal EMG and a neurologic deficit, 80% had abnormal EMG findings 4 years postinjury, although all returned to sports participation with minimal functional loss (1). Thus, both Bergfeld and Speer and Bassett conclude that a normal EMG should not be a criteria for return to activity following the burner syndrome.—J.S. Torg, M.D.

Reference

1. Bergfeld JA, et al: *Orthop Trans* 12:743, 1988.

Spinal Injuries in Ice Hockey Players, 1966–1987
Tator CH, Edmonds VE, Lapczak L, Tator IB (University of Toronto)
Can J Surg 34:63–69, 1991   7–3

Background.—A registry of spinal cord injuries established by the Committee on Prevention of Spinal Cord Injuries Due to Hockey lists 117 cases between January 1966 and March 1987. The committee monitors injuries, conducts research into the cause of the injuries, and develops preventive programs.

Findings.—Up to 15 hockey-related major spinal injuries were reported in Canada each year between 1981 and 1986. The injuries commonly resulted from the mechanism of axial loading as a push or check from behind caused the player to catapult head first into the boards. Small rinks may also be a factor because collisions are more frequent and the boards lack shock absorption. Teenagers and players younger than age 30 years playing in supervised games were the most commonly injured. Factors related to spinal cord injuries in hockey include the increased weight, speed, height, and aggressiveness of hockey players. The players' lack of strengthening of the neck muscles or knowledge of the hazards of the game are also factors.

Conclusion.—Preventive programs of the hockey associations, players, equipment manufacturers, health care professionals, researchers, and government are designed to be a prophylactic measure. The aim of the Canadian hockey program is to emulate the success of the United States football program and the European hockey program in reducing the incidence of spinal cord injuries by improving awareness and attitude and effecting rule changes.

▶ This paper clearly indicates that, similar to American football, the mechanism of cervical spine injury in ice hockey is that of axial loading. Specifically, "axial loading was found to be the most common mechanism causing cervical-spine and cervical-cord injury. Axial loading was applied to the head when the helmeted head struck another object, especially the boards. The

event that precipitated the injury was usually a push or check from behind
. . . ." Apparently, The Canadian Amateur Hockey Association introduced
specific rules against pushing or checking from behind in 1985. Unfortunately, this plus other measures apparently have not resulted in a decline of
spinal cord injuries, particularly those associated with paralysis. In view of
this, one must question the vigor with which coaching and officiating practices have been affected by the rules change. Also of note, previous reports
by these authors indicated that, similar to American football, an increase in
cervical spine injuries was noted with the advent of widespread use of
hockey helmets in Canadian Junior Hockey.—J.S. Torg, M.D.

**The Axial Load Teardrop Fracture: A Biomechanical, Clinical, and
Roentgenographic Analysis**
Torg JS, Pavlov H, O'Neill MJ, Nichols CE III, Sennett B (Univ of Pennsylva-
nia, Philadelphia; Hosp for Special Surgery, New York; Univ of Vermont, Bur-
lington)
Am J Sports Med 19:355–364, 1991   7–4

Background.—Schneider and Cann originally described an anteroinferior cervical vertebral body corner fracture as a "teardrop" fracture. The
biomechanical, clinical, and radiographic features of a series of these
fractures were analyzed.

Methods.—Fifty-five teardrop fractures registered with the National
Football Head and Neck Injury Registry were studied. These fractures
typically resulted when players attempted to make a tackle in which initial contact was made with the top or crown of the helmet.

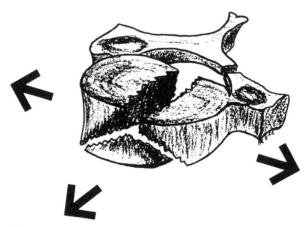

Fig 7–1.—Three-part, 2-plane fracture of C4 is identified on lateral and frontal roentgenograms.
There is anteroinferior corner fracture fragment and sagittal fracture through the entire vertebral body.
Posterior arch is fractured. (Courtesy of Torg JS, Pavlov H, O'Neill MJ, et al: *Am J Sports Med*
19:355–364, 1991.)

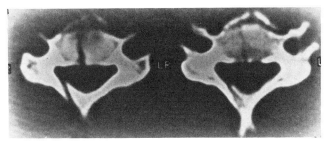

Fig 7–2.—A 3-part, 2-plane fracture of C6. Examination by CT shows sagittal fracture extending completely through vertebral body, with disruption of lamina on right. (Courtesy of Torg JS, Pavlov H, O'Neill MJ, et al: *Am J Sports Med* 19:355–364, 1991.)

Findings.—Two fracture patterns were associated with the anteroinferior corner fracture fragment. The first was an isolated fracture, which was usually not associated with permanent neurologic consequences. The second was the 3-part, 2-plane fracture associated with sagittal vertebral body fracture and fracture of the posterior neural arch. The second pattern was almost always associated with permanent neurologic sequelae, specifically quadriplegia. Axial loading of the cervical spine was a mechanism of injury in both types of fractures (Figs 7–1 and 7–2).

Conclusions.—Two fracture patterns are associated with the anteroinferior corner fracture. The mechanism of injury for both patterns is axial load. Seventy-three percent of these fractures in football occur while the player is attempting a tackle. Radiographic assessment must include both anteroposterior and lateral views with CT or tomography as needed to determine the presence of the sagittal vertebral body fracture and the integrity of the posterior neural arch.

▶ This paper corrects to 2 major flaws in Schneider's orginial description of what he termed the "hyperflexion teardrop fracture" (1). Specifically, on the basis of video analysis, it is quite clear that the mechanism of injury is that of axial load rather than hyperflexion of the cervical spine. Schneider's original paper relied solely on lateral x rays to the exclusion of other views, including anteroposterior projection. Thus, the sagittal vertebral body fracture was missed, as well as its significance with regard to neurological involvement. Emphasized is the fact that a complete radiologic examination should be performed and should include a lateral view to determine the extent of posterior displacement and angulation of the posterior vertebral body fragment, and an AP view with CT or tomography if necessary to determine the presence or absence of a sagittal vertebral body fracture as well as the integrity of the posterior arch. These views are essential in evaluating patients after cervical spine trauma. To be noted is the extensive bibliography that accompanies the original paper.—J.S. Torg, M.D.

Reference

1. Schneider RC, et al: *JAMA* 177:362, 1961.

Axial Loading Injuries to the Middle Cervical Spine Segment: An Analysis and Classification of Twenty-Five Cases
Torg JS, Sennett B, Vegso JJ, Pavlov H (Univ of Pennsylvania Sports Medicine Ctr, Philadelphia)
Am J Sports Med 19:6–20, 1991   7–5

Introduction.—There are few reports of injuries to the cervical spine at the C3–C4 level that involve the bony elements, intervertebral disks, and ligamentous structures.

Methods.—Data on 25 athletes with such injuries documented by the National Football Head and Neck Injury Registry were reviewed.

Results.—The response of energy inputs at the C3–C4 level differ from those involving the upper and lower cervical segments. The C3–C4 lesions appear to be unique in their infrequency of bony fracture, difficulty in effecting and maintaining reduction, and a better outcome after early, aggressive therapy. Injury at this level results from axial loading of the cervical spine in most patients. Lesion distribution was acute intervertebral disk herniation in 4 patients, anterior subluxation of C3 on C4 in 4, unilateral facet dislocation in 6, bilateral facet dislocation in 7, and

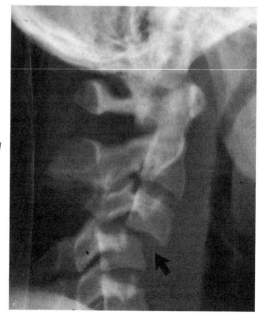

Fig 7–3.—Patient 19. Lateral roentgenogram of the cervical spine obtained shortly after the patient's injury demonstrates a bilateral facet dislocation at C3-C4. In addition to marked anterior translation of C3, there is an associated anterior angulation as well as increased distance between the spinous processes of C3 and C4. (Courtesy of Torg JS Sennett B, Vegso JJ, et al: *Am J Sports Med* 19:6–20, 1991.)

fracture of vertebral body C4 in 4. In 2 patients with unilateral facet dislocation reduced within 3 hours of the injury and subsequently fused anteriorly, there was significant neurologic recovery. The other 4 patients with this distribution remained quadriplegic. Although 4 patients with bilateral facet dislocation had successful reduction by closed or open methods and survived their injuries, they did not recover neurologically. The 3 patients with this type of injury who did not have successful reductions died (Fig 7–3).

Conclusion.—The response to axial loading energy inputs at the middle cervical level is different from those at the upper and lower cervical levels. Traumatic lesions to the cervical spine should be categorized accordingly. In patients with unilateral and bilateral facet dislocations, outcomes are much more favorable when immediate reduction is achieved.

▶ The material presented strongly supports the concept that traumatic lesions of the cervical spine should be classified as involving the upper (C1–C2), middle (C3–C4), and lower (C4–C7), segments. This is based on the following observations.

1. C3–C4 lesions generally do not involve fracture of the bony elements.

2. Acute intervertebral disk herniations are frequently associated with transient quadriplegia.

3. Reduction of anterior subluxation of C3–C4 is difficult to maintain.

4. Reduction of unilateral facet dislocation is difficult to maintain by skeletal traction and is best managed by closed manipulative reduction under general anesthesia.

5. Reduction of bilateral facet dislocation is difficult to obtain by skeletal traction and is best managed by open methods.

Also, to be emphasized is the more favorable result of immediate reduction of both unilateral and facet dislocations.—J.S. Torg, M.D.

Radiographic Findings of Degeneration in Cervical Spines of Middle-Aged Soccer Players
Kurosawa H, Yamanoi T, Yamokoshi K-i (Hokkaido Univ, Sapporo, Japan; Hokkaigakuen Univ, Sapporo)
Skeletal Radiol 20:437–440, 1991   7–6

Background.—Soccer players receive numerous blows to the head and loads to the neck, mainly because of heading. There have been few reports of the chronic cervical signs or symptoms in these athletes. The cervical radiographic findings were studied in 12 soccer players with symptoms of the head and neck.

Patients.—Twelve patients with an average age of 40.1 years were admitted with symptoms suggestive of cervical spondylosis. They had been playing soccer for an average of 15 years. All 12 underwent cervical radiography and classification of any abnormal shadows. Stress distribution analysis by using the finite element method was used to show the stress in heading the ball.

Findings.—Several types of abnormal radiographic findings were observed. Three patients had calcification of the anterior longitudinal ligament. Nine had anterior and 9 had posterior vertebral spurs. Nine had ossicles between spinous processes and 7 had calcification of the nuchal ligament. Three patients had ossicles on a spinous process and 10 had a bony spur on Luschka's joints. Stress analysis showed that forces were applied mainly to the lower parts of the cervical spine, which correlated well with some of the radiographic findings.

Conclusions.—Early degenerative changes may be seen in the cervical spines of middle-aged soccer players. These radiographic changes appear to result from acute or chronic trauma in conjunction with spondylosis of middle age. The changes observed were slight and not correlated with symptoms.

▶ It appears that the conclusion to be drawn from the material presented in this paper is that the cervical spondolytic changes that occur in the population in general are also experienced by those who have played soccer.—J.S. Torg, M.D.

Catastrophic Rugby Injuries of the Spinal Cord: Changing Patterns of Injury
Scher AT (Tygerberg Hosp, Republic of South Africa; University of Stellenbosch, Tygerberg)
Br J Sports Med 25:57–60, 1991   7–7

Background.—It has been reported in both England and New Zealand that the incidence of rugby injuries to the cervical spinal cord has decreased and that injuries from the tackle have also decreased. This has not been reported for South Africa. An analysis of spinal cord injuries sustained by 40 rugby players from 1985 to 1989 was undertaken to determine the true incidence and pattern of such injuries in South Africa.

Methods.—The radiological appearance on admission was correlated with the circumstances of injury, associated orthopedic injury, and neurologic deficit. The cases were subdivided into groups according to the phase of the game during which the injuries were sustained.

Results.—The tackle was responsible for most of these injuries. Tackles were also responsible for most cases of complete, permanent quadriplegia. The most common cause of injury in those being tackled was the high tackle around the neck. The most common cause of injury in players making the tackle was the dive tackle.

Conclusions.—The incidence and pattern of rugby cervical spinal cord injury has not improved in recent years in South Africa. The technique of safe tackling must be taught and rules against unsafe tackling practices must be enforced to prevent, as much as possible, these crippling avoidable injuries.

▶ This study indicates that the tackle is now the major cause of spinal cord injuries in South African rugby, in contrast to earlier reports in which the scrum was identified as the most common cause. In contradistinction to the significant reduction of catastrophic cervical spine injuries that has occurred in American football, "this survey has shown that despite the numerous changes in the laws of rugby, intensive media interest, and high level of public awareness, the situation as regards cervical spinal cord injuries in South Africa has not improved in recent years." The situation can also be contrasted to the experience in England (1) and New Zealand (2), where decreases in the incidence of spinal cord injuries resulting from rugby have occurred.—J.S. Torg, M.D.

References

1. Silver JR: *BMJ* 288:37, 1984.
2. Burry HC, Gowland H: *Br J Sports Med* 15:56, 1981.

Eye Injuries—Prevention, Evaluation, and Treatment
Erie JC (Mayo Clinic and Found, Rochester, Minn)
Physician Sportsmed 19:108–122, 1991   7–8

Background.—Sports-related ocular trauma has increased. Baseball, basketball, and racquet sports are the leading causes of sports-related

TABLE 1.—Postinjury Ocular Findings That Require Immediate
Ophthalmologic Referral

Embedded corneal foreign body

Haze or blood in the anterior chamber (hyphema)

Decreased central or peripheral vision

Irregular, asymmetric, or poorly reactive pupil

Diplopia

Laceration of the lid margin or impaired lid function

Suspected globe perforation

Broken contact lens or shattered eyeglasses

Note: Adapted from Vinger, PF, Hoerner, EF: Sports Injuries: The Unthwarted Epidemic.
(Courtesy of Erie, JC: *Physician Sportsmedicine,* 19:108–122, 1991.)

TABLE 2.—On-Site First Aid Equipment for Evaluating and Treating Eye Injuries

Telephone number of local hospital and covering ophthalmologist or physician

Near-vision card

Penlight

Hard metal or plastic protective eye shield

Eye patches (sterile)

Tape (transparent or micropore)

Skin closure strips (sterile)

Irrigating solution (sterile)

Cotton swabs (sterile)

Fluorescein strips (sterile)

Cobalt blue light

Antibiotic ophthalmic ointment, such as erythromycin, 0.5% (Ak-mycin, Ilotycin)

Anesthetic eye drops (sterile unit dose), such as proparacaine, 0.5% (various)

Note: Adapted from Vinger, PF, Hoerner, EF: Sports Injuries: The Unthwarted Epidemic. Littleton, MA PSG Publishing Co., Inc., 1986, p. 118.
(Courtesy of Erie, JC: *Physician Sportsmedicine*, 19:108-122, 1991.)

eye injuries. Most of these injuries could be prevented by the use of adequate eye wear. A thorough, 5-step first aid examination and appropriate treatment or referral can prevent long-term damage.

Discussion.—Eye injuries are categorized as either blunt or penetrating. Most sports-related injuries are in the blunt trauma category. Penetrating injuries to the globe may result from eyeglass breakage. An immediate on-site examination should include these 5 steps. After a near-vision check is completed, the pupil should be examined with a penlight. Pupil irregularity in the absence of surgical manipulation is almost always pathologic. Careful corneal inspection with a penlight may reveal an embedded foreign object, edema, hyphema, or iritis. The conjunctiva should be examined for scleral perforation or foreign bodies. Eye motility should be observed in all positions of gaze. Many sports-related ocular injuries may be treated on-site but certain types of eye injuries, such as blunt trauma, should be referred to an ophthalmologist (Tables 1 and 2). When used properly, protective devices that meet American Society for Testing and Materials and other industry standards can significantly reduce the risk and severity of sports-related eye injuries. These devices include polycarbonate eyeguards for racket sports, injection-molded polycarbonate face protectors for hockey, carbon steel rod batter's guard, or mylar-covered polycarbonate football eyeguards.

Conclusions.—Immediate attention is required for any sports-related eye injury. Following a 5-step protocol for eye examination should help the attending physician, coach, or trainer determine when and how to treat injuries on-site and when an injury should be referred to an ophthalmologist. The most important factor is prevention of injuries through the use of protective devices that meet American Society for Testing and Materials and other industry standards.

▶ Permanent eye damage can be prevented in many instances by the use of proper protective eye wear. Athletic trainers must be prepared for eye injuries and recognize those that need immediate referral to an opthomologist. Please refer to Tables 1 and 2, and remember that the goal we should be seeking regarding eye injuries is *prevention.*—F.J. George, A.T.C., P.T.

The Contribution of the Rectus Abdominis and Rectus Femoris in Twelve Selected Abdominal Exercises: An Electromyographic Study
Guimaraes ACS, Vaz MA, de Campos MIA, Marantes R (Federal University of Rio Grande do Sul, Brazil)
J Sports Med Phys Fitness 31:222–230, 1991   7–9

Introduction.—The importance of the abdominal muscles in human beings has been previously demonstrated. The effect of 12 selected abdominal exercises on the muscle action potentials (MAPs) of the rectus abdominis (upper and lower portions) and rectus femoris was studied.

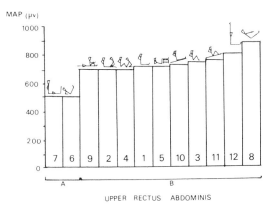

Fig 7–4.—Mean muscle action potentials (MAP) for the upper portion of the rectus abdominis are shown in microvolts for 12 exercises. Exercises not enclosed within the same bracket were significantly different. *Numbers within each column* identify exercises. (Courtesy of Guimaraes ACS, Vaz MA, de Campos MIA, et al: *J Sports Med Phys Fitness* 31:222–230, 1991.)

Methods.—The 12 exercises were performed by students of physical education.

Results.—Elevation of the lower limbs from the long lying and forearm supported positions elicited significantly lower MAPs for the upper rectus abdominis than all other exercises. Elevation of the lower limbs with the body suspended by hands and the V-sit exercises produced significantly higher MAPs for the lower rectus abdominis than all other exercises. Upper and lower rectus abdominis MAPs were not affected by extended or flexed knees with supported or unsupported feet in a horizontal or inclined plane. Rectus femoris results showed 5 significantly different groups of exercises. The curl-up produced the lowest MAP. The highest resulted from the elevation of the lower limbs with the body suspended by hands and sit ups with extended or flexed knees in an inclined plane (Fig 7–4).

Conclusion.—Considering the study limitations, the results should be considered suggestive rather than conclusive. An important finding was that the curl-up required the least activity of the rectus femoris, whereas the lower limbs elevation from a suspended position exercise along with inclined sit-ups with extended and flexed knees demanded the most of this muscle.

▶ The modified sit-up, which we now call a "curl-up," is used in our abdominal strengthening and back rehabilitation programs. It may be found in the 1989 YEAR BOOK OF SPORTS MEDICINE, (1). We have found this to be a very safe and effective method of strengthening the abdominal muscles. The following is a summarization of how the exercise is performed:

1. The athlete lies supine with the knees bent and the feet flat on the floor (hook lying position).

2. The arms are folded across the upper chest.

3. The low back is flat (pelvic tilt).

4. A curl-up or partial sit-up is done and held for a count of 6 (when doing this type of sit-up, the shoulders raise about 12 inches off the floor. The chin is brought to the chest in a curling motion).

There are related abstracts and figures in the 1991 YEAR BOOK OF SPORTS MEDICINE (2). These abstracts also indicate exercises that should be avoided.—F.J. George, A.T.C., P.T.

References

1. 1989 YEAR BOOK OF SPORTS MEDICINE, pp 221–222.
2. 1991 YEAR BOOK OF SPORTS MEDICINE, pp 325–330.

Results of a Multicenter Trial Using an Intensive Active Exercise Program for the Treatment of Acute Soft Tissue and Back Injuries
Mitchell RI, Carmen GM (Workers' Compensation Board of Ontario, Canada)
Spine 15:514–521, 1990   7–10

Background.—The traditional methods for the nonsurgical treatment of acute soft tissue and back injuries among workers have proved disappointing. Prompted by the encouraging results of early intervention, rapid mobilization, and an aggressive active exercise program for the treatment of sports injuries, a study was undertaken to assess the effects of an intensive exercise program among workers with these injuries.

Study Design.—In a multicenter trial involving 12 clinics, 1,072 workers with acute soft tissue and back injuries were treated using a protocol involving intensive time-limited exercises emphasizing mobility, muscle strengthening, work conditioning, sequence training, and appropriate education sessions. Return to full-time work was considered proof that the patient had made a full and complete recovery. Results were evaluated in terms of time off work and compensation costs, and were compared with those of 2,172 matched controls treated elsewhere in the community with a variety of conventional methods of managing soft tissue injuries.

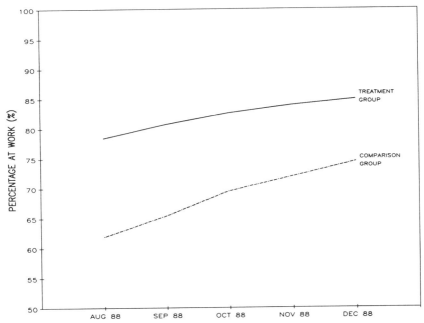

Fig 7–5.—A linear graph comparison of the monthly percentage at work of patients belonging to the treated and comparison groups. The trend shows a narrowing of the difference between the groups as time passes. (Courtesy of Mitchell RI, Carmen CM: *Spine* 15:514–521, 1990.)

Results.—Among the 703 patients treated at 5 clinics that participated in the program for more than 12 months, 79.8% returned to full-time work. In contrast with the comparison group, the treatment group returned to work earlier; but with passage of time, this advantage diminished, possibly from the spontaneous recovery of soft tissue injuries (Fig 7–5). Although the treatment group showed an increase in health care costs initially as a result of the intensity of treatment, these costs were more than offset by the savings in wage loss resulting from the earlier return to work. Substantial savings were realized in the number of days absent from work and compensation benefits.

Conclusion.—An intensive, time-limited program of active exercise is superior to the conventional methods of treatment currently used in the treatment of acute soft tissue and back injuries.

▶ Treating work-related soft-tissue and back injuries may be more effective using a model most of us follow when treating athletic injuries. The authors recommend "intensive time-limited exercises emphasizing mobility, muscle strengthening, work conditioning, sequence training, and appropriate education sessions." With the addition of early intervention, which the authors state occurs in their sports medicine centers, the above is the basic model we use when treating injured athletes. I am a strong believer in the effect that a proper first aid program has on limiting the consequences of an injury.—F.J. George, A.T.C., P.T.

Avulsion of the Anterior-Inferior Iliac Spine in Young Soccer Players
Tegner Y, Henriksson A, Lorentzon R, Lysholm J, Tegner S-O (Central Hospital, Boden, Sweden; University Hospital of Umeå, Umeå, Sweden; Vimmerby Hospital, Vimmerby, Sweden)
Clin Sports Med 2:143–148, 1990   7–11

Background.—Avulsion fractures of the pelvic apophyses are rare and occur mainly in adolescent athletes. Young soccer players who sustained avulsion fractures of the anterior-inferior iliac spine after minor indirect trauma were studied.

Patients.—The patients were 4 males and 1 female. Four of the athletes were aged 15–16 years, and the remaining patient was aged 23 years. Three of the patients tried to kick the ball but missed when the injury occurred. Radiographs showed an avulsed fragment from the anterior-inferior iliac spine. Nonoperative treatment was given in all patients.

Case Report.—Boy, 15, was making a penalty shot when he felt a snap in the right groin and sudden pain. He could not stand on the leg and had groin tenderness. An avulsion fracture was seen on a radiograph (Fig 7–6), and the patient was given crutches and placed in a rehabilitation program. He was able to resume playing soccer 8 weeks later. At 6 months, he had no strength deficit and normal healing of the fragment.

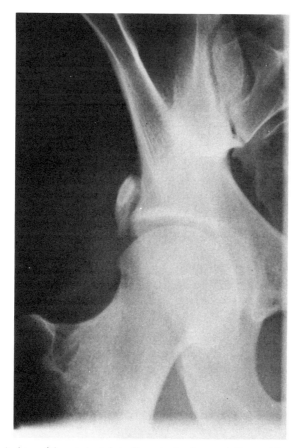

Fig 7–6.—Avulsion of the anterior-inferior iliac spine in a boy, aged 15 years. (Courtesy of Tegner Y, Henriksson A, Lorentzon R, et al: *Clin Sports Med* 2:143–148, 1990.)

Conclusions.—Five soccer players with avulsion fracture of the anterior-inferior iliac spine were evaluated. A history of powerful quadriceps contraction with subsequent pain should suggest the diagnosis, which is made radiographically. Treatment is nonoperative, and the prognosis is excellent.

▶ A graphic report on a relatively rare but fairly distinctive soccer injury. All 5 athletes here had the sudden onset of sharp pain in the groin, sometimes with a "snap," after either kicking the ball or attempting to kick it but missing. X-rays were diagnostic. Nonoperative treatment (crutches and then rehabilitation) worked well; several of these athletes were playing soccer again within 2–4 months.—E.R. Eichner, M.D.

Shoulder and Arm

The Normal Shoulder During Freestyle Swimming: An Electromyographic and Cinematographic Analysis of Twelve Muscles
Pink M, Perry J, Browne A, Scovazzo ML, Kerrigan J (Centinela Hosp Med Ctr, Inglewood, Calif)
Am J Sports Med 19:569–576, 1991   7–12

Introduction. —Swimming is the most popular participation sport in the United States. Competitive swimmers often practice most of the year, 6–7 days a week, covering 8,000–20,000 meters a day, which amounts to approximately 18,000 shoulder revolutions per week. The reported rates of shoulder problems in competitive swimmers range from 42% to 67%. The biomechanics of swimming have not been defined. A biomechanical study examined the muscle activity patterns in 12 muscles of the normal, pain-free shoulder during freestyle swimming.

Methods. —Twenty competitive swimmers with an average of 9 years of competitive swimming experience who were currently training 2,500–4,000 yards a day agreed to undergo electromyographic (EMG) testing while swimming. Before the swim data were recorded, a resting EMG of the 12 selected shoulder muscles was recorded while the swimmers did a prone float. Motion was recorded from the lateral projection with 2 high-speed motion cameras, with the underwater camera filming the pull-through phase of the stroke cycle and the surface camera filming the recovery phase.

Findings. —The patterns of muscular activity at hand entry and exit were similar. The 3 heads of the deltoid and the supraspinatus functioned in synchrony to place the arm at hand entry and exit. The function of the rhomboids and the upper trapezius was to position the scapula for the arm. The pectoralis major and the latissimus dorsi propelled the body. The subscapularis and the serratus anterior were active throughout the stroke cycle, and thus were susceptible to fatigue. The teres minor worked with the pectoralis major. The infraspinatus served only to rotate the arm externally at midrecovery.

Remark. —The findings provide a biomechanical framework for the development of muscle conditioning programs and specific rehabilitative muscle strengthening programs.

The Painful Shoulder During Freestyle Swimming: An Electromyographic Cinematographic Analysis of Twelve Muscles
Scovazzo ML, Browne A, Pink M, Jobe FW, Kerrigan J (Centinela Hosp Med Ctr, Inglewood, Calif)
Am J Sports Med 19:577–582, 1991   7–13

Objective.—This biomechanical study was designed to examine the patterns of activity of 12 shoulder muscles in the painful shoulder during freestyle swimming and to compare those patterns to those of the normal shoulder. The same 12 muscles as were examined previously in normal shoulders were recorded by electromyography and filmed by cinematographic analysis.

Methods.—Fourteen competitive swimmers with painful shoulders as determined by questionnaire replies and confirmed by physical examination participated in the study. The swimmers had an average of 11 years of competitive swimming experience and were currently training up to 4,000 yards per day, 3–5 days per week.

Findings.—The patterns of 7 of the 12 muscles studied differed significantly from those described for normal shoulders. The differences were seen for the anterior deltoid, middle deltoid, infraspinatus, subscapularis, upper trapezius, rhomboids, and the serratus anterior. The patterns of the latissimus dorsi, pectoralis major, teres minor, supraspinatus, and the posterior deltoid did not differ from those observed in normal shoulders.

▶ These 2 papers (Abstracts 7–12 and 7–13) represent the results of a study designed to compare painful and normal shoulders during freestyle swimming. Combined they are a well designed, well implemented work that provides information that the authors believe will contribute to the development of conditioning programs, optimize performance, and contribute to scientific rehabilitation and strengthening. It should be noted however that "painful shoulder" is not a diagnosis. Also, whether implementation of the information gained will be clinically useful remains to be seen.—J.S. Torg, M.D.

The Contribution of the Glenohumeral Ligaments to Anterior Stability of the Shoulder Joint

O'Connell PW, Nuber GW, Mileski RA, Lautenschlager E (Northwestern Univ, Chicago)
Am J Sports Med 18:579–584, 1990   7–14

Objective.—The cause of recurrent anterior shoulder instability remains uncertain. The ligamentous stabilizing processes that prevent anterior instability in the glenohumoral joint were investigated.

Methods.—Six unembalmed cadaver shoulders were dissected, preserving the joint capsule, the glenohumeral and coracohumeral ligaments, and the subscapularis tendon. Strain transducers then were placed on the glenohumeral ligaments and the humerus and scapula were placed in an apparatus allowing up to 90 degrees of glenohumeral joint abduction. An Instron device applied external rotation torque to the humerus.

Observations.—At zero-degree abduction, the superior and middle glenohumeral ligaments developed the most strain. The middle and inferior ligaments developed the most strain at 45 degrees of joint abduction, whereas at 90 degrees the inferior ligament, particularly its antero-superior band, was most involved.

Discussion.—Considerable individual variation was noted in the pattern of strain developing at different degrees of glenohumeral joint abduction. A better understanding of the functional anatomy of the intact shoulder should improve the diagnosis and repair of shoulder instability.

▶ This is an excellent study that supports the earlier findings of Turkel et al. (1). There are, however, several limitations. No attempt was made to evaluate the dynamic contribution of the subscapularis muscle to anterior stability of the shoulder. Also, it is pointed out that "despite the patterns seen, there was considerable variation from shoulder to shoulder."—J.S. Torg, M.D.

Reference

1. Turkel SJ, et al: *J Bone Joint Surg* 63A:1208, 1981.

The Coracohumeral Ligament: Anatomy of a Substantial But Neglected Structure
Edelson JG, Taitz C, Grishkan A (Poriya Government Hospital, Tiberias, Israel; Sackler School of Medicine, Tel Aviv, Israel)
J Bone Joint Surg 73-B:150–153, 1991   7–15

Introduction.—The area of the coracohumeral ligament is not well visualized and has not been considered important in clinical practice until recent years. The structure and clinical relevance of the coracohumeral ligament were studied.

Methods.—Shoulders of 10 cadavers (20 shoulders) were examined within 24 hours after death, and an additional 40 shoulders from preserved bodies were also used. Gross anatomic and histologic examinations were performed of sections from the coracohumeral ligament, coracoacromial ligament, and shoulder capsule. Figure 7–7 shows the dissection and the relationship of the coracohumeral ligament to the rotator cuff.

Observations.—Not a typical ligament, the coracohumeral ligament lacked superficial sheen and the taut feel of a bone-to-bone structure. Microscopically, it had the layered pattern of sheets and bundles of collagenous tissue interspersed with strands of loose connective tissue and vascular channels characteristic of the shoulder capsule. The coracohumeral ligament was found in all specimens at all ages and was a substantial and clearly defined structure.

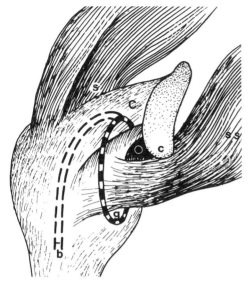

Fig 7–7.—Diagram of anterosuperior view of the shoulder. Abbreviations: g, glenoid; o, rotator interval between subscapularis and supraspinatus; C, coracohumeral ligament; c, coracoid process; s, supraspinatus; ss, subscapularis; b, biceps tendon. (Courtesy of Edelson JG, Taitz C, Grishkan A: *J Bone Joint Surg* 73-B:150–153, 1991.)

Conclusions.—With its strength and strategic position, the coracohumeral ligament is a central element in the suspension of the humerus. Because it is difficult to approach, it has not been fully appreciated in clinical practice.

▶ On the basis of this report, the coracohumeral ligament must be considered somewhat of an enigma. The authors specifically state that "the coracohumeral ligament is not a true ligament" and that "orthopaedic surgeons do not consider the role of the coracohumeral ligament because they do not see it." They further state that "although not fully appreciated at present and difficult to approach, the coracohumeral ligament may well become relevant to clinical practice." Although the structure is nicely described, the question of its clinical relevance is left unanswered.—J.S. Torg, M.D.

Electromyographic Analysis of the Glenohumeral Muscles During a Baseball Rehabilitation Program
Townsend H, Jobe FW, Pink M, Perry J (Centinela Hosp Med Ctr, Inglewood, Calif)
Am J Sports Med 19:264–272, 1991   7–16

Background.—There have been limited studies on the exercises used to strengthen the glenohumeral muscles. The optimal exercises for the glenohumeral muscles as part of a shoulder rehabilitation program for the throwing athlete were determined.

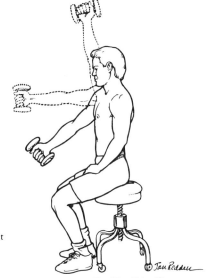

Fig 7–8.—Elevation of the arm in the sagittal plane
(flexion). (Courtesy of Townsend H, Jobe FW, Pink M, et
al: *Am J Sports Med* 19:264–272, 1991/)

© Baylor College of Medicine 1989

Fig 7–9.—Elevation of the arm in the
scapular plane (scaption) with the arm
internally rotated (thumbs down). (Courtesy of
Townsend H, Jobe FW, Pink M, et al: *Am J
Sports Med* 19:264–272, 1991.)

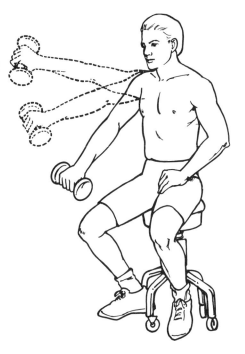

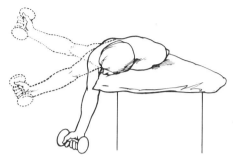

Fig 7–10.—Horizontal shoulder abduction with the arm externally rotated. (Courtesy of Townsend H, Jobe FW, Pink M, et al: *Am J Sports Med* 19:264-272, 1991.)

Methods.—Fifteen normal male volunteers performed 17 shoulder exercises derived from a shoulder rehabilitation program used by professional baseball clubs. The 4 rotator cuff muscles and other positioners of the humerus, including the pectoralis major, latissimus dorsi, and 3 portions of the deltoid, were studied with dynamic, fine wire, intramuscular electromyography (EMG). The latter was synchronized with cinematog-

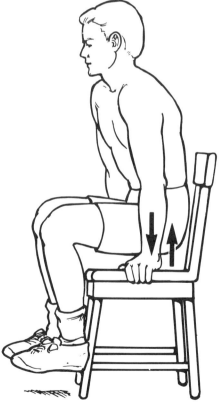

Fig 7–11.—Press-up. (Courtesy of Townsend H, Jobe FW, Pink M, et al: *Am J Sports Med* 19:264-272, 1991.)

raphy and averaged over 30-degree arcs of motion. An exercise was considered to be a significant challenge if the EMG activity generated was greater than 50% of its predetermined maximum contraction over 3 consecutive arcs (e.g. a 90-degree range).

Findings.—Fifteen shoulder exercises met the qualifying criterion for at least 1 muscle, but only 4 exercises were consistently found to be among the most challenging exercises for every muscle. Elevation of the arm in the subscapular plane with thumbs down generated the greatest EMG activity for the anterior and middle deltoids and subscapularis and second highest for the supraspinatus (Fig 7–8). Flexion involved a similar pattern of muscle activity to scaption in internal rotation (Fig 7–9). Horizontal abduction in external rotation was the leading exercise for the infraspinatus and second for the teres minor and posterior deltoid (Fig 7–10). Press-up was the leading exercise for both pectoralis major and latissimus dorsi (Fig 7–11).

Conclusion.—Scaption in internal rotation or flexion, horizontal abduction in external rotation, and press-up account for the highest level of EMG activity in all glenohumeral muscles. The minimum criterion for an effective and succinct rehabilitation protocol for the glenohumeral muscles should include these exercises.

▶ After reviewing this article, we now include these basic 4 exercises in all of our shoulder rehabilitation programs (See Figs 7–9, 7–10, 7–11, and 7–12). Please read abstract 7–17 to understand the important role the scapula plays in shoulder rehabilitation programs.—F.J. George, A.T.C., P.T.

Role of the Scapula in the Overhead Throwing Motion
Kibler WB (Lexington Clinic Sports Med Ctr, Lexington, Ky)
Contemp Orthopaedics 22:525–532, 1991   7–17

Background.—Arthroscopy and better techniques of high speed video analysis and EMG recording have provided a better understanding of complex shoulder mechanics, but the mechanics are still not completely understood. Previous investigations of the shoulder have shown that, as a bony joint, the shoulder is inherently unstable. Coordinated muscle firing patterns are necessary for efficient performance of the shoulder complex and for modification of the risk of injury to the components of the joint complex. In addition, a basic prerequisite in efficient throwing motion is congruent glenohumeral joint stability throughout the full range of motion of the arm during the act of throwing. Full motion of the entire shoulder joint complex and balance of all the muscles of the kinetic chin, which starts at the spine and hips and goes out to the finger, is necessary for efficient force production and minimal risk of injury. The role of the scapula in the overhead throwing motion was studied.

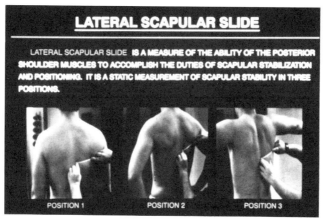

Fig 7–12.—Measurement of lateral slide. In position 1, a position of relative rest, one of the arms is in neutral rotation at the side. Position 2 is achieved by placing the hands on the hips with the thumbs pointing posteriorly. This position requires some shoulder internal rotation and upper trapezius muscle activity. Position 3 is one of maximum challenge to the scapular stabilizers. The arm is abducted 90 degree and maximally internally rotated. Stabilization requires upper and lower trapezius and serratus anterior function. (Courtesy of Kibler WB: *Contemp Orthop* 22:525–532, 1991.)

Methods.—Loss of the anchoring position of the scapula results in decreased muscle efficiency of the fibers of the muscles that normally attach to the scapula. The lateral slide measurement test can be used to clinically estimate this loss of anchoring position by measuring the ability of the scapular stabilizers to control the medial border of the scapula under varying load positions (Fig 7–12). Measurement from the spine to the medial border of the scapula is done bilaterally in 3 positions. In the normal asymptomatic athlete, the function of the scapular stabilizing muscle is very symmetrical, with less than 1 cm difference between sides. In symptomatic individuals, differences of more than 1 cm in the second and third positions are statistically significant and are associated with the onset of pain and decrease in shoulder function.

Discussion.—The normal role of the scapula in throwing includes its role as a site of muscle attachment, providing a stable glenohumeral articulation, retraction and protraction around the thoracic wall during phases of motion, and elevation of the acromion. Rehabilitation for shoulder disability should start with the base of the kinetic chain at the back and hip and work outward into the extremity. In most cases, using rotator cuff strengthening exercises as a starting point for rehabilitation will result in further pain and soreness if the scapular stabilizing musculature is weak.

Conclusions.—The scapula has central roles in muscle attachment, joint stability, and normal motion of the glenohumeral joint and is a central pivot in the throwing motion. Tests for the position and motion of the scapula should be incorporated into the routine examination of the painful shoulder. Rehabilitation must start at the base of the kinetic chain at the back and hip and work outward into the extremity.

▶ The authors explain the important role that the scapula plays in the throwing motion. They describe a measurement of lateral scapula slide that can be used when evaluating shoulder problems (Fig 7–12). They also explain the importance of not beginning shoulder rehabilitation programs using rotator cuff exercises as a starting point. Rather, dysfunction of the back, hip, and scapula must first be addressed.—F.J. George, A.T.C., P.T.

Shoulder Positioning for Optimal Treatment Effects
Lovinger A, Mangus BC, Ingersoll CD (Seattle Mariners Baseball Club; Univ of Nevada, Las Vegas)
Athletic Training JNATA 26:81–82, 1991   7–18

Background.—When the arm is in the resting position, adducted and rotated neutrally, the blood vessels are in traction and compression as they follow the tendon to the greater tuberosity of the humerus. This vascular pattern also occurs when the long head of the biceps tendon moves superiorly to its insertion on the supraglenoid. This traction and compression causes a "wringing out" of the blood vessels, creating an avascular area called the critical zone. Degenerative changes and chronic inflammation are common in this area. Thus, treatment of shoulder pathology in this "sling position" may be self-defeating because the critical zone becomes avascular with this position.

Treatment.—Proper positioning of the shoulder during treatment can enhance therapeutic effects. When performing therapy in this area, the arm should be placed in abduction (30–70 degrees) with neutral rotation

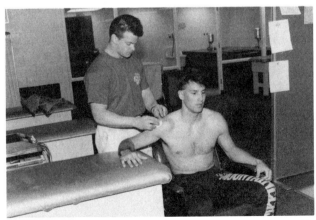

Fig 7–13.—Preferred treatment position can be maintained by using a treatment table and a chair. (Courtesy of Lovinger A, Mangus BC, Ingersoll CD: *Athlet Train*, JNATA 26:81–82, 1991.)

and slight extension. This position can be achieved using a small box or foot stool placed on the treatment table, having the athlete sit in the chair with the arm resting on the table (Fig 7-13), or having the athlete lie supine with a folded towel under the scapula of the affected shoulder. With this position, the tendons are relaxed, the blood vessels can fill, and increased blood flow to the area is achieved.

Conclusion.—Placing the arm in the abducted position during therapy can enhance the therapeutic effects of procedures used for the treatment of shoulder pathology.

▶ After reading Abstract 7-18, we have been careful to use the positioning method described by the authors when treating shoulder injuries. We attempt to avoid positions that cause a "wringing out" of the blood vessels and may defeat the purpose of our treatment.—F.J. George, A.T.C., P.T.

Complications of Shoulder Arthroscopy
Bigliani LU, Flatow EL, Deliz ED (Columbia Univ; New York Orthopedic Hosp)
Orthop Rev 20:743–751, 1991   7–19

Introduction.—The increased frequency of shoulder arthroscopy as a therapeutic and diagnostic technique is expected to lead to a high rate of complications. The anatomy, pathology, indications, and technique of arthroscopic shoulder surgery were reviewed to reduce the rate of complications.

General Considerations.—The patient with shoulder problems should undergo a complete history, a physical examination, basic shoulder roentgenographic studies, and appropriate laboratory tests. The differential diagnosis should be thorough, and both intraarticular and extraarticular pathology considered. In addition, it is important to distinguish between joint and bursal pathology.

Methods.—Irrigation fluid may result in edema of the shoulder, making the arthroscopic procedure more difficult. All landmarks and portals should be marked before the procedure begins. A closely monitored pump may be used to maintain a more constant distension pressure. Instead of a lateral decubitus position, a standard "beach chair" semirecumbent position is used to avoid potential neuropraxias. This position allows for better orientation and precise and continuous repositioning of the patient's arm for optimum visualization during the procedure. Intraoperative bleeding can be minimized by means of electrosurgical instruments plus adequate distension pressure. Strict adherence to antiseptic techniques will contribute to a low infection rate.

Conclusion.—It has been recommended that orthopedists perform open procedures before the more complicated arthroscopic repairs of the shoulder. With practice, proper patient selection, and attention to technical considerations, shoulder arthroscopy will continue to develop as a valuable and safe tool.

▶ Except for a complication rate of 5.3% associated with staple capsulorraphy as reported by the Committee on Complications of the Arthroscopy Association of North America (1), the relatively low rate of complications for other shoulder arthroscopic procedures is impressive. There are, however, reports by other authors of a 10%–30% incidence of transient neuropraxia associated with the lateral decubitus position. The use of perioperative antibiotic prophylaxis "with a first-generation cephalosporin" is emphasized.—J.S. Torg, M.D.

Reference

1. Small NC: *Arthroscopy* 2:253, 1986.

Suprascapular Nerve Lesions at the Spinoglenoid Notch: Report of Three Cases and Review of the Literature
Liveson JA, Bronson MJ, Pollack MA (Albert Einstein College of Medicine)
J Neurol Neurosurg Psychiatry 54:241–243, 1991   7–20

Background.—Entrapment of the suprascapular nerve can occur at either the suprascapular notch (SSN) or the spinoglenoid notch (SGN). Failure to distinguish between the 2 lesions can result in surgery to the wrong region. Three cases and a literature review of SGN lesions are presented.

Cases.—All patients were athletic males in their 20s. In 1, an isolated incident resulted in weakness in the dominant shoulder, which gradually subsided. His right scapula appeared to be losing bulk during this time. He had no numbness or radicular symptoms, but atrophy was evident in the region of the right infraspinatus, with tenderness below the scapular spine. Manual muscle examination showed no weakness and, as in all 3 cases, sensation was intact. As in all 3 patients, cranial nerves appeared normal, with no Horner's sign. A second patient noted a right shoulder ache, without numbness, symptoms of root involvement, or weakness detectable by examination. The last patient had unilateral scapular atrophy on the dominant side, without numbness or cervical symptoms. The external rotation of the humerus on the affected side was weak, and atrophy in the infraspinatus region was evident. In all cases, electrodiagnostic studies showed isolated denervation in the infraspinatus. These consisted of fibrillation potentials, positive sharp waves, and single-unit recruitment of normal motor unit potentials. Extensive electromyography showed no other abnormalities. Motor unit potentials did not suggest myopathy, nor was a diffuse condition of peripheral nerves detected. In 2 cases, the abnormalities were primarily axonal.

Results.—Conservative treatment resulted in normal or near-normal strength and functioning in all cases.

Conclusions.—The supraspinatus muscle should be examined to distinguish between lesions at the SSN and the SGN. Involvement of the supraspinatus marks the lesion at the SSN, while sparing of this muscle places it at the SGN. Clinically, pain was always the initial complaint in SSN lesions described in the literature, but had little involvement in SGN lesions.

▶ Suprascapular lesions, although rare, require an exacting diagnosis. Included in the differential are C5, C6 radiculopathy, brachial plexopathy, and rotator cuff injury. To be noted, weakness may not be a major feature and the clinical examination must include careful examination of the supra and infraspinatus under tension. With regard to a clear cut definition of the causes of these lesions, they remain an enigma. It should be pointed out that many suprascapular nerve lesions do not resolve with conservative treatment and surgical exploration of the nerve and decompression of the suprascapular or spinoglenoid notch may be necessary.—J.S. Torg, M.D.

Complete Acromioclavicular Dislocations: Treatment With A Dacron Ligament
Stam L, Dawson I (University of Limburg, The Netherlands)
Injury 22:173–176, 1991   7–21

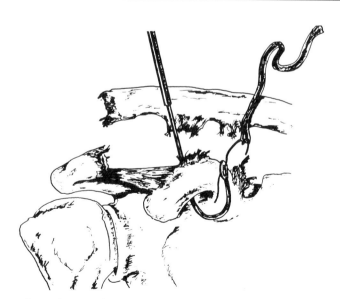

Fig 7–14.—Dacron ligament is brought under coracoid process before crossing clavicle. (Courtesy of Stam L, Dawson I: *Injury* 22:173–176, 1991.)

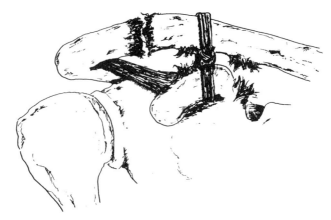

Fig 7–15.—Complete reduction of clavicle; Dacron ligament is knotted on anterior side. (Courtesy of Stam L, Dawson I: *Injury* 22:173–176, 1991.)

Background.—Operative treatment for complete acromioclavicular dislocations (ACD) must restore the anatomy so the best prospects for normal function are obtained with no loss of strength. Cerclage of the coracoid process and clavicle with a Dacron ligament was used in 23 patients to maintain dynamic fixation of the clavicle.

Procedure.—In these cases a Dacron ligament was pulled under the base of the coracoid process and over the clavicle (Fig 7-14). The distal clavicle was reduced and the Dacron ligament was knotted and the ends were sutured to prevent loosening (Fig 7-15). After 1 week in a sling after operation active function was permitted.

Outcome.—Nineteen of 20 patients who were followed up for a mean period of 3.9 years reported good or excellent results. Sick leave for the patients averaged 3.3 weeks, considerably shorter than with other operative or nonoperative methods. Operative treatment by the Phemister and Bosworth method is not recommended because cerclage provided better results, used no pins, and required only a 1-week immobilization.

Conclusions.—Cerclage with a Dacron ligament for ACD had a low complication rate and a high percentage of anatomic reduction. Recovery of shoulder function was quicker than with conservation methods and necessitated an average of only 3.3 weeks of sick leave. The operative technique of Phemister and Bosworth should not be used for reduction of ACD because of complications with infection and breakage of pins and screws.

▶ Although the authors claim that 19 out of 20 patients had good or excellent results, it should be noted that 7 patients complained of postoperative pain. All patients with an intact Dacron ligament had limitation of internal rotation. Nine patients had persistent dislocation on postoperative roentgenograms and 14 of the 19 patients had radiographic evidence of a "fissure in the clavicle at the point of the Dacron ligament graft crossed the bone." It is interesting that in 6 patients it was necessary to divide the Dacron ligament to prevent deepening of the fissure in the clavicle. Also, the conclusions of the authors that "the method of Phemister and Bosworth with a high complication and failure rate should be abandoned" and that "cerclage with a Dacron ligament is a simple operation with a low complication rate" does not appear to be supported by their data.—J.S. Torg, M.D.

Evaluation of the Painful Shoulder: A Prospective Comparison of Magnetic Resonance Imaging, Computerized Tomographic Arthrography, Ultrasonography, and Operative Findings
Nelson MC, Leather GP, Nirschl RP, Pettrone FA, Freedman MT (Georgetown Univ)
J Bone Joint Surg 73-A:707–716, 1991   7–22

Introduction.—The basis for pain in the shoulder is often difficult to determine accurately by noninvasive means. Plain and special radiographs, ultrasonography, MRI, and CT arthrography have all been useful in evaluating specific abnormalities. To determine the single best imaging modality for the preoperative assessment of patients whose shoulder pain had resisted nonoperative treatment, 21 patients with a mean age of 42 years who had shoulder pain of more than 3-months' duration were studied.

Methods.—All were evaluated by both MRI and CT arthrography; 19 had ultrasonography. Treatment consisted of 20 arthroscopic and 3 open operative procedures (2 patients required a second procedure). Findings from preoperative imaging were compared with those obtained at surgery (Fig 7-16). For each diagnosis the sensitivity, specificity, and accuracy of the 3 imaging techniques were calculated.

Results.—Disease of the rotator cuff was confirmed by operative findings in 19 patients. Twelve of the 21 patients had major abnormalities of the labrum; 8 of these abnormalities were detected with MRI and 9 with CT arthrography. Neither imaging modality detected a Bankart lesion in 1 patient.

Conclusion.—Both MRI and CT arthrography helped to demonstrate the presence and size of a full-thickness tear and to differentiate it from a partial tear. In addition, both techniques aided in the identification of a partial-thickness tear and subacromial impingement. Magnetic resonance imaging may not be feasible for large patients with massive shoulder bulk or for those with claustrophobia. In addition, the test is extremely expensive. Computed tomographic arthrography is costly and time consuming and uses ionizing radiation. Ultrasonography was judged

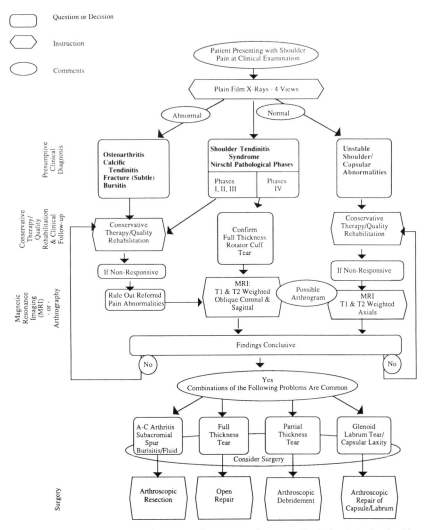

Fig 7–16.—Algorithm showing diagnosis and treatment of patients who had pain in the shoulder. (Courtesy of Nelson MC, Leather GP, Nirschl RP, et al: *J Bone Joint Surg* 73-A:707–716, 1991.)

useful as a screening test for persons who are obese, allergic to contrast medium, or claustrophobic.

▶ Clinical history and the experience of the radiologists with regard to the specific imaging modality are the key factors that should be considered when determining which study is to be done. The history "shoulder pain" is not helpful to determine what study will yield useful information nor does it identify how the chosen study should be performed. The specific study and the way it is performed is dependent on the clinical focus. Communication between the referring physician and the radiologist will facilitate a more rapid learning curve for both parties and provide a more accurate diagnostic yield.—J.S. Torg, M.D.

Luxatio Erecta: The Inferior Glenohumeral Dislocation
Mallon WJ, Bassett FH III, Goldner RD (Duke Univ Med Ctr, Durham, NC)
J Orthop Trauma 4:19–24, 1990   7–23

Introduction.—Inferior glenohumeral dislocation (luxatio erecta) is a rare disorder involving fewer than 1% of all glenohumeral dislocations. The patient typically lies with the arm abducted and externally rotated and a painful mass, the humeral head, is felt in the axilla. Extreme trauma to the arm and shoulder causes the injury.

Methods.—This injury was treated in 6 men with a mean age of 31 years, who were followed for up to 4 years. Hyperabduction force was responsible in all patients; 3 had football injuries. Immobilization averaged 4 weeks. In 3 patients, there were concurrent fractures of the shoulder region, and 3 had neurologic deficits that resolved spontaneously.

Case Report.—Man, 54, had his left arm forced over his head when working on a truck and was seen in the emergency room with the arm lying overhead and with a firm axillary mass. Radiographs confirmed an inferior glenohumeral dislocation and showed a fracture of the greater tuberosity. Reduction was achieved by overhead traction in line with the humeral shaft. A shoulder immobilizer was placed for 4 weeks. Deltoid weakness was noted at 3 weeks and mild weakness persisted at 3 months. There also was reduced sensation in the axillary nerve distribution.

Conclusion.—Inferior glenohumeral dislocation usually is reduced without difficulty. Fluoroscopic control may be helpful. Immobilization is maintained for 2–4 weeks after reduction. Overnight observation can exclude vascular injury. Patients with a fracture of the greater tuberosity should be observed for evidence of a rotator cuff tear.

▶ There are several points worth emphasizing regarding luxatio erecta. As pointed out by the authors, in 80% of the patients, it is associated with a fracture of the greater tuberosity or a rotator cuff tear. Also, 60% of the patients reviewed sustained some degree of neurologic compromise involving the axillary nerve, and 3%–4% have associated vascular compromise. A rare lesion, reduction is easily obtained with straight line overhead traction.—J.S. Torg, M.D.

Modification of the Bankart Reconstruction With a Suture Anchor: Report of a New Technique

Richmond JC, Donaldson WR, Fu F, Harner CD (Tufts Univ, Boston; Univ of Pittsburgh)

Am J Sports Med 19:343–346, 1991   7–24

Background.—The need to drill curved holes in the glenoid rim can make the Bankart procedure technically difficult. The technique was modified by using a small suture anchor to reattach the capsulolabral complex to the glenoid rim.

Patients.—Thirty-two patients at 2 centers had a modified Bankart shoulder reconstruction using the suture anchor technique. Twenty-six were men and 6 were women, mean age 25 years. All had recurrent, traumatic glenohumeral anterior instability. Follow-up was 12 months or more in 17 patients.

Technique.—The suture anchor is used in patients with avulsion of the capsulolabral complex from the glenoid. The surgeon drills 3 straight holes in the

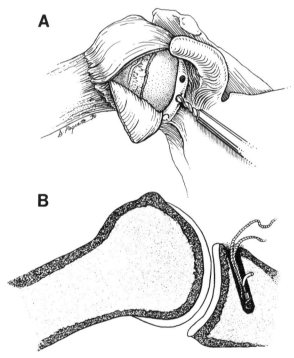

Fig 7–17.—A, 3 drill holes are placed on the glenoid rim in approximately the 1, 3, and 5 o'clock positions in this right shoulder. **B,** the drill holes start at the articular surface rim and angle into the body of the glenoid. The suture anchors are placed with the arcs directed away from the articular surface. (Courtesy of Richmond JC, Donaldson WR, Fu F, et al: *Am J Sports Med* 19:343–346, 1991.)

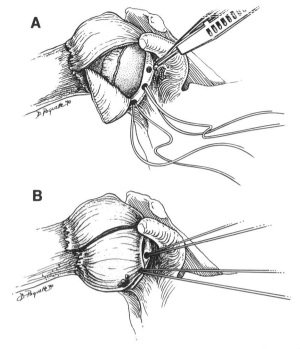

Fig 7–18.—A, double-armed sutures are used on each anchor. **B,** anatomical repair of the capsulola-bral complex to the glenoid is performed. Reefing of the interior capsule is carried out if it is redundant. (Courtesy of Richmond JC, Donaldson WR, Fu F, et al: *Am J Sports Med* 19:343–346, 1991.)

glenoid just off the articular surface, angled away from the glenoid (Fig 7–17). The anchors are then inserted, directing the arc away from the subchondral bone of the glenoid; and the capsule is repaired (Fig 7–18). The fixation has a strength of 67 N when a number 0 anchor is used and 82 N when a number 2 anchor is used.

Outcome.—There was no incidence of glenoid rim fracture related to the use of the anchor. The Bankart lesion was large in several patients, and the classic reconstruction would have been very difficult. In the 17 patients followed for at least 1 year, mean Bankart rating score was 94. Eighty-two percent had an excellent score, and 12% had a good score. Forward flexion increased by a mean of 4 degrees. One patient, a football player, had a recurrent dislocation.

Conclusions.—The use of a suture anchor as a modification of the Bankart reconstruction is examined. This method makes exposure and fixation easier, and the hardware is completely buried in bone, which prevents migration. Long-term follow-up is pending.

▶ It is important to note that the authors state "this paper represents a preliminary report on a new means of fixing sutures to bone . . . although the early results (1 year follow-up) are promising, long-term follow-up of these and other patients is necessary to determine the effectiveness of this procedure".—J.S. Torg, M.D.

Anterior Capsulolabral Reconstruction of the Shoulder in Athletes in Overhand Sports

Jobe FW, Giangarra CE, Kvitne RS, Glousman RE (Inglewood, Calif; Camarillo, Calif)

Am J Sports Med 19:428–434, 1991   7–25

Introduction.—Surgical procedures can correct anterior glenohumeral instability in athletes participating in sports that require overhand throwing, but many of these patients do not regain their previous level of throwing skill.

Methods.—A modified anterior capsulolabral reconstruction (ACLR) to restore preinjury level of function was evaluated in 25 athletes, 13 of whom competed at the professional level. All patients had documented anterior shoulder instability and shoulder pain that failed to improve with conservative therapy. The average patient age at the time of operation was 21 years. All patients underwent ACLR followed by a formal program of rehabilitative exercises.

Results.—The exercise program was continued for at least 1 year. By 2½ months, full range of motion was achieved and most patients were free of pain. Results at follow-up were rated excellent in 68% of patients, good in 24%, fair in 4%, and poor in 4%. All patients had negative impingement signs; 18 were able to return to their previous level of competition for at least 1 complete season. The 7 remaining players were satisfied with the stability, almost full range of motion, and freedom from pain resulting from the procedure and rehabilitation program.

Conclusion.—Most athletes with anterior glenohumeral instability associated with repetitive throwing will respond to nonoperative treatment. This procedure offers excellent results for many of those who require surgery and is a significant improvement over previous methods.

▶ The authors present this report as a new procedure to manage glenohumeral instability in the overhand throwing athlete. They maintain that it is the first study to evaluate the ability to return to competition following reconstructive surgery in the population. Also presented is the concept that the injury pattern in the overhand and throwing athlete represents a sequence of events beginning with instability and progressing to impingement and, ultimately, rotator cuff tearing. The original article is recommended reading for those caring for overhead throwing and striking athletes.—J.S. Torg, M.D.

Arthroscopic Stapling for Detached Superior Glenoid Labrum

Yoneda M, Hirooka A, Saito S, Yamamoto T, Ochi T, Shino K (Osaka Kohsei-nenkin Hospital, Sumitomo Hospital, Osaka, Japan)
J Bone Joint Surg 73-B:746–750, 1991   7–26

Introduction.—Athletes who make repeated overhead arm motions, as in throwing a baseball or playing tennis or volleyball, may have injury of the superior glenoid labrum involving the biceps insertion. Sudden forced abduction of the arm also can cause this injury.

Methods.—In 1986–1988, 10 young athletes underwent arthroscopic stapling for a detached biceps tendon-labral complex (BLC). The mean patient age at surgery was 18 years. In 7 patients, the injuries were baseball-related. Symptoms had been present for 10 months on average despite conservative measures. Shoulder pain was reproduced by maximal forward elevation of the arm and by forced abduction and external rotation. Range of motion was slightly limited in 2 patients.

Technique.—A motorized suction débrider and abrader are used to trim the lesion. Stapling is performed using a ligament/capsule repair system. After trimming the torn edge of the detached BLC and abrading the adjacent glenoid rim, the BLC is fixed with a staple driven into the anterosuperior scapular neck.

Results.—In 3 patients, there was a partial tear of the rotator cuff as well as BLC detachment. The BLC was stabilized in all patients, and 4 demonstrated complete healing at second-look arthroscopy at the time of staple removal 3–6 months postoperatively. Only 1 patient had significant synovitis. Pain was severe in 1 patient and moderate in another; 5 patients were free of pain. All patients but 1 had a full range of shoulder motion. The overall clinical results were excellent or good in 8 patients, fair in 1, and poor in 1. No infections or neurovascular complications occurred.

Conclusion.—Arthroscopic stapling is an effective approach to the detached BLC and is indicated in very active adolescent athletes.

▶ It should be emphasized that 6 of the 10 reported cases had "incomplete" healing of the lesion at second-look arthroscopy. I personally question the wisdom of inserting a metallic staple in the glenohumeral joint.—J.S. Torg, M.D.

Complications of a Failed Bristow Procedure and Their Management

Young DC, Rockwood CA Jr (Univ of Texas, San Antonio)
J Bone Joint Surg 73-A:969–981, 1991   7–27

Background.—When the Bristow procedure for reconstruction of the shoulder fails, the subsequent management can be very difficult. Forty such cases were reviewed to identify the complications, define the processes leading to failure, and assess the results of the subsequent treatment.

Patients.—Forty treatment failures in 39 patients were treated over a 10-year period. Average follow-up was 4.4 years. Mean age at presentation was 30 years. Each patient had undergone an average of 2 previous operations, including 23 anterior reconstructions in 17 patients. The presenting complaint was chronic painful anterior instability in 28 of 40 shoulders and pain with no subjective instability in 6 shoulders. All shoulders were started on a shoulder rehabilitation program, and those who had continued signs or symptoms had surgery (78% of cases). A special anterior capsular shift was done in 16 shoulders, capsular release in 4, total shoulder arthroplasty in 4, and other procedures in 7 shoulders. Complications of the initital procedure included recurrent painful anterior instability, articular cartilage injury, nonunion of the coracoid bone-block and the glenoid, loosening of the screw, neurovascular injury, and posterior instability. The main cause of failure was excessive laxity of the capsule in 80% of shoulders affected with chronic, painful anterior or posterior instability. The remaining 20% had an untreated Perthes-Bankart lesion. Outcome was judged as good or excellent in only 50% of patients.

Conclusions.—The results suggest that the Bristow procedure should not be used for primary treatment of the shoulder with symptomatic anterior instability. The anterior reconstruction described is a difficult procedure that requires meticulous technique. The Bristow procedure carries no better rate of success than other standard operations, and it causes a wide range of minor and serious complications.

▶ This paper bears credence to the thesis that "there is no condition that cannot be made worse by surgery." It should be noted that the authors did not present their reported complications from the Bristow procedure in terms of complication rates. Thus, their conclusion that the Bristow procedure should not be used for primary treatment of symptomatic anterior instability of the shoulder is not supported by their data.—J.S. Torg, M.D.

Quadrilateral Space Syndrome: Diagnosis and Operative Decompression Technique
Francel TJ, Dellon AL, Campbell JN (Johns Hopkins Univ, Baltimore)
Plast Reconstr Surg 87:911–916, 1991   7–28

Introduction.—The quadrilateral space syndrome is an uncommon injury that was first described in 1983. In 5 patients, the syndrome followed trauma to the upper extremity or shoulder. A surgical treatment was developed that does not require division of the deltoid or teres minor muscle.

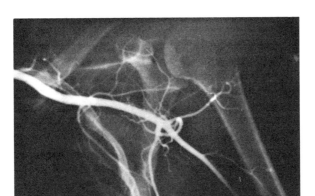

Fig 7-19.—Arteriogram with shoulder in neutral position showing the posterior circumflex humeral artery originating with the subscapular artery and the anterior circumflex artery from the axillary artery. (Courtesy of Francel TJ, Dellon AL, Campbell JN: *Plast Reconstr Surg* 87:911–916, 1991.)

Patients.—The patients were aged 31–50 years. All patients had shoulder pain, point tenderness over the quadrilateral space, paresthesia over the lateral aspect of the shoulder and upper arm, and difficulties in arm abduction. Clinical deltoid muscle weakness was noted in all of the patients. An arteriogram in 1 of the patients revealed compression of the posterior circumflex humeral artery (Figs 7-19 and 7-20).

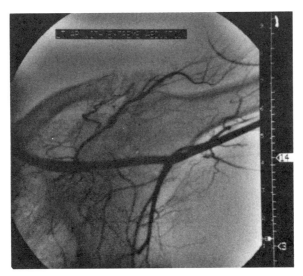

Fig 7-20.—Digital subtraction arteriography showing complete absence of posterior circumflex humeral artery with shoulder abduction. (Courtesy of Francel TJ, Dellon AL, Campbell JN: *Plast Reconstr Surg* 87:911–916, 1991.)

Technique.—The quadrilateral space (the point of maximum tenderness) is determined preoperatively with the patient standing. At surgery, a vertical or S-shaped incision is made at this location, with skin flaps raised to expose the inferior border of the deltoid muscle. The deltoid is then retracted superiorly, exposing the teres muscle. When the quadrilateral space is entered, sharp division of the fibrous bands will decompress the space. Complete decompression is confirmed by the protrusion of axillary fat into the space and the surgeon's ability to easily pass an index finger through the quadrilateral space and into the axilla.

Conclusion.—In all of the patients, shoulder pain improved, with improved active range of motion of the shoulder. This technique minimizes scarring and allows early exercise of the shoulder.

▶ What had the potential of being a good paper is significantly flawed by the authors' failure to present objective data corroborating their results. Although they report improved active range of motion of the shoulder and admit that 3 patients had limited motion, no preoperative and postoperative measurement data are offered. The presence of deltoid weakness was not only observed in all patients but also served as an integral diagnostic parameter. Not only have the authors failed to present objective data regarding deltoid strength preoperatively, but also no mention of its response to surgery is made.—J.S. Torg, M.D.

Ball Thrower's Fracture of the Humerus: A Case Report
Linn RM, Kriegshauser LA (Washington Univ, St Louis)
Am J Sports Med 19:194–197, 1991   7–29

Introduction.—Humeral shaft fracture may be an unusual result of overhand throwing, possibly caused by torsional stress concentrated at the middle and distal humeral diaphysis.

Case Report.—Man, 34, who was a recreational softball player, hurt his right arm while throwing a softball from centerfield to the infield. As he brought his arm forward in throwing motion, he heard and felt a loud snap with immediate pain and deformity in the distal arm. He had no history of injury to the arm. In the emergency room, the distal upper arm was swollen with painful gross motion at the junction of the middle and distal thirds of the arm. His skin and neurocirculatory status were intact. On radiography, a comminuted, displaced fracture of the right distal humerus with a 10-cm long butterfly fragment was seen. After fitting with a hanging posterior splint, residual apex anterior and varus angulation were seen. Several adjustments were necessary to achieve a satisfactory reduction, both before discharge and again at a few days of follow-up. The patient complained about the hanging cast and opted for open reduction and internal fixation. Closed antegrade Ender nailing of the fracture was performed under fluoroscopic control. The patient returned to full activity with full range of motion 3 months after the injury. The Ender nails were removed on an outpatient basis after 6 months.

Conclusion.—Minimally displaced and angulated spiral fracture of the middle or distal humeral diaphysis, with or without a butterfly fracture, is the most common fracture configuration. Hanging cast or humeral fracture brace-type device is the treatment of choice, although there are possible indications for surgery.

▶ Although rare, "ball thrower's fracture of the humerus" has been described to have occurred as a result of overhead throwing motion without external contact in individuals throwing baseball, softballs, snowballs, shotputs, javelins, and hand grenades. Also, the fracture has been described in arm wrestlers and handball players. Typically, there is a spiral fracture involving the middle or distal humerus with or without a butterfly fragment and with minimal displacement on angulation. The presented case in which there was marked displacement on angulation requiring internal fixation is the exception.—J.S. Torg, M.D.

Avulsion of the Medial Epicondyle of the Humerus in Arm Wrestlers: A Report of Five Cases and a Review of the Literature
Lokiec F, Velkes S, Engel J (Sheba Medical Centre, Tel Hashomer, Israel)
Injury 22:69–70, 1991   7–30

Introduction.—Although rare, the medial epicondyle of the humerus may avulse as a result of muscular action. Data on 5 patients with avulsion of the medial epicondyle of the humerus resulting from arm wrestling were reviewed.

Methods.—Four of the patients felt sudden sharp pain at the medial side of the elbow during arm wrestling, with severe tenderness and swelling over the medial epicondyle and weakness and pain on wrist flexion. Radiographs showed avulsion of the medial epicondyle (Fig 7–21). The other patient complained of persistent medial elbow pain of 6 months' duration. As in the other patients, the problem was first noted during an arm-wrestling match. Patients were treated with posterior plaster splint for 10 days, followed by gradual mobilization of the elbow for 3 weeks. Patients were asymptomatic with full function at 1 year, although nonunion of the medial epicondyle was seen on radiographic examination.

Conclusion.—This injury may be more common than previously thought. Open treatment should be reserved for patients with ulnar nerve palsy or an intraarticular fragment.

▶ The accepted criteria for open reduction and internal fixation of avulsion fractures of the medial epicondylar apophysis is when displacement is more than 5 mm. Presumably, this is to prevent the development of tardy ulnar neuropathy. In the 5 cases presented, there occurred an avulsion fracture

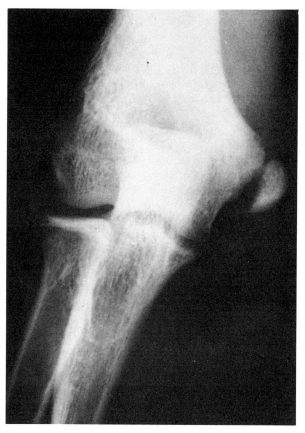

Fig 7–21.—Patient 1. (Courtesy of Lokiec F, Velkes S, Engel J: *Injury* 22:69–70, 1991.)

through what appears to have been mature medial epicondyles. Although nonoperative treatment resulted in nonunion of the respective fragments, the authors report such treatment having resulted in asymptomatic elbows with full function at 1 year. I question whether or not the follow-up was long enough to make a definitive recommendation.—J.S. Torg, M.D.

Surgical Treatment of Medial Epicondylitis: Results in 35 Elbows
Vangsness CT Jr, Jobe FW (Univ of Southern California School of Medicine, Los Angeles; Kerlan-Jobe Orthopaedic Clinic, Inglewood, Calif)
J Bone Joint Surg 73-B:409–411, 1991   7–31

Background.—Medial epicondylitis at the elbow, a relatively uncommon condition, usually responds to conservative treatment. When such treatment fails, however, and pain persists after 6 to 12 months, surgery

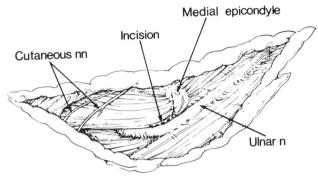

Fig 7–22.—Medial skin incision, showing the deep structures. (Courtesy of Vangsness CT Jr, Jobe FW: *J Bone Joint Surg* 73-B:409–411, 1991.)

must be considered. There have been no reports in the literature on the surgical treatment of medial epicondylitis.

Patients.—Between 1974 and 1984, 38 patients at 1 center required surgery (Figs 7–22, 7–23, and 7–24) for medial epicondylitis after conservative treatment failed. Thirty-five of those patients were reviewed. They had a mean age of 43 years, and were followed up for a mean of 85 months.

Outcomes.—At surgery, residual tears with incomplete healing were found consistently in the flexor origin at the medial epicondyle. Microscopy showed reactive fibrous connective tissues with various degrees of inflammation. The mean subjective estimate of elbow function improved from 38% to 98% after surgery. Isokinetic and grip strength testing after surgery showed no improvement in 16 cases. The results were classified

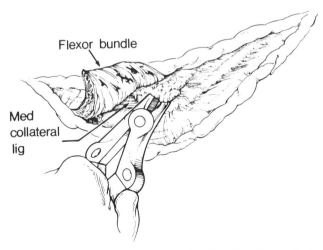

Fig 7–23.—Reflection of the common flexor origin and excision of the degenerative tissue with rongeurs. (Courtesy of Vangsness CT Jr, Jobe FW: *J Bone Joint Surg* 73-B:409–411, 1991.)

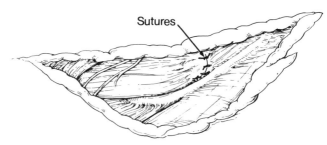

Sutures

Fig 7–24.—Reattachment of the forearm flexors. (Courtesy of Vangsness CT Jr, Jobe FW: *J Bone Joint Surg* 73-B:409–411, 1991.)

as excellent in 25 patients, good in 9, and fair in 1. Eighty-six percent of the patients had no limitation in elbow use.

Conclusions.—Surgery for medial epicondylitis after conservative treatment fails is predictably effective. It relieves pain and restores strength. After such surgery, patients can return to their previous levels of daily activity and sports participation.

▶ It is interesting to note that this paper, which emanated from the Jobe-Kerlan Orthopaedic Clinic in Inglewood, California, was published in the *British Journal of Bone and Joint Surgery.* The authors state that indication for the described surgery was "failure of conservative treatment." That the authors did not delineate what the conservative treatment was constitutes a major flaw in the paper.—J.S. Torg, M.D.

Acute Grade III Ulnar Collateral Ligament Ruptures: A New Surgical and Rehabilitation Protocol
Lane LB (North Shore Univ Hosp, Manhasset, NY)
Am J Sports Med 19:234–238, 1991   7–32

Introduction.—The thumb metacarpophalangeal joint is frequently injured in sports. The ulnar collateral ligament (UCL) is involved in most cases. A new treatment for acute grade III UCL injuries was compared to traditional treatment methods.

Data Analysis.—Thirty-two patients with acute grade III (unstable) sports-related sprains of the thumb metacarpophalangeal joint received surgical treatment. The first 7 were treated with traditional methods of pullout suture and K-wire fixation, casting for 4 weeks, and gradual mobilization over an additional 4 weeks. The remaining thumb injuries were treated with a new method (Fig 7–25) that involved suturing avulsed UCL to the tendinous insertion of the adductor pollicis or to a soft tissue remnant with strong sutures. Casting was done for 2 weeks and mobilization was rapid.

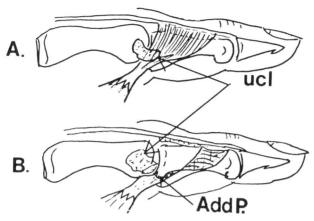

Fig 7–25.—A, Stener lesion with the avulsed UCL outside of the extensor mechanism/adductor aponeurosis; **B,** the extensor mechanism/adductor aponeurosis reflected, showing the proximity of the UCL to the tendinous insertion of the adductor pollicis (*Add P*) at the volar-ulnar corner of the proximal phalanx. (Courtesy of Lane LB: *Am J Sports Med* 19:234–238, 1991.)

Results.—Of the 7 patients receiving traditional treatment, 3 had excellent results with full motion and strength and no pain; 4 had good results with good strength, incomplete motion, and occasionally mild pain. Among patients receiving the new treatment, 21 of 25 had excellent results, 3 had good results, and 1 with midsubstance rupture had a good result. Both methods improved pain and restored stability and strength. Restoration of strength was significantly more rapid with the new method as was patients' ability to return to their previous sport.

Conclusions.—Both methods have similar outcomes, but the newer treatment seems to allow quicker return to sports and more rapid return of strength.

Rehabilitation Following Ulnar Collateral Ligament Reconstruction of Athletes

Seto JL, Brewster CE, Randall CC, Jobe FW (Kerlan-Jobe Orthopaedic Clinic, Inglewood, Calif)
J Orthop Sports Phys Ther 14:100–105, 1991   7–33

Background.—In athletes involved in sports that include throwing activity, the elbow is often subjected to repeated valgus forces. The ulnar collateral ligament (UCL) can get torn and may require reconstructive surgery. The anatomy and biomechanics of the elbow joint were studied, and a rehabilitation program was examined that can be followed after UCL reconstruction of the elbow with an emphasis on return to the throwing activity.

Rehabilitation Program After Ulnar Collateral Ligament Reconstruction

TIME PERIOD (postoperation)	EXERCISE PROGRAM
0 to ½ mo:	— Elbow immobilized.
	— Gripping exercises.
½ to 1 mo:	— Splint removed.
	— PROM and active-assisted elbow ROM.
	— Active shoulder ROM exercises (if necessary).
1 to 1½ mos:	— Active elbow and shoulder ROM exercises.
	— Strengthening exercises: wrist flexion and extension, forearm pronation and supination.
1½ to 3 mos:	— Continue shoulder and elbow ROM exercises.
	— Continue wrist and forearm strengthening exercises.
	— Add elbow strengthening exercises.
	— May add resistive radial and ulnar deviation.
3 to 5 mos:	— Avoid valgus stress to elbow and ballistic movement in terminal elbow ranges.
	— May begin shoulder strengthening exercises with light resistance, with emphasis on rotator cuff muscles.
	— Start total body conditioning exercises.
	— May begin easy tossing at 30 feet, progressing to 50 feet, no wind-up, 2–3 times/week, 10–15 min/session.
5 to 5½ mos:	— Continue upper extremity strengthening exercises.
	— Continue easy tossing, 50–60 feet, no wind-up, 2–3 times/week, 10–15 min/session.
5½ to 6 mos:	— Add shoulder internal rotation exercise in sidelying position.
	— Continue strengthening exercises and total body conditioning program.
	— Lob ball on alternate days, no more than 30 feet, 10–15 min/session.
6 to 6½ mos:	— Lob with easy wind-up, 40–50 feet, 15–20 min/session, 2–3 times/week.
6½ to 7 mos:	— Lob with occasional straight throw at ½ speed, 60 feet, 20–25 min/session, 2–3 times/week.
7 to 7½ mos:	— Increase throwing distance to 100 feet at ½ speed, 20–25 min/session, 2–3 times/week.

(continued)

Anatomy and Biomechanics.—Valgus stresses that occur during throwing cause a compression force on the laterally located radiocapitellar joint in the elbow. Loose bodies can form in the joint as the medial aspect of the olecranon process is compressed against the medial wall of the olecranon fossa. The UCL is the primary resistive force to valgus stresses among the soft tissue structures. The UCL is the structure that is usually torn by a valgus force.

Rehabilitation Program.—A program was designed to return athletes to their competitive level of throwing about 1 year after surgical reconstruction. The program focuses on increasing strength and endurance of the musculature around the elbow and restoring the elbow's functional range of motion (table). About 1 year is needed for the tendon graft to remodel and for the surrounding tissues to gain the strength and endur-

Table *(continued)*

TIME PERIOD (postoperation)	EXERCISE PROGRAM
7½ to 8 mos:	— Long easy throws from 150 feet with ball back to home plate on 5–6 bounces, 20–25 min/session. Begin 12-Day Throwing Cycle: Throw 2 days/rest one day, repeat 4 times.
8 to 8½ mos:	— OUTFIELDERS: Increase throwing distance to 200–250 feet, with ball reaching home plate on numerous bounces, 20–25 min/session, 12-Day Throwing Cycle. — PITCHERS AND INFIELDERS: In and Out Drill: Begin throwing at ¾ speed, gradually increasing the throwing distance until 150 feet. Gradually decrease throwing distance until reaching normal throwing position distance. Perform this drill 30–35 minutes on the 12-Day Throwing Cycle.
8½ to 9 mos:	— OUTFIELDERS: Increase throwing distance to 300–350 feet, with ball reaching home plate on 1–2 bounces at ¾ speed–full speed, 30–35 min/session, 12-Day Throwing Cycle. — PITCHERS AND INFIELDERS: In and Out Drill: Gradually reduce time throwing "in and out" and increase throwing time from normal playing position, ¾ speed–full speed, 30–35 min/session, 12-Day Throwing Cycle.
9 to 9½ mos:	— OUTFIELDERS AND INFIELDERS: Short, crisp throws from 100–150 feet, ¾–full speed, 30 minutes, 12-Day Throwing Cycle. — PITCHERS: Throw batting practice at ¾–full speed, 30 minutes, 12-Day Throwing Cycle.
9½ to 10½ mos:	— ALL PLAYERS: Return to throwing from normal playing position, ¾–full speed with emphasis on technique and accuracy, 25–30 min/session, 12-Day Throwing Cycle.
10½ to 11 mos:	— ALL PLAYERS: Continue throwing from normal playing position, ⅞–full speed, gradually increase throwing time.
11 to 12 mos:	— ALL PLAYERS: Simulate game day situation. — PITCHERS: warm up with appropriate number of pitches and throw for an average number of innings, taking the usual rest breaks between innings. Repeat this simulation 2–4 times with a 3–4 day rest period in between.

Courtesy of Seto JL, Brewster CE, Randall CC, et al: *J Orthop Sports* 14:100–105, 1991.)

ance required for a return to sports. Time must be allowed for tendon vascularization to occur and to promote its viability. Careful patient supervision is also needed to avoid complications, (e.g., inflammation, tendinitis, or undue stress on the ligament substitute).

Conclusions.—As with all rehabilitation programs, the exercises in this program should be tailored to the specific needs of the patient. The program described, designed mainly for baseball pitchers, is easily adapted to other types of athletes.

▶ The table in Abstract 7–33 describes a program of rehabilitation and return to throwing activities following a UCL reconstruction. Please note the times stated and level of activity are to be used as a guideline. The program should be individualized according to each patient's rate of recovery and progress made.—F.J. George, A.T.C., P.T.

Risks of Neurovascular Injury in Elbow Arthroscopy: Starting Anteromedially or Anterolaterally?
Verhaar J, van Mameren H, Brandsma A (University Hospital, Maastricht, The Netherlands; State University Limburg, Maastricht)
Arthroscopy 7:287–290, 1991   7–34

Introduction.—Arthroscopy of the elbow can be a valuable adjunct to diagnosis of elbow pathology, but the technique is demanding. The risks for severing neurovascular structures in elbow arthroscopy are greater than in arthroscopy of most other joints. The usual method involves use of the anterolateral portal as starting portal. The risks of injuring the neurovascular structures when starting with an anteromedial portal were assessed in 5 fresh cadaver elbows.

Methods.—Arthroscopy was performed using the portal sequence: anteromedial, anterolateral, and posterolateral. The anteromedial portal was made 2 cm distal and 1 cm anterior to the medial epicondyle. The anterolateral portal was placed 2 cm distal and 2 cm anterior to the lateral epicondyle. The posterolateral portal was placed 3 cm proximal to the tip of the olecranon and lateral to the triceps tendon.

Results.—The risk of injury to the radial nerve was higher with the anterolateral approach than was the risk of injury to the medial nerve with the anteromedial approach. Starting medially may aid in accurate placement of the anterolateral portal and may further reduce the risk of injuring the radial nerve. In addition, most elbow pathology is localized in the lateral compartment, which is visualized best from the anteromedial approach.

Conclusion.—In elbow arthroscopy, the safety margin is increased by placing the medial portal less anteriorly. This finding is in contrast to those of previous studies, which have recommended the anterolateral approach.

▶ Although a matter of semantics, it is interesting to note that the authors state that "our results indicate that there may be a decreased risk of damaging neurovascular structures in the anteromedial approach compared with the anterolateral one." To be noted, no mention is made about whether a sharp or dull trochar was used. It is my opinion that use of a dull trochar substantially decreases the risk of injury to neurovascular structures whether or not an anteriomedial or anterolateral portal is used.—J.S. Torg, M.D.

Fatigue Fracture of the Ulna Occurring in Pitchers of Fast-Pitch Softball

Tanabe S, Nakahira J, Bando E, Yamaguchi H, Miyamoto H, Yamamoto A
(University of Tokushima, Japan)
Am J Sports Med 19:317–321, 1991   7–35

Introduction.—Fatigue fracture of the ulna is infrequently seen but can be associated with various sports. Data on 3 patients with fatigue fracture of the ulna in male pitchers of fast-pitch softball were reviewed, along with CT evaluation of the ulna and high-speed cinematography of the pitch to help delineate the cause of the injury.

Methods.—The patients, aged 16-20 years, complained of worsening pain on throwing. Examination revealed tenderness, swelling, and pain on motion of the ulnar shafts; the sites of this pain were correlated with fractures detected radiographically. There was no history of violent force, so the diagnosis of fatigue fracture was made. Well-trained college athletes were studied to elucidate the mechanism of injury. High-speed cinematography, at a speed of 64 frames per second, was performed to record their body movements during the windmill delivery. Computed tomographic scanning sections of the forearms were also obtained to investigate the shapes and areas of the ulna and its cortical and cancellous bones from the elbow to the hand joints.

Results.—High-speed cinematography showed slight elbow flexion during wind-up, hand dorsiflexion on release of the ball, and extreme forearm pronation during follow-through. The CT sections showed shapes significantly different from circles at around the center of the ulna. Cross-sectional areas were smaller in the middle third than in other parts.

Conclusion.—Fatigue fractures of the ulna may occur in pitchers of fast-pitch softball. These injuries appear to be torsionally induced and to occur mainly in the middle third of the bone, which must be distinguished from the lifting mechanism of injury.

▶ It is interesting to note that there had only been 16 prior cases of fatigue fractures of the ulna reported in the literature. As the authors point out, most of these fractures are related to the patient's activities. Specifically, they include tennis, softball, volleyball, fencing, and weightlifting. They point out that in activities in which the forearm is stressed during full supination, (i.e., weightlifting), repeated stress results in a fracture involving either the proximal one third of the distal two thirds of the bone. However, when stress occurs with the forearm pronated (i.e., tennis and softball), repetitive torsional forces result in a fracture of the midthird of the bone.—J.S. Torg, M.D.

Radial Tunnel Syndrome: An Etiology of Chronic Lateral Elbow Pain
Lutz FR Jr (North Hills Sports Medicine, Pittsburgh)
J Orthop Sports Phys Ther 14:14–17, 1991   7–36

Introduction.—Radial tunnel syndrome (RTS) is a rare disorder in which the posterior interosseous branch of the radial nerve is trapped in the radial tunnel. It is important to distinguish between RTS and tennis elbow in patients who are seen with lateral elbow pain.

Mechanisms.—Compression usually occurs between the head of the radius and the supinator muscle. Fibrous tethering bands anterior to the radial head may compress the nerve when the elbow is fully flexed. A radial fan of vessels crossing the radial nerve or the fibrous arcade of Frohse also may produce nerve compression, as may a tendinous margin of the extensor carpi radialis brevis muscle. Less often, compression results from edema of adjacent structures or thickened tissue about the nerve near its bifurcation.

Clinical Features.—Tenderness on palpation of the radial tunnel anterior to the radial head suggests RTS rather than tennis elbow. Symptoms of RTS are reproduced by flexing the elbow to 90 degrees with full pronation of the forearm and resisting active supination. Resisted extension of the middle finger with the elbow extended also is suggestive.

Management.—Such conservative measures as ultrasound, splinting, resistive and stretching exercises, and steroid injection have not proved very helpful in patients with RTS. Decompression of the radial nerve in the radial tunnel has given quite satisfactory results. Release of the extensor carpi radialis brevis is an alternative procedure. Surgery should be considered if conservative measures fail for longer than 6 months.

▶ This author reports that most cases of radial tunnel syndrome are satisfactorily treated by radial nerve decompression. He said that 114 of 123 cases showed significant relief from pain and symptoms 1 to 2 weeks after radial nerve decompression. Follow-up studies show that the relief from RTS symptoms appears to be permanent.—Col. J.S. Anderson, PE.D.

8 Knee

Lidocaine Local Anesthesia for Arthroscopic Knee Surgery
Dahl MR, Dasta JF, Zuelzer W, McSweeney TD (Ohio State Univ Hosp, Columbus)
Anesth Analg 71:670–674, 1990   8–1

Objective.—Local anesthesia by periarticular infiltration and intra-articular (IA) instillation may be used as an alternative to regional anesthesia for arthroscopic knee surgery. In the present study the dose-response relationship was determined when lidocaine was used as a local anesthetic for knee arthroscopy. The serum concentrations of lidocaine were measured after extra-articular and IA administration.

Methods.—Forty-five patients were randomized to receive 20 mL of .5%, or 1.5% lidocaine with epinephrine intra-articularly. Patients verbally ranked intraoperative discomfort on an 11-point linear pain scale.

Results.—During the first 45 minutes of surgery, the .5% lidocaine group had significantly higher pain scores than the 1 or 1.5% groups. Pain scores on the last intraoperative measurement were not statistically different among the groups. In the 1.5% lidocaine group 94% of the patients were willing to repeat the anesthetic technique, compared with 83% of those in the 1% group and 75% of those in the .5% group. Serum concentrations of lidocaine in the 1.5% lidocaine group were higher than in the .5% or 1% groups. The duration of postoperative analgesia was similar in all groups and no patients had symptoms of toxicity.

Conclusions.—Based on the patients' verbal assessments of intraoperative discomfort, the use of 1% or 1.5% lidocaine with epinephrine is appropriate for knee arthroscopy. There was no lidocaine toxicity in any patient.

▶ This paper emphasizes the efficacy of local anesthesia for arthroscopic procedures on the knee. Our preference is to instill 40 mL of 100% xylocaine and 1:200,000 epinephrine solution for 5 minutes before complete joint suspension and local infiltration of the portal sites (1). The importance of waiting 5 minutes before beginning the procedure so that the local anesthetic has an opportunity to take affect must be emphasized. Procedures that can be performed using this method of anesthesia without tourniquet include meniscectomies, meniscal repairs, removal of loose bodies, arthroscopic lateral retinacular release, and abrasion arthroplasties.—J.S. Torg, M.D.

Reference

1. Yacobucci GN, et al: *Arthroscopy* 6:311, 1990.

Medial Dislocation of the Patella
Miller PR, Klein RM, Teitge RA (Hutzel Hosp, Detroit; Wayne State Univ, Detroit)
Skeletal Radiol 20:429–431, 1991   8–2

Introduction.—Although lateral patellar dislocation and subluxation of the patella are well recognized, there have been no reports of medial dislocation of the patella. Three cases of such injury were revealed by CT or by double-contrast arthrography with CT (DCCT).

Patients.—The 2 women and 1 man were aged 21 to 26 years. All had undergone previous and repeated treatment, including lateral retinacular release, for injuries to the left knee sustained 1 to 3 years previously. Lateral release was done for either chronic knee pain or recurrent lateral patellar subluxation. All patients were able to dislocate their patella medially at the time of CT or DCCT and reduce it before leaving the radiology department. Clinical atrophy of the distal thigh was present in all 3 cases. One patient also had patella alta and a shallow trochlear groove in the distal femur. Both CT and DCCT proved capable of demonstrating the injury; DCCT showed marked loss of patellar articular cartilage resulting from the recurrent dislocation in the patient with a shallow trochlear groove.

Conclusions.—A potential complication of lateral retinacular release is medial patellar dislocation. This may result from loss of the extensor mechanism provided by the vastus lateralis, leading to unbalanced forces on the patella. The disorder may be disabling, occasionally requiring hospital reduction. Double contrast arthrography with CT with or without rotational analysis has become a standard imaging examination for patients with medial or lateral displacement of the patella.

▶ Hughston and Deese have previously reported a series of 18 patients who had medial subluxation of the patella as a complication of lateral retinacular release surgery (1). This paper by Miller et al. would be more appropriately titled "Medial Dislocation of the Patella Following Multiple Surgeries for Lateral Dislocation." Specifically, 1 patient had an extensor realignment plus 2 lateral retinacular releases, the second patient had 9 surgical procedures for anterior knee pain, and the third patient had 2 lateral retinacular releases before medial dislocation.—J.S. Torg, M.D.

Reference

1. Hughston J, Deese M: *Am J Sports Med* 16:383, 1988.

Reflex Sympathetic Dystrophy of the Patellofemoral Joint

Finsterbush A, Frankl U, Mann G, Lowe J (Hadassah University Hospital, Jerusalem)
Orthop Rev 20:877–885, 1991   8–3

Introduction.—The number of cases of reflex sympathetic dystrophy (RSD) involving the knee is increasing as clinicians become more aware of the disorder. Data were reviewed on 18 patients in whom RSD of the patellofemoral joint was diagnosed.

Patients.—The average age when the "triggering" injury occurred was 34 years, and at the time of final evaluation, 39 years. Symptoms were present for 5.4 years on average. In 6 patients, RSD was diagnosed retrospectively after several operations had failed. In 4 patients there was previous pathology in the involved knee joint. In 11 patients, there was direct injury to the knee; 12 patients had compensation or liability cases pending.

Clinical Features.—Pain was out of proportion to trauma and was prolonged. It tended to be severe and constant at first, and later initiated by activity. The patients with late diagnoses tended to have an unstable knee or uncontrolled knee motion. Regional osteoporosis was a nearly universal finding. Scintigraphy usually showed increased technetium uptake about the knee. Arthroscopy usually revealed synovitis and minor changes in the articular surface of the patella.

Treatment and Outcome.—Patients received continuous epidural nerve block with lidocaine or regional sympathetic block with reserpine, which temporarily relieved pain. Aggressive physical therapy was then instituted. Patients in whom RSD was diagnosed at a relatively early phase had the best outcome. The chance of improvement decreased when surgery was performed, and patients with late diagnoses remained disabled.

Conclusion.—Confidence in the physician is critical in the treatment of RSD. Initially, a block is used to reduce pain, and regular physical therapy is then started.

▶ The findings presented in this paper are similar to those reported by Ogilvie-Harris et al. (1) and Katz et al. (2). Specifically, salient clinical features of reflex sympathetic dystrophy of the knee are the following:

1. Onset of pain after minor injury or arthroscopic surgery
2. Marked hypersensitivity to touch
3. Quadriceps atrophy
4. Flexion contracture
5. Unsuccessful attempts at rehabilitation
6. Patchy demineralization and generalized osteoporosis on roentgenograms

7. Characteristic bone scan findings of increased nuclide uptake involving both sides of the joint

8. Cutaneous temperature decreases in excess of 1°C in a dermatomal pattern of tomography.

Oglivie-Harris noted that "the cinequinone for diagnosis as well as the mainstay of treatment in our series was lumbar sympathetic block." Also, the importance of a high index of suspicion for RSD involving the knee is that all authors agree that when treatment is implemented at an early stage there is a better response to therapy. That 6 of the patients in this report had multiple operations clearly underlines the importance of a prompt and accurate diagnosis.—J.S. Torg, M.D.

References

1. Ogilvie-Harris DJ, Roscoe M: *J Bone Joint Surg* 69-B:804, 1987.
2. Katz MM, Hungerford DS: *J Bone Joint Surg* 69-B:797, 1987.

Ultrasonography in the Detection of Partial Patellar Ligament Ruptures (Jumper's Knee)
Kälebo P, Swärd L, Karlsson J, Peterson L (University of Gothenburg, Sweden; Gothenburg Medical Center)
Skeletal Radiol 20:285–289, 1991   8–4

Background.—Sports activities such as jumping and kicking, which place repeated strain on the knee, may produce chronic localized pain that arises from the proximal part of the patellar ligament or the distal quadriceps tendon. Degenerative and necrotic tendon tissue and granulation tissue with neovascularization follow multiple partial ruptures of collagen fibers. Most often the patellar ligament is affected at the inferior pole of the patellar.

Study.—Eighty-one athletes with chronic pain localized to the patellar ligament were examined ultrasonographically, along with 20 asymptomatic nonathletes. Twenty-five partial tendon ruptures were proved surgically. A real-time linear-array probe with a 7.5 MHz transducer was used for the studies. Patients were examined while in a supine position with the knee in 30 degrees of flexion.

Findings.—A cone-shaped, poorly echogenic area more than .5 cm long in the center of the patellar tendon was a reliable indicator of jumper's knee. Other abnormalities included localized thickening of the patellar tendon, prepatellar extension of the lesion, and erosion of the tip of the patella. There were no false negative or false positive studies but in 1 case there was a true negative result. Sonography was able to demonstrate lack of healing after surgery. Soft-tissue radiographs showed only localized swelling.

Discussion.—Sonography is the best way of evaluating jumper's knee. It is inexpensive, noninvasive, accurate, and repeatable. The study is helpful in distinguishing between jumper's knee, chondromalacia, meniscal injury, tendinitis, and bursitis. A negative study can prevent unnecessary tendon surgery.

▶ The diagnostic yield of an ultrasound study depends on the expertise of the individual performing and interpreting the examination. Knowledge of the expected pathology is extremely helpful. A good ultrasound examination is preferable compared to MR examination because it is more cost-effective, more comfortable for the patient, and should be more readily available. Clinical information should be provided by the referring physician so that the appropriate imaging examination can be performed given the clinically anticipated pathology.—J.S. Torg, M.D.

Partial Rupture of the Patellar Ligament: Results After Operative Treatment
Karlsson J, Lundin O, Lossing IW, Peterson L (University of Göteborg, Sweden)
Am J Sports Med 19:403–408, 1991   8–5

Introduction.—"Jumper's knee" describes several peripatellar disorders that involve the patellar ligament and, less often, the quadriceps tendon. It is found most often in athletes who incur repeated knee strain because of jumping or kicking.

Patients.—Eighty-six patients had surgery for partial rupture of the patellar ligament in 1971–1988. Seventy-eight of the 86 were followed up for a mean of 5 years. All but 3 of the patients were active in sports. The mean age at time of surgery was 25 years. All patients had constant pain at rest and on activity and were unable to participate at their previous level of activity. Treatment lasted at least 6 months before surgery.

Operation.—All patients had abnormalities in the ligament near its junction with the distal pole of the patella. Abnormal tissue was radically resected longitudinally, and the margins were closed with resorbable sutures. Two patients also had ligament calcifications removed. The extremity was immobilized in a knee plaster cast for 4 weeks after operation.

Results.—Ninety-one percent of patients had excellent or good results. Seven patients were unable to return to their preinjury level of sports activity. The reasons for the unsatisfactory results in these cases were unclear.

Recommendations.—Conservative treatment is appropriate initially in these cases. Perhaps 1 in 3 patients will require surgery for partial rupture of the patellar ligament. Resection is a relatively simple approach and has given satisfactory results in most patients.

▶ I would certainly agree with the authors' conclusion that "surgical treatment for partial rupture of the patellar ligament, or jumper's knee, is recommended only after a prolonged and well supervised conservative treatment program fails." Their description of the procedure involving "radical resection" of the affected tissue deserves comment. Our practice is to perform the procedure with local anesthetic infiltrated in the area of the skin incision and without a tourniquet. With this method, the patient can identify the involved area of the tendon when the surgeon applies pressure with a point of a dull instrument. Precise localization of the lesion is achieved and its excision is then performed with actual relief of pain while the patient is on the table. Subsequently, no lengthy immobilization is necessary and rehabilitation is quite rapid.—J.S Torg, M.D.

Repair of Peripheral Meniscal Tears; Open Versus Arthroscopic Technique
Hanks GA, Gause TM, Sebastianelli WJ, O'Donnell CS, Kalenak A (Hershey Med Ctr, Hershey, Pa; Univ of Rochester, NY)
Arthroscopy 7:72–77, 1991   8–6

Introduction.—Both open and arthroscopic techniques have been used successfully for repair of peripheral meniscus tears, but no previous study has compared the 2 techniques in terms of difficulty, efficacy, and safety. In addition to addressing this question, the role of anterior cruciate ligament stability in meniscus repair was investigated.

Methods.—During the study period (1978–1986), 71 meniscal repairs were performed in 68 knees. Sixty of the patients were men; the average age was 24 years. In 19 cases the anterior cruciate ligament was intact; the remainder had an associated acute or chronic tear of the anterior cruciate ligament in addition to the meniscus tear. Twenty-six patients underwent meniscus repair by open arthrotomy and 45 had arthroscopic repair. Open repair was performed by a posteromedial arthrotomy incision. Arthroscopic repair was done using the double-lumen guide system with a limited posterior incision for retrieval of needles. A formal rehabilitation program followed the postoperative period of bracing.

Results.—At an average follow-up of 50 months, the overall failure rate was 9.8% and was not significantly different for the 2 techniques. The failure rate was higher, again not significantly so, in the anterior cruciate-deficient knees (13%) than in the cruciate-stable knees (8%). No neurologic or vascular injuries occurred with either procedure. The arthroscopic technique was easier to perform than open repair because some tears were too far inside the rim to lend themselves to open suture.

Conclusion.—Both open and arthroscopic meniscus repair techniques can yield good results, with few complications, in both stable and unstable knees. Although anterior cruciate ligament stability is desirable, it is not required for a successful outcome.

Magnetic Resonance Imaging of the Surgically Repaired Meniscus: Six-Month Follow-Up

Kent RH, Pope CF, Lynch JK, Jokl P (Yale Univ, New Haven, Conn)
Magn Reson Imag 9:335–341, 1991   8–7

Introduction.—Recent evidence suggests that meniscectomy increases the risk of early damage to hyaline cartilage, and that the extent of damage relates to the amount of meniscus removed.

Methods.—Magnetic resonance imaging was used to assess sutured meniscal repairs in 17 patients who had 18 operations; 12 medial and 6 lateral menisci were repaired, usually with polydioxanone sutures. There was a complete anterior cruciate ligament tear in 8 patients. Initial MRI was performed after an average of 7 weeks and follow-up studies were obtained for 11 patients.

Results.—All patients had abnormal areas of increased meniscal signal at the repair site when examined at 7 weeks. All those restudied at 6 months had persistent meniscal defects, which often were unchanged from the initial appearances. The 3 patients who had 2 follow-up MR assessments had no significant change in their defects.

Conclusion.—Complete healing may not occur as early after meniscal repair as previously thought. Nonabsorbable suture material therefore may be best suited to repairing the meniscus.

▶ The value of MR to evaluate postoperative meniscal healing has not yet been established. As stated by the authors, "defects may be present for relatively long periods of time following meniscal repairs and caution must be exercised when attempting to diagnose new or recurrent tears."—J.S. Torg, M.D.

Arthroscopic Meniscal Repair With Fibrin Glue

Ishimura M, Tamai S, Fujisawa Y (Nara Medical University; Nara Sinohmiya Seikeigeka, Nara, Japan)
Arthroscopy 7:177–181, 1991   8–8

Objective.—Thirty-two patients who underwent 40 arthroscopic repairs of meniscal tears since 1984 with the use of fibrin glue were studied. Most of the patients also had cruciate ligament lesions. Eighteen meniscal tears were treated within 3 weeks of injury.

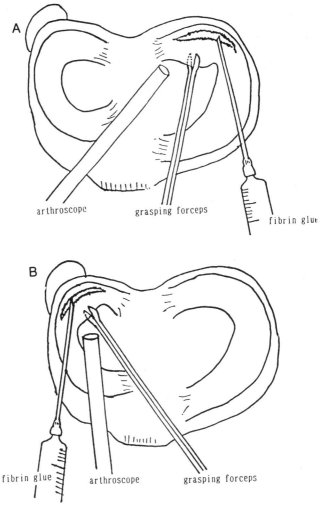

Fig 8–1.—Arthroscopic meniscal repair with fibrin-adhesive systems for medial meniscal tear (**A**) and lateral meniscal tear (**B**). (Courtesy of Ishimura M, Tamai S, Fujisawa Y: *Arthroscopy* 7:177–181, 1991.)

Technique.—A lateral infrapatellar approach is taken for visibility to repair a medial meniscal tear. After refreshing the tear by a medial infrapatellar approach, fibrin glue is placed using a 20-gauge needle inserted from around the anterior border of the medial collateral ligament. After glue injection, the torn meniscus is reduced with forceps and held in place for 1–2 minutes (Fig 8–1). A lateral meniscal tear is treated by inserting the needle around the anterior border of the lateral collateral ligament.

Results.—Only 2 patients had meniscal symptoms during a mean follow-up of 3½ years. In 20 patients with 25 tears who underwent repeat arthroscopy an average of 5½ months after repair, 73% of the old tears had a good outcome with firm adhesion over the full length of the tear even under traction by grasping forceps. Medial meniscal tears achieved a better overall outcome than tears of the lateral meniscus.

Conclusion.—Arthroscopic repair using fibrin glue can produce good clinical results even when a long tear is seen. Presently, glue is most useful for repairing posterior segment tears, which are difficult to suture without arthrotomy.

▶ According to the authors, the fibrin adhesive system used consist of fibrinogen, thrombin, aprotinin, calcium chloride, and factor VII. Presumably, when fibrinogen is converted to fibrin and polymerized it has tissue adhesive qualities. Also, the fibrin glue apparently facilitates tissue healing. Attractive as these properties appear, it should be pointed out that fibrin glue does not have DEA approval. More importantly, the presence of factor VII in its conversion raises the spectrum of HIV transmission! Need more be said?—J.S. Torg, M.D.

Meniscus Repair in the Anterior Cruciate Deficient Knee
Hanks GA, Gause TM, Handal JA, Kalenak A (Pennsylvania State Univ, Hershey)
Am J Sports Med 18:606–613, 1990   8–9

Background.—In patients with both a meniscal tear and anterior cruciate ligament (ACL) injury, most surgeons suggest concurrent repair of these structures, but some patients prefer to undergo meniscal repair alone.

Methods.—Twenty-five repairs of meniscal tears in the peripheral vascular zone were performed in 24 patients having ACL insufficiency. Twenty-two patients with 23 repaired menisci were followed for 56 months on average. Twelve patients underwent open meniscal repair by posteromedial arthrotomy. Five of those tears extended into the middle third of the meniscus. Arthroscopic repair was undertaken in 11 patients using the double-lumen cannula system.

Results.—Three of 4 patients who had new pain of moderate degree postoperatively had a new or recurrent tear. Eight patients had symptoms of instability and, in 4 of them, moderate restriction of activity resulted. Nine patients in all had some reduction in level of activity after meniscal repair, but in 4 cases this was the result of graduation. Several recreational athletes remained active despite participating less often.

Conclusions.—Meniscal repair was successful in 87% of the ACL-deficient knees, compared with a success rate of 94% in cruciate-stable knees. Ensured ACL stability is preferable, but meniscal repair alone should be undertaken in a patient who does not wish to have ligament repair or reconstruction.

▶ The rationale for concomitant anterior cruciate ligament reconstruction at the time of meniscal repair is not to facilitate meniscal healing but rather to prevent meniscal reinjury. Another, and perhaps more reasonable, interpretation of the data would be that in view of the fact that 26% of the patients had subsequent giving way episodes and 13% were known to have failed repairs or retear, anterior cruciate ligament reconstruction should have been performed in all patients.—J.S. Torg, M.D.

Active Knee Joint Subluxation: Its Influence on the Prognosis of Ligament Reconstruction

Robinson D, Halperin N (Assaf Harofeh Medical Center, Zerifin, Israel)
Acta Orthop Scand 62:264–265, 1991   8–10

Background.—After a tear of the anterior cruciate ligament, some patients can actively subluxate the joint. This has been classified as an "active pivot shift" or a grade 4 positive Lachman sign. Combined reconstruction including an intra-articular reconstruction of the anterior cruciate ligament and an extra-articular reefing of the posteromedial corner has been recommended by Gurtler et al. The present study was designed to evaluate whether voluntary subluxation is of prognostic significance in knee-ligament surgery.

Methods.—Sixty-one patients who underwent intra-articular reconstruction of the anterior cruciate ligament were compared to 7 patients who were treated for anterior cruciate ligament insufficiency and demonstrated active subluxation of the knee joint.

Results.—The 2 groups had similar preoperative clinical knee scores, but the postoperative score was worse in the smaller group. All 7 patients had limited function, a more rapid development of arthrosis, and subjective complaints. In all 7 cases, the ability to voluntarily subluxate the joint reoccurred despite a stable knee immediately after operation.

Conclusion.—The active pivot shift sign appears to be prognostic for a high failure rate in anterior cruciate ligament reconstruction surgery.

▶ The authors have provided us with what appears to be an effective noninvasive prognosticator for helping to determine the efficacy of anterior cruciate ligament reconstruction.—J.S. Torg, M.D.

Functional Anatomy of the Anterior Cruciate Ligament: Fibre Bundle Actions Related to Ligament Replacements and Injuries

Amis AA, Dawkins GPC (Imperial College of Science, Technology, and Medi-

cine, London)
J Bone Joint Surg 73-B:260–267, 1991   8–11

Background.—Controversy remains as to the anatomy and function of the anterior cruciate ligament (ACL), particularly the fascicular anatomy. None of the many reports on measuring changes in ACL length have measured the lengths of the actual fibers themselves. One study of the fiber bundle anatomy of the ACL, including measurements of the actual fiber bundles, was reviewed.

Methods.—The study material consisted of 27 cadaver knees prepared to provide good access to the ACL without disturbing the meniscus. Fibrous structure was identified by careful dissection. Fine wires were passed from the origins of the individual fibers along the ACL and through the tibia. The specimens were mounted on a special device that rotated the tibia, which was attached to a stroke displacement transducer, around a vertical axis with the femur maintained at particular angles of flexion.

Findings.—Most knees showed 3 distinct fiber bundles, the anteromedial, intermediate, and posterolateral. None of these bundles was isometric. The posterolateral bundle increased in length in extension and the anteromedial bundle stretched in flexion; these findings suggest that they contribute to knee stability and were likely to rupture in these positions. No significant effect of tibial rotation was noted. The anteromedial and posterolateral bundles appeared to have a reciprocal action in anterior drawer resistance.

Conclusions.—Three functional but not necessarily separate fiber bundles appear to make up the multifascicular structure of the ACL. They are not isometric in flexion and extension; rather, they stretch in correlation with their changing participation in total ACL action. These findings may help explain and diagnose partial ACL ruptures and provide data for the design of more sophisticated implants.

▶ The classic study on ACL fiber bundle length as it relates to anatomic placement and isometry was performed by Sapega et al. (1). Instrumented tibia femoral excursion wires were implanted in the midsubstance of the an terior medial, central, and posterior fiber regions of fresh cadaver knees. I was pointed out that in both operative testing conditions and in the cadaver studies, "the anatomical areas of insertion of the anterior cruciate ligament normally exhibit characteristic patterns on non-isometric behavior." On the basis of this work, it was concluded that "a limited deviation with the specific physiometric pattern might even be desirable, due to its close correspondence to the form of a normal anterior laxity profile of the knee" and "the acceptability of any deviation from isometry should be judged by its direction and overall pattern throughout the range of motion of the knee, and not just by its absolute magnitude."—J.S. Torg, M.D.

Reference

1. Sapega AA, et al: *J Bone Joint Surg* 72-A:259, 1990.

Does Tourniquet Use During Anterior Cruciate Ligament Surgery Interfere With Postsurgical Recovery of Function? A Review of the Literature

Gutin B, Warren R, Wickiewicz T, O'Brien S, Altchek D, Kroll M (Hosp for Special Surgery, New York)
Arthroscopy 7:52–56, 1991   8–12

Introduction.—Some surgeons use a tourniquet during surgical repair of the anterior cruciate ligament (ACL), whereas others do not. No randomized, controlled trials have directly reported the effects of tourniquet use during ACL surgery. A review of the pertinent literature was undertaken to help surgeons weigh the costs and benefits of the available approaches.

Background.—Increasing sports participation has led to an increased number of injuries. Knee injuries, including tears of the ACL, are very common. Substantial disruption of the ACL was reported in 250,000 patients in 1984. Many of those patients undergo surgery and a rehabilitation program to return to their previous level of activity.

Tourniquet Use.—A tourniquet is used in surgery of the extremity to provide a bloodless field and enable the surgeon to visualize the joint clearly. However, recent reports have noted neuropathies, muscle weakness, and atrophy in patients after tourniquet-aided knee surgery. Animal studies also provide evidence of long-term muscle and nerve damage with use of a tourniquet. Yet randomized trials of tourniquet use during arthroscopic meniscectomy have reached contradictory conclusions.

Conclusion.—The application of a tourniquet for 1 to 2 hours during ACL surgery appears to have a damaging effect on muscles and nerve and may interfere with early rehabilitation exercises. Until definitive information regarding tourniquet use becomes available, pressure gauges should be monitored so that the minimum pressure needed to occlude the circulation can be applied. If use of the tourniquet is prolonged, the patient may need more time for strength recovery.

▶ Although no definitive answers are provided by this paper, the questions presented concerning the routine use of tourniquets during knee surgery are not only pertinent but are a long time in coming. I would certainly agree with the authors that "there is reason to believe that the routine use of tourniquets during knee ligament surgery needs to be re-evaluated."—J.S. Torg, M.D.

Anterior Cruciate Ligament Replacement: A Review

Silver FH, Tria AJ, Zawadsky JP, Dunn MG (UMD-Robert Wood Johnson Med School, Piscataway, NJ)

J Long-Term Effects Med Implants 1:135–154, 1991   8–13

Purpose.—The anterior cruciate ligament (ACL) is a multifasciculated structure composed of crimped aligned collagen fibers. It is the major intra-articular mechanical element that limits motion of the tibia with respect to the femur. Failure of the ACL leads to excessive joint mobility and instability, which, if left untreated, limits fine cutting motions and leads to osteoarthritis. The literature on ACL repair that incorporates biologic and synthetic grafts was reviewed.

Current Status.—Because of an increase in athletic activities in the United States and improved diagnostic accuracy, ACL injuries of the knee are more commonly identified. Successful repair of the ACL is routinely accomplished with the use of autografts of bone-patellar-bone complexes. Although the use of autografts requires a second surgical site and sacrifices other soft tissue structures in the knee, it results in progressive revascularization and subsequent ligament remodeling, leading to an increase in the failure load of the neoligament. Revitalization of the implanted autografts occurs by 8 weeks and is complete by 20 weeks after implantation. At 1 year after operation, autografts have 80% of the tensile strength and 52% of the maximum load present before transfer.

Outlook.—The mechanical properties of the autograft can be enhanced with the use of a ligament augmentation device (LAD). The device must be designed to support, but not stress shield the neoligament. Autografts provide scaffolding materials that stimulate revitalization and repair, whereas the synthetic polymers of the LADs provide strength. The next generation of ACL replacements will most likely contain scaffolding materials in addition to high-strength biodegradable fibers analogous to LADs. By combining the advantages of autografts and LADs, a new generation of materials with the advantages currently provided by the combined use of autograft tissue and LADs is feasible. These new materials will undoubtedly lead to the development of a new generation of ACL replacement procedures.

Prospective Evaluation of Arthroscopically Assisted Anterior Cruciate Ligament Reconstruction: Patellar Tendon Versus Semitendinosus and Gracilis Tendons

Marder RA, Raskind JR, Carroll M (Univ of California, Davis)

Am J Sports Med 19:478–484, 1991   8–14

Background.—Some studies have suggested that autogenous patellar tendon is the best available replacement for the anterior cruciate ligament (ACL) in patients with chronic laxity caused by a torn ACL. However, other reports reveal nearly comparable results with other autogenous tissues. The clinical outcome was evaluated prospectively after reconstruction of the ACL using either autogenous patellar tendon or doubled gracilis and semitendinosus tendons.

Methods.—A group of 80 consecutive patients were studied. Of these, 40 had reconstruction with autogenous middle third patellar tendon bone complex (PTBC) and 40 had reconstruction with double-looped semitendinosus and gracilis tendons (STG). The 2 treatment groups were similar with respect to age and sex. Most of the patients had been injured during skiing or basketball. All complained of recurrent giving way of the knee with activities requiring pivoting. Rehabilitation after surgery consisted of immediate passive knee extension, stationary cycling, and protected weightbearing for 6 weeks. In addition, the patients were to avoid resisted terminal knee extension for 6 months and return to activity at 10 to 12 months postoperatively.

Results.—A total of 72 patients were available for follow-up at a mean period of 29 months. The majority (65 of 72 patients) did not experience any postoperative episodes of giving way, and most (64%) returned to their preinjury level of activity. A group of 17 patients reported anterior knee pain with activity, whereas 2 complained of significant swelling. The 2 treatment groups showed no statistical difference with regard to return to activity. In addition, they did not differ significantly with respect to objective laxity evaluation.

Conclusion.—Comparable results were demonstrated for arthroscopically assisted ACL reconstruction performed with autogenous patellar tendon or combined semitendinosus and gracilis tendons. However, there was a statistically significant weakness in peak hamstring torque at 60 degrees per second with the latter graft.

▶ The conclusion of this well controlled prospective study is that comparable results for arthroscopically assisted ACL reconstruction can be obtained with either autogenous patellar tendon or combined semitendinosus and gracilis tendons. In my own experience, there are several notable exceptions to this. Specifically, in the chronic ACL-deficient knee, in large individuals returning to vigorous physical activities and in those with any degree of valgus laxity, autogenous infrapatella bone tendon bone preparation is the preferable graft material.—J.S. Torg, M.D.

Anterior Cruciate Ligament Reconstruction Using Freeze-Dried, Ethylene Oxide-Sterilized, Bone-Patellar Tendon-Bone Allografts: Two Year Results in Thirty-Six Patients
Roberts TS, Drez D Jr, McCarthy W, Paine R (Univ of Mississippi Med Ctr, Jackson; Knee and Sportsmedicine Ctr, Lake Charles, La; Louisiana State

Univ, Lake Charles; and Louisiana Med Ctr, New Orleans)
Am J Sports Med 19:35–41, 1991   8–15

Introduction.—Anterior cruciate ligament (ACL) reconstruction with locally harvested allografts that have been freeze dried and ethylene oxide sterilized was evaluated and followed for 2 years in a group of patients. Functional activity levels were assessed and radiographic evaluations were made.

Methods.—Of 44 patients who had ACL reconstruction with freeze-dried, ethylene oxide-sterilized bone-patellar tendon-bone allographs, 36 (82%) were evaluated by all or some of the following methods: Lysholm knee scoring scale, Tegner activity scale, physical examination, instrumental testing, and roentgenographic evaluation.

Results.—Only 17 of the 36 patients were functioning at a desirable activity level. The Lysholm scores in the failures averaged 61.1, compared to a mean score of 92.2 in the 17 patients at a desired activity level. Knee symptoms caused loss of activity in the failure group. Complete dissolution of the graft was noted in 8 patients (22%) undergoing repeat surgery; large femoral cysts were detected roentgenographically in these patients.

Discussion.—Another point of investigation involved whether the method of sterilization was effective against AIDS. Before allograft reconstruction is accepted as routine, these methods should be closely monitored. It was concluded that ethylene oxide-sterilized bone-patellar tendon-bone allografts have a high failure rate and a significant rate of graft dissolution. Careful evaluation of knee reconstruction, including subjective, objective, functional, and roentgenographic analyses, should continue.

► This paper sets forth 2 important conclusions: (1) Ethylene oxide-sterilized, bone-patellar tendon bone allografts cannot be recommended for use in humans; and (2) careful evaluation of methods of sterilization, especially their effectiveness against the AIDS virus, should be completed before allograft reconstruction is accepted as a routine procedure. It should be noted, however, that significantly better success rates have been reported using fresh frozen allografts for ACL reconstruction.—J.S. Torg, M.D.

The Gore-Tex Anterior Cruciate Ligament Prosthesis: Two Versus Three Year Results

Woods GA, Indelicato PA, Prevot TJ (Univ of Florida, Gainesville)
Am J Sports Med 19:48–55, 1991   8–16

Introduction.—Prosthetic replacements are growing in popularity for the treatment of patients with a ruptured anterior cruciate ligament (ACL). The Gore-Tex polytetrafluoroethylene ligament has had successful short-term results. To determine whether these results will be maintained with time, a cohort of patients with a minimum of 3 years of follow-up was examined and results were compared with those at 2-year follow-up.

Methods.—Forty-one patients, 85% of whom injured their knee during sports, underwent ACL reconstruction with the Gore-Tex prosthesis between November 1983 and May 1985. All but 2 were available for 2-year follow-up. At that time 4 of these patients had failed results. Twenty-nine of the 35 patients with successful results underwent follow-up at a minimum of 36 months (mean, 48 months) after implantation. Outcome was determined by both subjective and objective methods.

Results.—After the 2-year postoperative examination, there were 7 additional cases of failure. All the failed cases involved chronic ACL-deficient knees, and 3 of the 11 failures occurred after a specific traumatic event. The failure rate did not differ significantly between patients who required notchplasty and patients who did not. Knee swelling was the only significant finding before implantation that appeared to predispose patients to failed results. Subjective symptoms of giving way at 2 years and increased anterior drawer sign in 90 degrees of flexion may also be predictive of failure.

Conclusion.—There was a tendency for deterioration with time after replacement of a ruptured ACL with the Gore-Tex prosthesis. At the minimum 3-year follow-up 90% of the patients believed their knee was either normal or improved from its pre-operative condition. The modified Hughston knee score, however, found only 66% with good or excellent results. More time is required to judge long-term outcome with the Gore-Tex prosthesis.

▶ I certainly agree with the authors that success with implantation of the Gore-Tex polytetrafluoroethylene ligament is certainly "technique sensitive." Their conclusion that "better design and instrumentation are likely to improve the performance of this implant" would more appropriately read "must improve the performance." In its current form, because of its propensity to wear and demonstrate an early nonprogressive shift towards loosening, its role in the management of ACL deficiency appears to be limited.—J.S. Torg, M.D.

Reconstruction of the Anterior Cruciate Ligament With a Dacron Prosthesis
López-Vázquez E, Juan JA, Vila E, Debón J (Hospital de Sagunto, Valencia, Spain)
J Bone Joint Surg 73-A:1294–1300, 1991   8–17

Introduction.—Use of autogeneous grafts from the patellar ligament provides good results in the reconstruction of knees with a torn anterior cruciate ligament (ACL), but such grafts may require a long period of time to be incorporated. The use of synthetic materials to replace the ACL provides the advantage of immediate stability. Results with the Dacron prosthesis as a substitute for the torn ACL are reviewed.

Methods.—Fifty-four patients met the study criteria between October 1984 and October 1987. Nineteen had an acute injury of the ACL and 35 had a chronic injury. The patients were randomized to reconstructive treatment either by arthrotomy (28) or by arthroscopy (26). In each patient, the implanted synthetic ligament was 8 mm in diameter and 70 cm long. The majority of patients (80%) were followed up for 30 to 50 months. Thirty-one patients underwent a second arthroscopy of the knee at follow-up.

Results.—During the first 2 postoperative years, the degree of stability was encouraging. Ruptures of the Dacron began to occur, however, and only 23 of the 54 patients had a satisfactory result. At the latest follow-up, 15 patients had a negative Lachman test, 16 had a sign of 1+, and 23 had a sign of more than 1+. There were no differences in results between patients who had a closed procedure and those who had an open procedure, nor between those with acute injury and those who had a chronic rupture. Most ruptures of the Dacron prosthesis occurred at the femoral insertion of the ligament and during the third postoperative year.

Conclusion.—The use of a Dacron prosthesis in reconstruction of the ACL is associated with problems at long-term follow-up. Although the prosthesis does allow an early return to physical activity, problems occur after the second year. The authors believe the cause of the ruptures to be mechanical.

▶ To be emphasized, the authors "concluded that a free Dacron prostheses that is used to replace or supplement a torn anterior cruciate ligament is not a durable substitution for that ligament."—J.S. Torg, M.D.

Reconstruction of the Chronically Insufficient Anterior Cruciate Ligament With the Central Third of the Patellar Ligament
O'Brien SJ, Warren RF, Pavlov H, Panariello R, Wickiewicz TL (Hosp for Special Surgery, New York)
J Bone Joint Surg 73-A:278–286, 1991   8–18

Introduction.—There have been few studies of the factors that determine the clinical outcome after reconstruction of the anterior cruciate ligament (ACL) with the central third of the patellar ligament as a free autogenous graft. From 1980 to 1985, a total of 120 patients had this procedure and 79 of them (80 reconstructions) were available for follow-up.

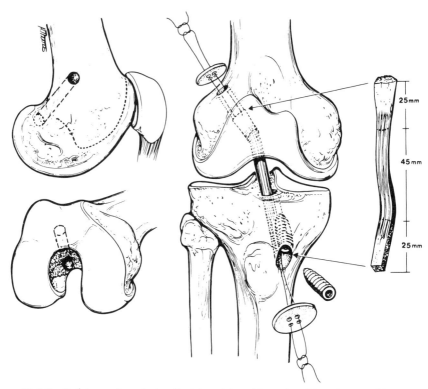

Fig 8–2.—Graft is passed proximal to distal through lateral femoral condyle and intercondylar notch and into tibia, and tibial bone-block is fixed distally with Hewson ligament-button over tibia. Concept interference screw is shown on lower right. Although screw is now used routinely, that was not the case at the time of this study. (Courtesy of O'Brien SJ, Warren RF, Pavlov H, et al: *J Bone Joint Surg* 73-A:278–286, 1991.)

Patients.—These 58 men and 21 women had an average age of 24 years at the time of operation. Clinical instability was the indication for surgery in 79 knees. The remaining knee was operated on because of pain and swelling. In 60% of the knees reconstruction was augmented with an extra-articular lateral sling of iliotibial band.

Technique.—A slightly oblique anterior approach is used to reconstruct the ACL. The central third of the patellar tendon is taken as a bone-tendon-bone, free, autogenous, nonvascularized graft with a trapezoid-shaped section of bone from the patella and a rectangular graft from the tibia. The ligamentous portion of the graft is passed from proximal to distal and fixed with a Hewson ligament-button (Fig 8–2). A modified Bosworth technique is used when the medial collateral ligament must be reconstructed. Patients wear a plaster cast for 6 weeks after operation, then a hinged knee-brace during physical therapy. They are advised to wear an ACL brace for 1 year.

Results.—Only 6 patients were dissatisfied with the results, usually because of pain in the anterior aspect of the knee. The remaining patients were either very satisfied (45) or satisfied (28) with the outcome. After operation, 76 (95%) knees no longer gave way.

Conclusion.—Overall, these patients had excellent results. Many returned to sports activities, but often at a lower level of competition because of fear of injury. Major associated ligamentous instability appears to predict failure and should be corrected at the time of reconstruction.

Retrospective Direct Comparison of Three Intraarticular Anterior Cruciate Ligament Reconstructions
Holmes PF, James SL, Larson RL, Singer KM, Jones DC (Orthopaedic Surgery and Athletic Medicine, San Antonio; Orthopedic and Fracture Clin of Eugene, Ore)
Am J Sports Med 19:596–600, 1991   8–19

Introduction.—Clinicians currently use several types of treatments for the anterior cruciate ligament (ACL) deficient knee, depending on patient age, length of time since injury, future requirements, patient rehabilitation possibilities, and physician outlook. A retrospective study was made of patients undergoing 3 different kinds of intra-articular reconstruction 5 or more years after the operations. The 3 types of intra-articular reconstructions included semitendinosus use in chronically unstable knees (CST) and in acutely unstable knees (AST), and use of the middle third-patellar tendon in chronically unstable knees (CMT).

Methods.—Of the 90 consecutive patients fulfilling the entry criteria, 75 knees in 73 patients were studied. Patients had surgery between 1977 and 1982. At follow-up they underwent objective tests of the ACL, including the Lachman test, the pivot-shift test, and KT-1000 measurements. Patients also participated in 3 subjective assessments of preinjury sports activity, present sports activity, and a present symptom rating.

Findings.—Of the 27 chronic ACL-deficient knees reconstructed with CMT, 16 had an excellent outcome, 7 good, and 3 poor after an average of 68 months post surgery; there was 1 failure. The patients' self-rating was 6.4 of 10 possible points, and the present activities averaged 120 of 200 points. Of the 28 chronic ACL-deficient knees that underwent surgery, outcomes were excellent in 4, good in 10, poor in 7, and failure in 7 after an average of 84 months post surgery. The self-rating score was 6.2 of 10 points, and the average present activity score, 105 of 200. The 20 acute SCL-deficient knees reconstructed with AST had 8 excellent outcomes, 9 good, and 3 poor, there were no failures. These patients had an average self-rating score of 7.9 of 10 and 144 of 200 for present activity. The objective ratings were significantly different between the AST and the CST groups and between the CST and the CMT groups.

For the subjective tests, the AST groups faired significantly better than the CST and the CMT groups.

Conclusions.—These results indicate that the use of the middle third-patellar tendon remains superior to that of the semitendinosus tendon in chronically unstable knees. Patients with acute reconstructed ACLs using the semitendinosus tendon were more active than those with chronic reconstructed ACLs.

A Prospective, Randomized Study of Three Surgical Techniques for Treatment of Acute Ruptures of the Anterior Cruciate Ligament
Engebretsen L, Benum P, Fasting O, Mølster A, Strand T (Trondheim University Hospital, Trondheim; University of Oslo; University of Bergen, Bergen Norway)
Am J Sports Med 18:585–590, 1990   8–20

Introduction.—Repair of complete ruptures of the anterior cruciate ligament (ACL) is often performed during the acute stage of injury to avoid stretching the secondary restraints. There is evidence that nonoperatively treated patients have a high frequency of poor results, and that primary repair seems to lead to deterioration over time.

Methods.—Primary repair, biologic augmentation, and synthetic augmentation were compared in a randomized, prospective study of 150 patients with acute ACL tears. The patients were divided into 3 surgical groups of 50 patients each. One group was treated with primary repair, 1 with the Kennedy Ligament Augmentation Device (LAD), and 1 with patellar tendon augmentation. All patients followed identical rehabilitation protocols including a long leg cast for 2 weeks and a brace with limited motion for 6 weeks. The patients were followed-up for 2 years.

Results.—All groups had significantly reduced activity levels 1 year after surgery. By 2 years, the LAD group had not achieved the preinjury level of activity, although activity had increased compared with the 1 year level. The patellar tendon group also had activity levels near preinjury values at 2 years. The repair group did not change activity level between 1 and 2 years. All groups functioned similarly at 1 year based on the Lachman test, the pivot shift test, and KT-1000 testing. By 2 years, these test results indicated that the patellar tendon group had improved, the LAD group stayed the same, and the repair group deteriorated. Reoperations were required by 2 patients in the repair group and 3 in the LAD group to treat gross instability, and by 4 in the patellar tendon group to treat range of motion deficits.

Conclusion.—Patellar tendon augmented repair is superior in most respects to both direct repair and augmentation with the Kennedy Ligament Augmentation Device for the treatment of acute ACL ruptures. Patellar tendon augmentation results in significant reductions in extension compared with direct repair.

▶ These 3 papers (Abstracts 8–18, 8–19, and 8–20) clearly define autogenous infrapatella bone tendon bone graft as the gold standard for reconstruction of both the acute and chronic anterior cruciate ligament deficient knee.—J.S. Torg, M.D.

The Effect of an Extra-Articular Procedure on Allograft Reconstructions for Chronic Ruptures of the Anterior Cruciate Ligament
Noyes FR, Barber SD (Cincinnati Sportsmedicine and Orthopaedic Ctr; Deaconess Hosp, Cincinnati)
J Bone Joint Surg 73-A:882–892, 1991   8–21

Introduction.—The results of the use of an intra-articular allograft as a replacement for the anterior cruciate ligament (ACL) in patients with chronic rupture were evaluated. In some cases, an extra-articular procedure with a lateral iliotibial band was also performed at the surgeon's discretion. The 2 procedures were compared.

Patients.—In all, 104 patients underwent repair of chronic rupture of the ACL. The 64 patients in group 1 were treated with only an intra-articular replacement with an allograft; the 40 in group 2 were treated with both an intra-articular replacement with an allograft and the extra-articular procedure. All patients underwent the same postoperative program of immediate motion of the knee and rehabilitation and follow-up. Results were evaluated with a comprehensive subjective and objective rating system.

Findings.—Both procedures decreased functional limitations and symptoms and improved the level of sports activity and the overall scores, but results in group 2 were significantly better in tests done with the KT-1000 arthrometer, as well as in levels of sports activity and overall scores. The 2 groups had similar results on pivot-shift or isokinetic testing, patellofemoral crepitus, functional limitation, or symptoms. In only 4 knees was a 0- to 135-degree range of motion not restored. The rate of failure was 16% in group 1 and only 3% in group 2.

Conclusions.—Use of the intra-articular allograft alone did not satisfactorily reduce anterior-posterior displacement in all knees. The addition of the extra-articular procedure with a lateral iliotibial band reduced deleterious forces and tibial displacements and restored the secondary restraints provided by the lateral iliotibial band in the healing intra-articular allograft.

▶ This paper should be viewed within the context of a recent report by the authors in which they concluded "we caution against the widespread use of allografts at the present time and recommend that they be used only at centers that have the necessary personnel resources available" (1). The current study strongly indicates that the use of an intra-articular allograft alone does not satisfactorily reduce anterior-posterior displacement in those who have chronic rupture of the ACL. For this and other reasons, autogenous patella-bone-tendon-bone remains the gold standard for reconstruction of both the acute and chronic anterior cruciate ligament deficient knees. To be questioned is the practice of the authors to test for AP laxity with the KT-1000 arthrometer using only 89 newtons (20 lb.) of total anterior force. It is our experience that accurate determination of anterior translation with the KT-1000 arthrometer requires the use of maximal manual pull. Thus, it appears that this factor represents a major flaw in this study.—J.S. Torg, M.D.

Reference

1. Noyes FR, et al: *J Bone Joint Surg* 72-A:1125, 1990.

Reconstruction of the Anterior Cruciate Ligament Alone in the Treatment of a Combined Instability With Complete Rupture of the Medial Collateral Ligament: A Prospective Study

Ballmer PM, Ballmer FT, Jakob RP (University of Berne, Switzerland)
Arch Orthop Trauma Surg 110:139–141, 1991   8–22

Introduction.—Combined instability caused by anterior cruciate ligament (ACL) and medial collateral ligament (MCL) injuries can be treated several different ways. Reconstruction of the ACL alone in this type of combined injury was evaluated.

Methods.—Fourteen patients had complete rupture of both the ACL and the MCL, and instability was noted clinically and by stress roentgenograms. Treatment included reconstruction of the ACL only, followed by immediate mobilization and partial weight bearing for 6 to 8 weeks.

Results.—At 14-month follow-up, 11 patients had excellent results, 2 had good results, and 1 had fair results. Nearly all knees had full range of motion and almost normal stability in the frontal and sagittal planes. All patients had returned to their preinjury activity status.

Conclusions.—In ACL reconstruction, using the patellar tendon alone in treating combined instability from ACl and MCL injuries was successful. The early mobilization hastened knee rehabilitation without compromising stable ligamentous healing.

▶ Interestingly, the authors state that "there is a limit to the conclusions that can be drawn from the present study, because of its relatively short follow-up time and small number of patients, the results support some trends in the treatment of ligamentous injuries to the knee." I believe that this report presents yet another problem. Specifically, the authors refer to a "grade III MCL" injury as though it were 1 ligament. The medial collateral ligament in fact consists of 4 segments: (1) deep layer of the medial capsular ligament, (2) anterior capsular ligament, (3) posterior capsular or posterior oblique ligament, and (4) superficial or tibial collateral ligament. In those instances where

3 or more of the 4 segments are completely disrupted I question the wisdom of managing the problem with an "isolated" ACL repair.—J.S. Torg, M.D.

The O'Donoghue Triad Revisited: Combined Knee Injuries Involving Anterior Cruciate and Medial Collateral Ligament Tears
Shelbourne KD, Nitz PA (Methodist Sports Medicine Ctr, Indianapolis)
Am J Sports Med 19:474–477, 1991   8–23

Introduction.—The O'Donoghue triad indicates the association of anterior cruciate ligament (ACL), medial collateral ligament (MCL), and medial meniscus tears. To determine the frequency of the O'Donoghue triad, the records of 60 consecutive patients injured during athletic activities were retrospectively reviewed.

Methods.—The patient group with a combined ACL-MCL injury included 49 men and 11 women treated between January 1983 and April 1989. They represent 17% of all patients treated for acute ACl insufficiency during this period. Each underwent arthroscopy and ACl reconstruction within 30 days of the original injury. The 35 patients in group I had a second-degree sprain; the 25 patients in group II had a complete or third-degree injury.

Results.—Medial meniscus tears were rare finding and were outnumbered in both groups by lateral meniscus tears. In group I, tears of the medial meniscus were associated with a concomitant lateral meniscus injury. Group II patients were more likely than those in group I not to have any meniscal abnormality. No meniscal tears were found in 60% of group II patients or in 29% of group I patients.

Conclusion.—The use of arthroscopy has revealed that the combined ACL-MCL-medial meniscus injury is not as common as previously assumed. Athletes with knee injuries are, in fact, more likely to have a trial consisting of ACL, MCL, and lateral meniscus tears, especially when an incomplete tear of the medial collateral has occurred.

▶ The observations of the authors are in keeping with our own experience.—J.S. Torg, M.D.

The Semitendinosus: Anatomic Considerations in Tendon Harvesting
Ferrari JD, Ferrari DA (Univ of Massachusetts Med Ctr)
Orthop Rev 10:1085–1088, 1991   8–24

Objective.—Reconstruction of the anterior cruciate ligament (ACL) has used a number of tendon autograft harvest sites, including the semitendinosus tendon. Currently, harvesting of the semitendinosus graft can proceed through a small incision using tendon strippers. The length and course of the semitendinosus tendon was examined along with its rela-

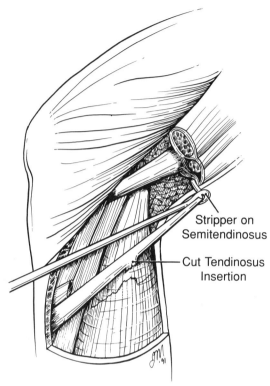

Stripper on
Semitendinosus

Cut Tendinosus
Insertion

Fig 8–3.—Stripper passing outside fascial band. (Courtesy of Ferrari JD, Ferrari DA: *Orthop Rev* 20:1085–1088, 1991.)

tionships to adjacent structures and how these relationships affect stripping and the length of the tendinous portion available for grafting. The semitendinosus tendons of 35 cadaveric specimens were studied.

Observation.—The mean length from insertion to the tendinous termination was 23 cm, and the average distance from distal insertion to the musculotendinous portion was 15.5 cm. Separation of the semitendinosus from other pes anserinus tendons occurred beneath the semimembranosus. An area of fascial thickening was noted where the gracilis and semitendinosus separate. The thickening seemed to interdigitate with the crural fascia, forming a sling that kept the semitendinosus tendon beneath the semimembranosus. This thickening occurred about 12–15 cm proximal to the semitendinosus insertion.

Technique.—In freeing the graft, sharp dissection is required to remove the attachments of the semitendinosus to the gracilis and gastrocnemius. At 7 cm proximal from the tibial insertion, a band inserted into the gastrocnemius can be palpated or, after a small incision, visualized. Dissection of this band facilitates passage of the tendon stripper proximally (Fig 8–3). Because difficulty in harvesting may occur at the thickened fascia of the semimembranosus that forms a sling for the semitendinosus, the stripper should not be passed blindly outside the tunnel consisting of the fascia medially and interiorly and the semimembranosus muscle above.

Implication.—If the attachment of the semitendinosus to the gastrocnemius and the thickened fascia of the semimembranosus that invests its tendon is not recognized, a graft of adequate length may not be obtained.

▶ The observation that the failure to recognize and section the fascial bands connecting the semitendinosus, semimembranosus, and gracilis when harvesting the tendons can result in inadequate graft length is accurate.—J.S. Torg, M.D.

Results of Knee Manipulations After Anterior Cruciate Ligament Reconstructions

Dodds JA, Keene JS, Graf BK, Lange RH (Univ of Wisconsin, Madison)
Am J Sports Med 19:283–287, 1991   8–25

Introduction.—The efficacy of intra-articular anterior cruciate ligament (ACL) reconstructions has been well documented as well as complications associated with this procedure. Knee manipulation for the treatment of patients who have limited knee motion after this procedure was evaluated in 42 knees with persistent flexion or extension deficits after intra-articular ACL reconstructions that were evaluable 6–56 months after manipulation.

Methods.—Manipulations were performed under general or spinal anesthesia an average of 7 months after the reconstruction. In 10 knees, adhesions were débrided by arthroscopy after the manipulation. In 6 knees, more than 1 manipulation was performed.

Results.—At manipulation, the average flexion increased from 95 to 136 degrees, and the average extension deficit was reduced from 11 to 3 degrees. At final follow-up, average flexion was 127 degrees and average extension 4 degrees. Increased range of motion was not accompanied by decreased joint stability. The final range of motion achieved was not a function of the time from reconstruction to manipulation, the severity of the premanipulation flexion deficit, nor whether débridement had been performed. In knees with premanipulation extension deficits of 15 degrees or greater, less extension was achieved after manipulation than in other knees. In most patients, hemarthrosis resulted, but never resulting in delays in initiating physical therapy. No complications from anesthesia, fractures, or clinically detectable ACL laxity occurred. Posterolateral laxity developed in 1 knee 6 weeks after a second manipulation.

Conclusion.—Manipulations were successful in improving both flexion and extension in 86% of the knees in this study. Such treatments seem to be safe and effective for improving range of motion in patients with restricted motion after ACL reconstructions.

▶ The results presented by the authors are in keeping with my own experience. In their report of 42 knees that had undergone ACL reconstructions using a patella-bone-tendon-bone graft, 9 had been done arthroscopically and 33 by an arthrotomy. Thus, the arthroscopically assisted procedures do not appear to be predisposed to flexion-extension deficits, and presumably this complication will be seen less frequently with more widespread use of minimally invasive techniques. I agree with the following points:

1. Knee manipulation is a safe and effective method for improving motion.
2. Joint stability is not affected.
3. Arthroscopic debridement of adhesions does not affect the final result.
4. Fracture of the femur and/or tibia does not occur.

It should be noted that the increase in motion is not observed immediately after manipulation but rather after several weeks of intensive physical therapy.—J.S. Torg, M.D.

Fracture of the Patella During Graft Harvest for Cruciate Ligament Reconstruction
Crosby LA, Kamins P (Creighton Univ, Omaha)
Comp Orthop July/Aug 104–107, 1991   8–26

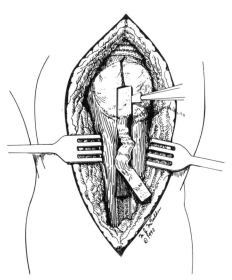

Fig 8–4.—Illustration representing harvest of central one third of patellar tendon resulting in longitudinal fracture. (Courtesy of Crosby LA, Kamins P: *Comp Orthop* July/Aug: 104–107, 1991.)

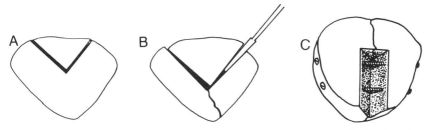

Fig 8–5.—**A,** cross-section of patella showing ideal depth of harvest cuts to half of total patellar thickness. **B,** cross-section showing excessive depth of cuts resulting in weakness and fracture propagation during osteotome removal of bone wedge. **C,** fixation of patellar fracture with 2 3.5-mm AO lag screws. (Courtesy of Crosby LA, Kamins P: *Comp Orthop* July/Aug:104–107, 1991.)

Introduction.—Although a review of the literature revealed no reports of patellar fracture during graft harvest for cruciate ligament reconstruction, intraoperative patella fracture occurred in 3 of 60 patients.

Case Report.—Man, 20, sustained a hyperextension injury while playing basketball. A partial tear of the medial meniscus and a complete tear of the anterior cruciate from its femoral attachment were seen on arthroscopy performed at the time of surgery. A longitudinal fracture, running the entire length of the patella, occurred during harvest of the central third of the patellar tendon as the graft was being removed from its seat (Fig 8–4). The fracture was stabilized with 2 3.5-mm A0 lag screws. The patient progressed steadily through a structured physical therapy program and achieved 90% normal strength at about 4 months. He had no discomfort at the end of rehabilitation, but discomfort over the screws developed during running at 6 months. The screws were removed, and the patient returned to unrestricted sports activity, 1 year postoperatively.

Conclusion.—Intraoperative patellar fracture during graft harvest for cruciate ligament reconstruction appears to result from excessive depth in the unguided cuts that make up the patellar wedge, along with levering against the patella (Fig 8–5). The corners of the graft should be gently released before the graft is lifted from its bed.

▶ Clearly, an ounce of prevention is worth a pound of cure! With regard to harvesting techniques, the authors state "during the standard technique of harvesting the central one third of the patellar tendon, it is common to cut the wedge into the patella to approximately one half its total anteroposterior depth. The fractures occur as the wedge is being lifted from its bed with a thin osteotome. The problem seems to be an excessive depth in unguided angular cuts made with the oscillating saw, which predisposes the patella to fracture during wedge removal. Care must be taken not to lever against the patella with the osteotome when lifting out the graft. It is important to gently release the corners of the graft with the osteotome before lifting the graft from its bed. We feel the patellar fracture is produced by the combination of excessive depth and levering against the patellar.—J.S. Torg, M.D.

Patellar Fracture and Avulsion of the Patellar Ligament Complicating Arthroscopic Anterior Cruciate Ligament Reconstruction
Bonatus TJ, Alexander AH (Naval Hosp, Camp Pendleton, Calif; Naval Hosp, Oakland, Calif)
Orthop Rev 20:770–774, 1991   8–27

Introduction.—An effective treatment for acute or chronic anterior cruciate ligament (ACL) insufficiency involves arthroscopic reconstruction using the middle third of the patellar tendon. A rare complication, patellar fracture, occurred during the early postoperative period.

Case Report.—Woman, 19, twisted her knee while playing football. Her torn ACL was arthroscopically reconstructed using the middle third of the patellar tendon. She was allowed immediate range of motion (ROM) and continuous passive motion postoperatively and discharged with an orthosis 4 days after the procedure. Eight days after arthroscopic reconstruction, the woman fell down a flight of stairs and sustained a displaced longitudinal fracture of the patella through the patellar tendon graft-donor site. An avulsion of the lateral third of the remaining patellar ligament from the tibia was noted at surgery. Both the patellar fracture and ligament avulsion were repaired with open reduction and internal fixation. Physical therapy was initiated at 6 weeks after removal of the 18-gauge wire used to splint the ligament. Arthroscopic débridement and manipulation, performed 5 months postoperatively because of incomplete range of motion, completely restored motion to the limb. The patient declined removal of the remaining patellar hardware.

Conclusion.—The initial procedure used in this patient provides the strongest type of ACL reconstruction. Patellar fracture or avulsion of the remaining patellar tendon occur but rarely, yet the surgeon should be aware of this possibility.

▶ It is difficult to determine whether the displaced patella fracture reported was the result of an intraoperative complication or the result of trauma incurred when the patient fell down the flight of steps 80 days after her surgery. Of note, however, is a report by the authors of a second case in which, despite "extreme care in harvesting the patella tendon graft", a longitudinal patella fracture was observed intraoperatively when mechanical stress was applied. Apparently the fracture was not visible with intraoperative roentgenography. This certainly raises the question of whether such fractures may occur more frequently but go undetected and heal without complication. At any rate, a word to the wise is sufficient.—J.S. Torg, M.D.

Continuous Passive Motion After Arthroscopically Assisted Anterior Cruciate Ligament Reconstruction: Comparison of Short- Versus Long-Term Use
Richmond JC, Gladstone J, MacGillivray J (Tufts Univ; New England Med Ctr

Hosp, Boston)
Arthroscopy 7:39–44, 1991   8–28

Introduction.—A number of clinical studies and animal experiments have demonstrated the benefits of continuous passive motion (CPM) in the immediate postoperative period after anterior cruciate ligament (ACL) reconstruction. Although CPM is commonly used, the duration of this protocol required for maximal therapeutic benefit is not known. The effects of using a CPM machine after ACL reconstruction for periods of 4 days and 2 weeks were compared.

Methods.—Twenty patients undergoing ACL reconstruction for chronic injury were randomly selected for the study. Half were allocated to the CPM 4-day group and underwent 6 hours per day of CPM for 4 days in hospital, followed by intermittent passive motion (IPM) at home. The remaining patients used a home CPM machine and underwent 6 hours of daily CPM for 14 days, together with IPM. Outcome was assessed on postoperative days 2, 7, 14, and 42.

Results.—The study sought to determine any increased benefit with the longer use of CPM in reduction of swelling, improvement of motion, and reduction of muscle atrophy. Girth measurements were obtained at 4 lower limb locations for joint swelling and muscle atrophy. Range of motion of the knee was measured goniometrically, and KT-1000 arthrometry was used to evaluate joint laxity. With the exception of KT-1000 laxity at 42 days, no statistically significant differences were apparent between the groups at 42 days. Despite an intensive exercise program, muscle atrophy occurred equally in both groups.

Conclusion.—No additional benefits were found with the additional 10 days of CPM after ACL reconstruction. Because home CPM machines rent for $50 per day, this finding could result in significant savings.

▶ The obvious deficiency of this study is that it did not include a group in which no continuous passive motion was instituted.—J.S. Torg, M.D.

Arthrofibrosis in Acute Anterior Cruciate Ligament Reconstruction: The Effect of Timing of Reconstruction and Rehabilitation
Shelbourne KD, Wilckens JH, Mollabashy A, DeCarlo M (Methodist Sports Medicine Ctr, Indianapolis)
Am J Sports Med 19:332–336, 1991   8–29

Introduction.—In patients who require acute reconstruction of the torn anterior cruciate ligament (ACL), arthrofibrosis (ankylosis, flexion contracture) can prevent the return of full motion after operation, especially of the terminal part of full extension. The development of arthrofibrosis was studied in 169 young athletes who had acute ACL reconstruction.

Findings.—Limited extension and scar tissue were more frequent in patients who had reconstruction within a week after injury than in those who were operated on after 3 weeks or longer. The latter patients had greater knee flexion and greater extension. Among patients operated on 1 to 3 weeks after injury, those who followed conventional rehabilitative procedures had arthrofibrosis as often as the patients treated in the first week. An accelerated rehabilitation program substantially lowered the risk of arthrofibrosis in these patients and also in those operated on 3 weeks or longer after injury.

Recommendations.—It appears that ACL reconstruction is best delayed for at least 3 weeks after injury. Accelerated postoperative rehabilitation will optimize the range of knee motion.

Limitation of Motion Following Anterior Cruciate Ligament Reconstruction: A Case-Control Study

Mohtadi NGH, Webster-Bogaert S, Fowler PJ (University Hospital, London, Ont)
Am J Sports Med 19:620–625, 1991   8-30

Background.—Limitation of motion is common after anterior cruciate ligament (ACL) reconstruction. No causative factors or characteristics have identified the patient at risk for this outcome. An attempt was made to identify patients with motion limitation after ACL reconstructive surgery, to define the causative factors for this problem in a case-control manner, and to outline prevention management for this postsurgical problem.

Methods.—A total of 527 ACL reconstructions were performed between 1983 and 1988, all with autogenous tissue. Initial rehabilitation after surgery included case immobilization for 4 weeks, cast bracing or rehabilitation bracing for 6 weeks, or early range of motion using cast or rehabilitation for 6 weeks. The case group was defined, and a control group was selected from the remaining patients.

Results.—Thirty-seven of the initial 527 patients comprised the cases; all had undergone manipulation under anesthesia because of loss of range of motion, for an overall incidence of 7%. These manipulations occurred at an average of 5.8 months after the initial surgery. The 37 patients, 17 females and 20 males, had an average of 24.2 years. The right knee was affected in 16 cases and the left in 21. The semitendinosus tendon was used in 17 cases and the quadriceps patellar tendon in 20. Cases and controls demonstrated no significant differences for any demographic parameter. A significant difference between the 2 groups was observed for time after surgery, with the cases experiencing stiffness before the controls did. Time to reconstruction was the only independent predictive variable for stiffness. At follow-up, the average loss of extension was 4 degrees and the loss of flexion was 5 degrees.

Implications.—These results indicate that patients experiencing stiffness after ACL reconstruction usually underwent the operation less than 2 weeks after injury. The avoidence of immediate surgery and the use of early motion and physiotherapy to ensure a full range of motion by 3 months post surgery are recommended.

▶ These 2 papers (Abstracts 8–29 and 8–30) call attention to the fact that arthrofibrosis after ACL reconstruction can be caused by a number of factors. It is important to note, as pointed out by Mohtadi et al., (Abstract 8–30) that "the odds of getting knee stiffness were 2.85 times higher if operations were performed within 2 weeks, with a corresponding trend for patients operated on within the first 6 weeks following injury. This is clearly an association and cannot be assumed to be causative". It is interesting to note that in the study by Mohtadi et al., other variables such as concomitant meniscal repair, MCL repair, open vs. arthroscopically assisted reconstruction, choice of autogenous tissue, synthetic augmentation, or postoperative rehabilitation protocol were eliminated as factors. On the basis of my own experience, it is quite apparent that these factors play a causative role in the development of postoperative arthrofibrosis. The observation by Shelbourne et al. (Abstract 8–29) that "an accelerated postoperative rehabilitation program can significantly decrease the incidence of arthrofibrosis in knees that are reconstructed sooner than 3 weeks after injury" is in keeping with my own experience.—J.S. Torg, M.D.

Operative Management of Acute PCL Injuries With Associated Pathology: Long-Term Results
Barrett GR, Savoie FH (Mississippi Sports Medicine and Orthopaedic Ctr, Jackson)
Orthopedics 14:687–692, 1991   8–31

Background.—The best treatment for acute isolated posterior cruciate ligament (PCL) injury continues to be debated. The results of early repair and augmentation by using the semitendinosus tendon and a synthetic stent were reviewed to define a consistent method of treatment for midsubstance PCL injuries.

Methods.—Subjects were 18 consecutive patients with PCL injury and associated conditions. The patients were followed up for 3.5 to 7.5 years (mean follow-up, 5.4 years). Six PCLs were repaired to the femur with multiple no. 2 nonabsorbable sutures. One "mop end" midsubstance tear was repaired with sutures in each stump. Seven midsubstance tears were repaired and augmented with the semitendinosus tendon. Four other midsubstance tears were repaired and augmented with the semitendinosus tendon and a Dacron stent. A medial meniscus was repaired, and 1 was partially excised. One lateral meniscus tear was also partially

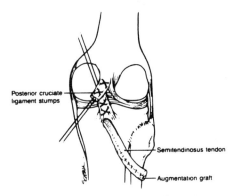

Fig 8–6.—Stitches passed in proximal and distal stumps of PCL. (Courtesy of Barrett GR, Savoie FH: *Orthopedics* 14:687–692, 1991.)

excised. The anterior cruciate ligament was repaired to the tibia in 2 knees, excised with extra-articular iliotibial band tenodesis augmentation in 5, and left alone in 2.

Results.—Arthrometer readings at follow-up were well correlated with clinical assessment. The 4 knees with Dacron stents had a 0 to 1 mm difference at 90 degrees. The failures had greater than 5 to 6 mm differences. Six were in the repair alone group, and 2 were in the repair with semitendinosus augmentation group. Radiographic changes, mainly in the medial compartment, were noted in 8 knees (44.5%). According to Hughston's criteria 55.5% of the results were good, 27.8% were fair, and 16.7% were poor or failed. According to Clancy's criteria, results were excellent in 22.2%, good in 22.2%, fair in 44.5%, and rated as failed in 11.1% (Figs 8–6, 8–7, and 8–8).

Conclusions.—In this series adequate stabilization did not result from either repair of the PCL alone or semitendinosus augmentation of the

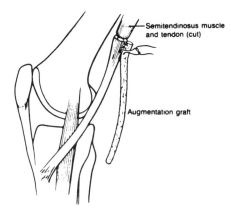

Fig 8–7.—Synthetic stent sutured to semitendinosus tendon with absorbable suture. (Courtesy of Barrett GR, Savoie FH: *Orthopedics* 14:687–692, 1991.)

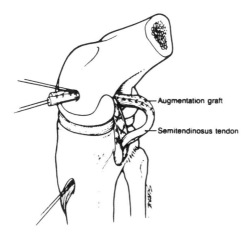

Fig 8–8.—Sutures from stump repair and synthetic augmentation graft passed through femoral and tibial tunnels. (Courtesy of Barrett GR, Savoie FH: *Orthopedics* 14:687–692, 1991.)

proximal one third or midthird substance tears. A synthetic stent appears to keep the tibia in a reduced position and improve results. It is not known what effect the patella tendon would have on the frequently affected patellofemoral joint during the rehabilitation phase of this type of injury.

Injuries to the Posterior Cruciate Ligament of the Knee
Kannus P, Bergfeld J, Järvinen M, Johnson RJ, Pope M, Renström P, Yasuda K (Univ of Vermont, Burlington; The UKK-Institute for Health Promotion Research, Tampere, Finland; Hokkaido University, Sapporo, Japan)
Sports Med 12:110–131, 1991   8–32

Introduction.—Posterior cruciate ligament (PCL) tears, thought to be 5%-20% of all knee ligament tears, may be more commonly diagnosed with new techniques. Although it is the strongest ligament of the knee, the PCL can be injured by a direct blow to the anterior tibia with the knee flexed.

Data Analysis.—Approximately 95% of the strength to resist posterior displacement of the tibia is provided by the PCL, which is twice as strong as the anterior cruciate ligament. About 50% of the injuries to the PCL are from motor vehicle accidents, 40% involve sports, and 10% are caused by other activities. Diagnostically, the main characteristic in a knee with PCL rupture is a posterior sag sign. Magnetic resonance imaging can verify the PCL tear, as can examination under anesthesia and arthroscopy. Surgical intervention is recommended when PCL avulsion fragment has been dislocated. Additionally, if PCL injury disrupts other major ligaments or capsular structures, surgery is usually indicated. However, most studies recommend conservative treatment for isolated complete midsubstance tears of the PCL consisting of intensive quadriceps exercises, 2 weeks or less of immobilization, and early return to controlled activities and weight bearing. When giving-way symptoms persist, reconstruction with bone-patella-tendon-bone autograft or allograft may be considered.

Conclusions.—Injuries to the PCL are not common. Newer radiologic techniques have improved the diagnosis of PCL tears, yet treatment of complete ruptures is still controversial.

▶ Essentially, the PCL has replaced the anterior cruciate ligament as the enigma of the knee. Clearly, reports of consistently successful repair or reconstruction of the posterior cruciate deficient knee are nonexistent. We have previously published a paper on the natural history of the PCL deficient knee. On the basis of our own experience, it was established that the functional outcome can be predicted on the basis of the instability type. Specifically, those knees with PCL disruption without associated ligamentous laxity will probably remain symptom free. However, when PCL disruption is associated with combined instability a less than desirable functional result will probably occur. On the basis of the data analysis, our study supported the thesis that individuals with unidirectional posterior instability do not require repair or reconstruction. However, in view of a much less favorable prognosis for the PCL deficient knee with multidirectional instability, consideration should be given to surgical stabilization (1). As pointed out by Kannus et al. "acute phase surgery (primary PCL repair with augmentation or primary PCL reconstruction) is indicated in fresh injuries of the PCL associated with disruption of other major ligaments or capsular structures. Simultaneously with the PCL surgery, all the other damaged structures should also be repaired." They further point that at even with surgery, the prognosis is poorer than in isolated PCL tears. With regard to chronic PCL insufficiency "a reconstruction with bone-patella tendon-bone autograft or allograft can be considered, if the patient suffers from repeated giving way symptoms which are not resolved by rehabilitation".—J.S. Torg, M.D.

Reference

1. Torg JS, et al: *Clin Orthop* 246:208, 1989.

Rehabilitation Following Knee Surgery: Recommendations
Paulos LE, Wnorowski DC, Beck CL (Salt Lake City Knee and Sports Medicine)
Sports Med 11:257–275, 1991   8–33

Objective.—Rehabilitation of the knee surgery patient begins with patient selection, because a patient who is not compliant or ambitious may doom the procedure to failure despite the best techniques. A cooperative patient does not, however, assure a successful outcome. Given a satisfactory foundation, a well-conceived and executed rehabilitation plan is the final step in achieving a successful outcome.

Early Rehabilitation.—The period of immobility and bracing should be limited, with immobility restricted to 6 weeks at most. Passive range-of-motion exercises begin as soon as possible after surgery. Passive patient-initiated and active range-of-motion exercises are preferred. The time of initial weight-bearing is a procedure-specific judgment.

Exercise Regimen.—Isometrics are the earliest strengthening techniques. Electric muscle stimulation helps to restore motion after knee surgery and may retard atrophy. Isotonic (progressive resistance) exercises should be supervised. "Closed-chain" functional exercises usually are begun at the time early weight-bearing is allowed. Isokinetics generally are deferred for at least 20 to 24 weeks after reconstructive surgery. High speed settings will maximize strength and coordination.

Return to Sports.—The time of return to sports activity depends on the patient, the activity, and the surgery performed. No fixed time figure should be used. Typically, functional bracing is used for 2 years after surgery if all else is satisfactory.

Rehabilitation Concerns Following Anterior Cruciate Ligament Reconstruction
Frndak PA, Berasi CC (Doctor's Hosp, Columbus, Ohio)
Sports Med 12:338–346, 1991   8–34

Background.—Opinions vary as to the best rehabilitation program for patients who have had anterior cruciate ligament (ACL) reconstruction. These patients have particular problems, which have become more important as more ACL reconstructions are performed and arthroscopically assisted ACL reconstruction gains in popularity.

Rehabilitation Concerns.—A few basic themes underlie all rehabilitation programs for ACL reconstruction, but the most fundamental principle is the need for early motion. If postoperative immobilization is prolonged, serious complications will result. Another important consideration is the avoidance of positions or activities that put excessive strain on the newly reconstructed ligament. The graft will require varying protection depending on the type of graft and fixation. Non–weight-bearing, active resistance quadriceps exercises should be avoided; closed chain exercises may be begun relatively early. Postoperative recovery of quadriceps strength is obviously important; however, all the muscles of the knee must be strengthened to the greatest extent possible. Strength of the hamstring muscles is especially important, because they may actively support the reconstructed ligament. Before the patient returns to full sports participation, the problem of sensory loss in the knee must be addressed. He or she must have progressive neuromuscular reeducation exercises that rely on sensory input from the remaining intact pericapsular structures. Bracing is another important consideration. Braces are commonly used to limit postoperative knee motion, but their use during heavy athletic activity is not supported by the literature. The desire to prescribe a brace must be secondary to the need for strength and agility of the leg to protect the graft.

Conclusions.—In patients who undergo ACL reconstruction the goal of rehabilitation is to hasten recovery while achieving an optimal result. Questions persist as to the stress the reconstructed ligament can tolerate in the various phases of recovery.

Kinetic Chain Exercise in Knee Rehabilitation
Palmitier RA, An K-N, Scott SG, Chao EYS (Mayo Clinic and Found, Rochester, Minn)
Sports Med 11:402–413, 1991   8–35

Background.—There has been a great deal of research into the rehabilitation of anterior cruciate ligament (ACL) injuries in athletes. The sound scientific principles applied to this problem have improved the outcome of both surgical and nonsurgical treatment. One of the most important of these principles is the use of the kinetic chain exercise.

Principles.—The lower extremity kinetic chain comprises the hip, knee, and ankle. Exercises that recruit all 3 of these links in unison, such as the squat, are considered kinetic chain exercises. Exercises that recruit only 1 link, such as seated quadriceps extensions, are not kinetic chain exercises. Force diagram assessment shows that kinetic chain exercise decreases ACL strain because of the axial orientation of the applied load and muscular co-contraction. Kinetic chain exercise also takes advantage of specificity of training principles. An even more important effect is the ability to reproduce the concurrent shift of "antagonistic" biarticular muscle groups that occurs during simultaneous extension of each of the 3 links. Exercises that isolate the muscle groups may obstruct complete recovery.

Clinical Application.—Despite the soundness of these theoretical concepts, the use of kinetic chain exercise in rehabilitation has been met with skepticism. A strong, well-placed graft should be included in reconstruction to restore joint kinematics. Modifications of present leg press and isokinetic equipment are needed to allow reproduction of the squat movement. The machine must allow complete hip extension, the foot plate should move in an arc, and the footplate must be fixed perpendicular to the frontal plane of the hip. The knee movement arm will be decreased, thus keeping patellofemoral compression and knee shear forces low.

Discussion.—Rehabilitation and testing of the injured ACL ligament should include early kinetic chain exercise. The principles discussed can also facilitate treatment of other common problems such as anterior knee pain and low back pain.

▶ The above 3 articles (Abstracts 8–33, 8–34, and 8–35) present an excellent review of the current status of both the principles and controversies involving postoperative knee rehabilitation. The original articles are recommended reading for all those involved with knee surgery.—J.S. Torg, M.D.

The Effect of Tourniquet Use and Hemovac Drainage on Postoperative Hemarthrosis
Coupens SD, Yates CK (Oklahoma Med Ctr, Oklahoma City)
Arthroscopy 7:278–282, 1991   8–36

Background.—Although arthroscopic surgery has become a common means of diagnosing and treating pathologic conditions of the knee, few studies have addressed the complications related to arthroscopy. The effects of hemovac drainage and tourniquet use on the incidence of postoperative hemarthrosis, the most commonly reported complication of arthroscopic procedures, were assessed in 60 patients.

Methods.—Mean age of the patients was 29 years. All underwent arthroscopic knee surgery. The most common types of procedures were medial meniscectomies (25), lateral retinacular releases (16), lateral meniscectomies (16), and chondroplasties (16). Thirty-two patients had a tourniquet and 28 did not; a hemovac drain was used postoperatively in 24 patients. The patients were evaluated at 1 day, 1 week, and 3 weeks postoperatively.

Results.—At all periods of follow-up, patients who had a hemovac drain used postoperatively and those who did not have a tourniquet had fewer hemarthroses and a greater range of motion. The hemovac drain was also associated with a greater range of motion and fewer hemarthroses when the types of procedures were evaluated separately.

Conclusion.—The incidence of postoperative hemarthrosis can be reduced by placement of a hemovac drain after arthroscopic knee surgery. The routine use of a pneumatic tourniquet, however, should be avoided.

▶ The conclusions of the authors are sound. However, it would appear that the use of hemovac drainage in patients who have been operated on an outpatient basis might present somewhat of a logistical problem.—J.S. Torg, M.D.

Arthroscopic Treatment of Symptomatic Synovial Plica of the Knee: Long-Term Followup

Dorchak JD, Barrack RL, Kneisl JS, Alexander AH (Naval Hosp, Oakland, Calif)

Am J Sports Med 19:503–507, 1991   8–37

Introduction.—The diagnosis of symptomatic plica can be made when a thickened synovial band is palpated and reproduces a patient's symptoms. No other knee abnormality is present. Conservative treatment is often sufficient, although arthroscopic resection of the synovial plica may be necessary. The long-term results in a large group of patients were reviewed to determine factors predictive of outcome.

Methods.—Of nearly 2,000 patients who underwent diagnostic arthroscopies in 1981–1987, 76 had a postoperative diagnosis of plica, of whom 51 were available for follow-up. The patients' mean age at arthroscopy was 24.9 years. All patients initially had pain, 23 experienced giving way, and 16 had swelling. There was a history of trauma in 32 patients.

Results.—At an average follow-up of 47 months, the overall results were excellent in 22 patients, good in 16, and poor in 13. No patient was worse. Factors associated with good or excellent results included age younger than 20 years, onset after a specific episode of trauma or definite activity, a specific operative diagnosis that localized symptoms to the medial compartment, and a documented impingement lesion in the medial femoral condyle. A poor result was associated with an arthroscopic finding of chondromalacia of more than grade 1, preoperative symptoms of longer than 6 months' duration, and a nonspecific preoperative diagnosis.

Conclusion.—Arthroscopy should be considered when conservative management brings no improvement to patients with suspected diagnosis of plica syndrome. Although most previous reports of plica excision have had better results, the present study has to date the longest follow-up of any series.

▶ It is interesting to note that Patel (1) reported 100% excellent results, Hardaker et al. (2) reported 97% excellent or good results, Vaughn-Lane and Dandy (3) reported 84% excellent and good results, and Nottage et al. (4) reported 91% excellent or good results with arthroscopic plica excision. However, Dorchak et al. are reporting on a 4-year average follow-up compared with the above studies in which there was less than 2 years of follow-up. It should also be noted that they state that poor prognostic factors included associated chondromalacia and an unclear preoperative diagnosis. It appears that this paper, more than anything, emphasizes the importance of proper patient selection.—J.S. Torg, M.D.

References

1. Patel D: *Am J Sports Med* 6:217, 1978.
2. Hardaker W Jr, et al: *J Bone Joint Surg* 62:221, 1980.
3. Vaughn-Lane T, Dandy D: *J Bone Joint Surg* 64:475, 1982.
4. Nottage WM, et al: *Am J Sports Med* 11:211, 1983.

Thermal Injury Resulting From Arthroscopic Lateral Retinacular Release by Electrocautery: Report of Three Cases and a Review of the Literature
Lord MJ, Maltry JA, Shall LM (Univ of South Florida College of Medicine, Daytona Beach; Eastern Virginia Med School, Norfolk)
Arthroscopy 7:33–37, 1991   8–38

Patients and Methods.—A group of 85 patients underwent arthroscopic lateral retinacular release using electrocautery. Of the 85 patients, 3 incurred full-thickness thermal burns of the skin, a previously unreported complication. One of these injuries is shown in Figure 8–6. Of the 3 burn injuries, only 1 became infected.

Discussion.—The risk of a thermal burn injury occurring during lateral retinacular release by electrocautery may depend partly on the distending fluid used. A conductive solution such as Ringer's lactate requires a high power setting. However, 1.5% glycine was used in this study. The benefits of electrocautery in limiting the risk of hemarthrosis must be weighed against the chance of burn injury occurring.

► This appears to be the first report of thermal injury following arthroscopic lateral release performed by electrocautery. It is interesting to note that in all 3 cases, the procedure was performed with glycine, a comparatively noncon-

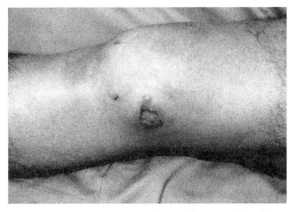

Fig 8–6.—Clinical photograph of resultant thermal injury. (Courtesy of Lord MJ, Maltry JA, Shall LM: *Arthroscopy* 7:33–37, 1991.)

ductive solution. Our own practice is to perform this procedure with local anesthesia, without tourniquet, and using normal saline solution. On occasion, the patients will relate having pain and at this point either the intensity of the cautery or the depth of the cautery tip are reduced. Using this method, we have not experienced this unfortunate complication.—J.S. Torg, M.D.

Thigh Muscle Function After Partial Tear of the Medial Ligament Compartment of the Knee

Kannus P, Järvinen M (University and University Central Hospital of Tampere, Finland)
Med Sci Sports Exerc 23:4–9, 1991   8–39

Introduction.—Thigh muscle atrophy from immobilization is a recognized sequel to treating knee ligament injuries. Long-term studies of the effects of second-degree knee ligament sprains on muscle function are lacking.

Methods.—Isokinetic and isometric strength and the power profile were recorded in 48 patients, with a mean age of 31 years, who had a second-degree sprain or partial tear of the medial ligament compartment. The patients were treated nonoperatively at first. Studies were performed using the CYBEX II isokinetic dynamometer an average of 8 years after injury.

Results.—The mean strength scores for the injured knee were in the range of excellence. The mean strength deficit was 4% in extension and 2% in flexion. Deficits in total work, average power, and peak torque acceleration energy were somewhat greater than those in strength, but not significantly so. The greatest circumferential deficit on the injured side was 1.5 cm.

Conclusion.—Long-term follow-up after partial tear of the medial ligament compartment of the knee demonstrates good general thigh muscle function on testing with low to moderate speeds. Greater deficits are noted as the speed of isokinetic movement increases. Selective atrophy of fast-twitch muscle fibers may mean that specific high-speed extension and flexion exercises will be most helpful.

▶ A well-designed and implemented study perhaps of some usefulness in programming therapy programs. It should be noted that the authors recognize that further research is needed to confirm their findings and to determine what the truly functional results are concerning different sporting activities.—J.S. Torg, M.D.

Analysis of Subjective Knee Complaints Using Visual Analog Scales

Flandry F, Hunt JP, Terry GC, Hughston JC (Hughston Orthopaedic Clinic;

Hughston Sports Medicine Found, Columbus, Ga)
Am J Sports Med 19:112–118, 1991   8–40

Introduction.—Treatment results can be difficult to measure and analyze, particularly when outcome is related to subjective factors such as pain and functional ability. A system using a possible 100-point numerical score is often used to evaluate knee problems, but such a method may have a low degree of sensitivity and interpretation bias. A visual analogue scale (VAS) was developed to bring a greater sensitivity and greater statistical power to the analysis of subjective knee complaints.

Methods.—The VAS (Fig 8-7) was tested on 117 consecutive patients who underwent knee surgery ranging from arthroscopy to total arthroplasty. The validity of the VAS was compared with that of 3 other established subjective evaluation methods: the Lysholm scale, the Noyes knee scale, and the Larson scale. After completing the VAS and 1 of the other scales, the patients were asked to rate the forms and state which form allowed them to best depict their symptoms.

Results.—User understanding was similar for the VAS, Lysholm, and Larson knee scales, but patients were less able to respond satisfactorily to questions posed by the Noyes scale. Of the patients who took the Noyes test, 80% found that the VAS was easier to complete. Of those who took the Lysholm knee scale, 43% found the VAS easier to complete and 43% believed there was no difference between the scales. The Larson scale was found more confusing than the VAS by 58% of the patients.

Conclusion.—The VAS, with its open structure of responses, does not force patients to interpret the definition of the terms mild, moderate, or severe, or to assign themselves to such categories. Because the responses can be converted to objective measures, bias is minimized and statistical power is increased. Patient affinity was greater for the VAS than for other scales.

▶ The authors state that their goal in developing the visual analogue scale was to create a method that would objectively record subjective data by "minimizing collection and interpretation bias and to facilitate statistical analysis by providing a means of converting a magnitude of subjective experiences to numeric values." What they appear not to appreciate is that subjective data is just that and, regardless of how it is handled, statistically remains subjective data.—J.S. Torg, M.D.

KNEE DISORDERS SUBJECTIVE HISTORY

NAME _____

CHART _____ DATE _____ SIDE: L R

INSTRUCTIONS:
For each question, shade in a box between the two descriptions which you think describes your knee **relative** to the two extremes. Please complete both sides of this form.

1. How often does your knee hurt?
never — daily even at rest

2. How bad is the pain at its worst?
none — severe, requiring pain pills every few hours

3. Do you have swelling in your knee?
never — daily, even at rest

4. Does your knee give way or buckle?
never — I must guard my knee to prevent giving way even with normal everyday activity

5. Does your knee lock up so you are unable to straighten it?
never — I must guard my knee to prevent locking even with normal everyday activity

6. Does your knee catch or hang up when moving?
never — I must guard my knee to prevent catching even with normal everyday activity

7. Is your knee stiff?
none — I can barely move my knee because of stiffness

8. Are you able to walk on level ground?
no problem — unable

9. Are you able to walk on rough ground, inclines, or negotiate curves?
no problem — unable

10. Do you need crutches, cane, or walker to walk?
never — always

11. Do you feel grinding when your knee moves?
none — severe

12. Do you have problems twisting or pivoting on your injured knee?
none — unable

13. Do you have problems carrying heavy objects because of your knee?
none — unable — not attempted

14. Do you have problems climbing stairs?
none — unable — not attempted

15. Do you have problems going down stairs?
none — unable — not attempted

16. Do you have problems running?
none — unable — not attempted

17. Do you have problems decelerating (slowing down) after running or jogging?
none — unable — not attempted

18. Do you have problems cutting (changing directions while running by pivoting on affected knee)?
none — unable — not attempted

19. Do you have problems jumping?
none — unable — not attempted

20. Do you have problems taking part in competitive sports?
none — unable — not attempted

21. Do you have night pain?
none — severe

22. Do you have problems kneeling?
no problem — unable — not attempted

23. Do you have problems squatting?
no problem — unable — not attempted

24. Do you have problem getting in and out of a car?
no problem — unable

25. Does your knee ache while you are sitting?
never — always

26. Do you have problems getting in or out of a chair?
no problem — unable

27. Do you have stiffness or discomfort when you first start to walk?
none — always

28. Do you have problems turning over in bed?
none — unable

HUGHSTON SPORTS MEDICINE FOUNDATION, INC. HUGHSTON SPORTS MEDICINE FOUNDATION, INC. HUGHSTON SPORTS MEDICINE FOUNDATION, INC.

Fig 8-7.—The VAS currently used is an adaptation of the original form. The continuous line has been converted to continuous boxes, thus allowing it to be read by automated data entry equipment. (Courtesy of Flandry F, Hunt JP, Terry GC, et al: *Am J Sports Med* 19:112–119, 1991.)

Magnetic Resonance Imaging of Traumatic Knee Articular Cartilage Injuries
Speer KP, Spritzer CE, Goldner JL, Garrett WE Jr (Duke Univ, Durham, NC)
Am J Sports Med 19:396–402, 1991   8–41

Objective.—When athletes have knee pain after acute trauma, the diagnostic problem can be difficult. Magnetic resonance imaging was carried out in 102 consecutive patients who had knee arthroscopy. Fortynine lesions of articular cartilage were found in 28 knees of 27 patients.

Methods.—Multiplanar MR imaging was carried out by using spin echo and gradient-refocused acquisition in a steady-state pulse technique. Studies were done within 4 weeks of arthroscopy in all cases.

Findings.—Magnetic resonance imaging detected 41% of full-thickness articular cartilage lesions before arthroscopy and 83% after arthroscopy. The respective sensitivities for partial-thickness chondral injuries were 15% and 55%. Intra-articular effusion helped in detecting chondral lesions by producing an "arthrographic" effect.

Conclusions.—Magnetic resonance imaging does not reliably rule out articular cartilage injury in athletes who have knee pain after acute injury. Hopefully improvements in MR imaging software will make it easier to evaluate injuries to the hyaline cartilage of the knee.

▶ There have been vast improvements in technique and the learning curve of MRI since this study was conducted in 1986 to 1989. Nevertheless, as the authors advise, patients should still be operated on for their clinical symptoms and not for the findings on an imaging study.—J.S. Torg, M.D.

Occult Osseous Lesions Documented by Magnetic Resonance Imaging Associated With Anterior Cruciate Ligament Ruptures
Rosen MA, Jackson DW, Berger PE (Southern California Ctr for Sport Medicine and Memorial Magnetic Resonance Ctr of Long Beach, Long Beach, Calif)
Arthroscopy 7:45–51, 1991   8–42

Objective.—Magnetic resonance imaging was carried out in 75 skeletally mature patients within 3 weeks of an anterior cruciate ligament (ACL) rupture. The patients (mean age, 30 years) had no bony abnormalities on radiographical examination. The MRI examinations were performed in the coronal and sagittal planes.

Findings.—Of the 75 patients, 64 had a total of 84 bony injuries; 19 patients had more than 1 area of involvement. Lesions of the lateral tibial plateau and lateral femoral condyle predominated; in 10 patients both of these structures were injured. A total of 8 lesions involved cortical disruption.

Pathology.—An exact correlation between MR abnormalities and underlying pathology has not been established. Some believe that the areas of low signal intensity on the T1-weighted images represent trabecular compression edema, whereas the increased signal intensity on the T2-weighted images reflects edema and hemorrhage. The term "fracture" was used only when cortical bone was involved because there is no proof that an altered medullary signal actually represents trabecular fracture or compression.

Conclusion.—Bony lesions may be present in more than 80% of all patients with acute ACL injury; some of these patients will have multiple lesions. If such lesions are present, the lateral compartment is likely to be involved. Bony lesions may increase the risk of arthritis. In addition, their frequent occurrence provides a reason for protected weight-bearing when rehabilitating more severely injured patients.

▶ The significance of the previously undetected pathology associated with ACL injuries as determined by MR "remains speculative and requires further study." Clearly, these injuries were occurring before they were detected by MR. The mechanism of injury, the time delay between the injury and ACL repair, the associated meniscal and ligamentous injury, the location, type and severity of occult osseous injuries identified, the type of surgery, and the success of the repaired anterior cruciate ligament all must be considered when evaluating the significance of these "osseous lesions" on the development of arthritis, etc.—J.S. Torg, M.D.

The Effects of Knee Brace Wear on Perceptual and Metabolic Variables During Horizontal Treadmill Running
Highgenboten CL, Jackson A, Meske N, Smith J (Orthopaedic Consultants, Dallas; Univ of North Texas, Denton)
Am J Sports Med 19:639–643, 1991   8–43

Introduction.—Selected knee braces are often used to provide stability to the knee after injuries to the anterior cruciate ligament. Selected braces can decrease speed and muscle strength and increase oxygen consumption and heart rate.

Methods.—The metabolic and perceptual effects of 4 different braces on treadmill running were investigated in 14 males, aged 18–35 years, all of whom were asymptomatic joggers or runners. Treadmill runs were performed for 5 minutes each at 6, 7, and 8 mph. Each person performed 1 run wearing each of the Generation II Poli-Axial Knee Cage, the Orthotech Performer, the CTi Brace, and the Lenox Hill Derotation Brace. Physiologic variables were measured and perceived exertion was rated during all runs, and the findings were compared with those obtained while running without a brace.

Results.—Significant brace effects of 3% to 8% were found for oxygen consumption, ventilation, and heart rate, although no significant differences were found among the different braces. Analysis of covariance showed that the weight of the brace accounted for the increase in oxygen consumption. A significant brace effect was found for peripheral ratings of perceived exertion, but no differences were found among braces in this regard.

Conclusion.—The use of all 4 braces increases the metabolic cost of treadmill running by 3% to 6%. This effect is related to the weight of the braces.

The Effects of a Supportive Knee Brace on Leg Performance in Healthy Subjects
Veldhuizen JW, Koene FMM, Oostvogel HJM, v Thiel ThPH, Vestappen FTJ
(University of Limburg, Maastricht, The Netherlands)
Int J Sports Med 12:577–580, 1991   8–44

Introduction.—Knee braces are often used prophylactically for support of symptomatic knee joint instability and after knee ligament injuries. The injury-preventive effect of these braces is questionable, and there is evidence to suggest that preventive bracing induces muscular atrophy and reduces lower leg performance.

Methods.—A supportive knee brace designed for use in sports was evaluated for the direct and long-term effects on leg performance in 8 healthy persons, all active in sports, with a mean age of 24 years. Each person wore a Push Brace 'Heavy' on 1 knee during the day for 4 weeks. Before, during, and after application of the brace, individuals were tested for isokinetic muscle strength measurements, performance in 60-m dash, vertical jump height, and treadmill running performance.

Results.—Some individuals complained of transient knee pinching during the first 3 days. Wearing the brace did not affect duration and level of performance in sports. In all strength measurements there were transient decreases on day 1 of brace wearing, but measured strength returned to baseline after 4 weeks of wearing. Similarly, there was a transient increase in the running time of the 60-m dash on the first day of brace wearing, but baseline values were regained after 4 weeks of wearing. Speed to volitional exhaustion decreased 6% on day 1 and 4% after 4 weeks. Heart rate did not change during brace wearing, but was slightly lower 1 day after removal of the brace than before the application of the brace. Oxygen uptake during treadmill running was not significantly changed while wearing the brace, but decreased below baseline after removal of the brace. Similarly, the mean plasma lactate concentration at submaximal exercise was slightly but not significantly increased during brace application, but after removal was slightly but not significantly lower than at baseline.

Conclusion.—The application of the Push Brace 'Heavy' seems to result in slightly impaired performance for 1 day only. Thereafter, only a slight mechanical hindrance and resistance training effect remain. Use of this supportive brace did not seem to result in muscular atrophy.

► These 2 studies (Abstracts 8–43 and 8–44) evaluate several other parameters relating to the controversy involving the use of prophylactic and functional knee bracing. Certainly they should be considered only in terms of the entire context of the bracing issue.—J.S. Torg, M.D.

Rapid Rehabilitation Following Anterior Cruciate Ligament Reconstruction
Blair DF, Wills RP (Wenatchee Valley Clinic Sports Medicine Ctr, Wenatchee, Wash)
Athlet Train, JNATA 26:32–43, 1991   8–45

Background.—Rehabilitation after anterior cruciate ligament (ACL) reconstruction is very controversial. A rapid rehabilitation protocol using early motion and weight bearing was assessed.

Methods.—The cornerstones of the program are early motion and weight bearing (table). Continuous passive motion starts immediately after surgery while the patient is under a long-lasting regional anesthetic. Five to 7 days after the operation, the formal rehabilitation begins. This includes passive extension and flexion, stationary bicycling, muscle stimulation, and a series of heavy rubber tubing exercises. The athlete progresses from partial to full weight bearing within 2 weeks of surgery. Closed kinetic chain activities and proprioceptive exercises are emphasized as the rehabilitation progresses (Fig 8–8). At 6 weeks, when the involved extremity reaches 70% of the uninvolved extremity on high-speed isokinetic testing, light agility activities and jogging may be started. Sport-specific drills and a more intensive strengthening program follow progressively.

Results.—Early results have been very encouraging. Athletes have returned to sports 4 to 6 months after surgery.

Conclusions.—A rehabilitation program including early motion and weight bearing enables athletes to return to sports quickly if certain functional criteria are met. Although the preliminary results are positive, a larger group of patients and longer follow-up are needed to establish its success.

► In the past 2 years, we have become more aggressive at earlier stages of our postoperative ACL rehabilitation program. We have not moved quite as fast as the authors of this abstract; however, there are many clinics that follow a routing very similar to this one and are reporting excellent results. We are moving away from isolated isometric, isotonic, and isokinetic type exer-

Rapid Rehabilitation Protocol

Immediately Following Surgery
- Continuous passive motion while under effects of long lasting regional anesthetic

2-3 Days Postoperatively
- Continue CPM; 0-90° ROM goal
- Prone leg hang; 3-4 times daily for 20-30 minutes
- Partial weight bearing with crutches and knee immobilizer as tolerated

5-7 Days Postoperatively
- Continue CPM; 0-95° ROM goal, continue prone leg hang
- Wall slides, towel pull, opposition bending, passive stationary biking for flexion
- Electrical muscle stimulation with co-contraction of quadriceps and hamstrings; patellar mobilization
- Heavy rubber tubing exercise; hip flexion, extension, abduction, adduction, (resistance above knee) closed kinetic chain terminal knee extensions; tubing hamstring pull-back; seated toe raises
- Partial weight bearing with progression to full weight bearing

10-14 Days Postoperatively
- Continue prone leg hang and add gentle joint mobilization; soft tissue release, if full extension has not been achieved at this time; continue flexion ROM 0-100° ROM goal
- Full weight bearing at this time, decrease use of knee immobilizer (depends on amount of walking and outdoor conditions)
- Continue above strengthening; add active cycling on stationary bike, leg press (tubing or weight), 2" step-ups, 1/4 squat with tubing, isotonic hamstring curls

3-4 Weeks Postoperatively
- Continue ROM as needed, 0-120° ROM goal
- Continue above strengthening; add toe raises, 4" step-ups, 1/4 squat with tubing on mini-trampoline, scooter drills. [All quadriceps strengthening performed through closed kinetic chain exercises. NO open chain quadriceps exercises (except isokinetic testing, with Anti-Shear) are performed in the first 4 months]

(continued)

Table *(continued)*

6 Weeks Postoperatively
- Continue as above; ROM should be full at this point
- Continue strenghtening as above
- Add intensive proprioception [one foot multi-directional balance board (also 1/4 squat with tubing on board), sport-specific drills, proprioceptive toe raises, balance board walking].
- Add slide board, Fitter, and Pogo Ball
- Isokinetic evaluation at 180°/sec. with a 20° extension stop with Anti-Shear is performed at this time; if strength is 70% of the uninvolved leg, the athlete may begin light functional drills (light jogging, agilities, jumping rope)

2–3 Months Postoperatively
- Continue strengthening as above
- Begin or add more agilities; important not to slack off at this time as the knee begins to feel more functional (a common occurrence)
- Isokinetic testing every two to four weeks; important not to do follow-up testing to find residual weaknesses

4–6 Months Postoperatively
- Athlete can return to activities at this time depending upon:
  Level of strength
  Absence of residual swelling
  Good stability (as measured by knee arthrometry)
  Functional abilities
  Amount of cutting required in sport
- Athlete continues to work intensively on strengthening, proprioceptive, and agility exercises

(Courtesy of Blair DF, Wills RP: *Athlet Train*, JNATA 26:32–43, 1991.)

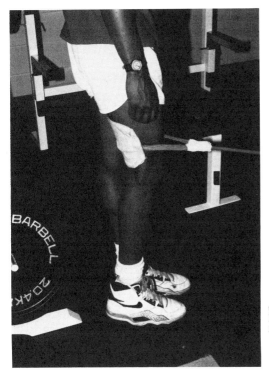

Fig 8–8.—Closed kinetic chain terminal extensions. (Courtesy of Blair DF, Wills RP: *Athlet Train, JNATA* 26:32-43, 1991.)

cises, and toward the more functional "closed kinetic chain" exercises (see Abstract 8–49). We do include some isolated muscle exercises. We continue to use a baseline of 90% strength of the uninvolved extremity when doing isokinetic testing before allowing running or agility activities.—F.J. George, A.T.C., P.T.

Prevention and Treatment of Patellar Entrapment Following Intra-Articular ACL Reconstruction
Tomaro JE (Sports Medicine Services, Pittsburgh)
Athletic Training, JNATA 26:11–18, 1991   8–46

Background.—Patellar entrapment can complicate intra-articular reconstruction of the anterior cruciate ligament (ACL). Postoperative adhesions forming at the patellofemoral joint lead to reduced patellar mobility, which causes a loss of knee extension with significant symptoms and functional limitations. This complication can require prolonged treatment with possible permanent residual effects. The best significant complications is by early detection and intervention. Principles and techniques for prevention of and rehabilitation after patellar entrapment were reviewed.

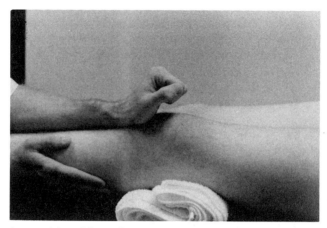

Fig 8–9.—Superior gliding of the patella to enhance knee extension. (*Courtesy of Tomaro JE: Athlet Train, JNATA* 26:11–18, 1991.)

Prevention.—Patellar entrapment after ACL can have surgical or non-surgical causes. Use of arthroscopy for ACL reconstruction should help reduce the occurrence of the syndrome. Recent research has identified optimal graft positioning and tensioning, which should also help prevent patellar entrapment. Postoperative rehabilitation procedures can also result in the syndrome. Current recommendations include performing range-of-motion exercises with a constant passive motion machine at 0 to 90 degrees starting the second day after surgery. There are exceptions, however. Isometric exercises for the hamstrings and quadriceps are also begun on the second day. Self-patellar mobilization begins within the first 5 days. If these guidelines are followed, the graft should not be affected, and the deleterious effects of immobilization should disappear.

Treatment.—Early intervention is important. Transverse friction massage and ultrasound are helpful in treating parapatellar adhesions and retinacular thickening. Patellar mobilization is important. It should be done with the knee in slight flexion to avoid pinching the synovial tissues (Fig 8–9). Constant passive motion can also be used to increase knee extension. Initiating quadriceps contraction is also important when treating patellar entrapment. A drop-out cast is sometimes used in the early stages. When conservative treatment fails, surgery may be needed.

Conclusions.—When treating an athlete after reconstruction surgery, clinicians must be aware of the clinical signs and symptoms of patellar entrapment. This complication can usually be prevented through proper surgical and postoperative procedures.

▶ Patella mobilization, especially superior patella gliding, is an important and significant portion of our early ACL rehabilitation program. Patients are taught self-mobilizing techniques and are instructed to do them frequently throughout the day. Knee flexion exercises are not forced before proper patella mobilization and function. Proper length of the patella tendon must be restored to ensure normal range of motion and to avoid patellofemoral joint problems.—F.J. George, A.T.C., P.T.

Functional Rehabilitation of the Cruciate-Deficient Knee
Markey KL (San Antonio Orthopaedic Group, San Antonio, Tex)
Sports Med 12:407–417, 1991   8-47

Introduction.—The traditional concepts of rehabilitation are motion and strength. Functional rehabilitation extends these concepts by adding the concepts of agility, proprioception, and finally the confidence to do whatever task the person wishes to undertake. The meaning of functional rehabilitation and its goals as they pertain to the cruciate-deficient knee were examined.

Determinants.—The patient is the most important determinant of the rehabilitation program. The second factor involved is the nature of the knee injury sustained. The stability provided by the repair is another major determinant. The final determinant is the effectiveness of the rehabilitation program, specifically the application and imagination of the rehabilitator.

Principles.—The overriding principle of functional rehabilitation is to return patients to the level at which they were previously functioning. Whether this may be achieved depends on the determinants outlined above. Rehabilitation involves joint motion and stability, as well as muscular endurance and strength. All 4 factors should be kept in mind during the immobilization phase, the surgical and postsurgical phases, and throughout the early, late, and final healing stages.

Treatment.—Conservative and surgical treatment programs for the cruciate-deficient knee are essentially the same, except for the time factors involved. The completion times for different levels of activity are generally longer for the surgical program.

Modalities.—Muscular development is accomplished by means of isometric activity of the quadriceps and hamstrings, a passive motion machine, passive flexion, progressive resistance exercises, and muscular stimulation. The bicycle should be used for the development of motion and endurance in the knee, but transfer to activities such as walking stairs, running backward and forward, and short leg squats should be prescribed to develop additional strength. This type of activity places the proper vertical orientation of the body in relationship to the knee and functional activities. Thereafter, jumping rope, agility training, and weight-training are appropriate.

Discussion.—The rehabilitator must advance activity to levels of ever increasing complexity while avoiding overtraining and too rapid a progression of activities. Progressing from less difficult to more difficult activities before the patient is ready usually results in injury or reinjury.

Constant assessment of the patient's performance level before advancing to more demanding activities is essential to effective rehabilitation.

▶ The author emphasizes the importance of avoiding pain in the rehabilitation program. Pain will prevent muscular development and cause a loss of range of motion. A number of functional activities are described to bring the patient back to full athletic activity. The author states that return to athletic activity is allowed if the patient has a "knee range of motion from 5 degrees to 10 degrees of extension to 110 degrees or more of flexion." We insist that our athletes regain full knee extension and have at least 130 degrees of flexion before returning to athletic activity.—F.J. George, A.T.C., P.T.

Functional Performance Tests for the Anterior Cruciate Ligament Insufficient Athlete
Lephart SM, Perrin DH, Fu FH, Minger K (Univ of Pittsburgh; Univ of Virginia, Charlottesville; Univ of Texas, Austin)
Athletic Training, JNATA 26:44–50, 1991   8–48

Introduction.—Three objective functional performance tests (FPTs) have been recommended previously to assess the anterior cruciate ligament insufficient athlete's readiness to return to preinjury levels of activity. The cocontraction semicircular test reproduces the rotational forces at the knee, necessitating control of tibial translation by the thigh musculature. The carioca crossover maneuver reproduces the pivot shift phenomenon, whereas the shuttle run test reproduces acceleration and deceleration forces that are common to athletic activity.

Methods.—Thirty male and 15 female healthy division 1 intercollegiate athletes performed all 3 FPTs, and mean values for all 3 FPTs were established.

Findings.—Football back, football line, and baseball athletes performed all 3 FPTs significantly faster than male gymnasts. Female basketball and volleyball players performed the FPTs in less time than the female gymnasts.

Conclusion.—Athletes who participate in sports that require lateral and running maneuvers as a dominant function of their sport perform better on FPTs that require such maneuvers. These preliminary mean scores on the 3 FPTs may serve as guidelines for clinicians in assessing the readiness of the ACL insufficient athlete to return to sports activity.

▶ The carioca and shuttle run have always been a part of our onfield testing to determine an injured athlete's readiness to participate. We have since added the test described by the authors as a cocontraction test. We also test the athletes in running figure eights and making cutting maneuvers similar to those of their sport. The last stages of testing are very sport specific and must be done successfully at a very low intensity before more advanced stresses are placed on the knee.—F.J. George, A.T.C., P.T.

Biomechanical Analysis of Rehabilitation in the Standing Position
Ohkoshi Y, Yasuda K, Kaneda K, Wada T, Yamanaka M (Hokkaido University, Sapporo, Japan)
Am J Sports Med 19:605–611, 1991   8–49

Introduction.—Rehabilitation after anterior cruciate ligament (ACL) reconstruction must take into consideration the shear force exerted on the joint during daily activities.

Methods.—A 3-phase study was conducted of 21 men with a mean age of 21.5 years who were free of knee pain and abnormalities. In the first phase, muscle torque and integrated EMGs were recorded in separate isometric contractions of the quadriceps and the hamstrings. For the second phase, the principal experiment, measurements were performed during standing (Fig 8–10). In the third phase, a sagittal model of the lower limb in a standing position with the knee flexed was established.

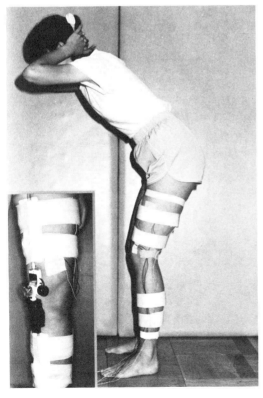

Fig 8–10.—Bipolar surface electrodes were attached at the sites of the rectus femoris, medial and lateral vastus, and medial and lateral hamstrings. The knee flexion angle was monitored using an electrogoniometer. (Courtesy of Ohkoshi Y, Yasuda K, Kaneda K, et al: *Am J Sports Med* 19:605–611, 1991.)

Results.—All EMGs showed simultaneous contraction of the quadriceps and hamstrings. Amplitude observed on EMGs of the hamstrings increased as the trunk flexion angle increased. At every knee flexion angle, the calculated average values of shear force were negative. And as the trunk flexion angle increased, posterior drawer force increased at knee flexion angles of 30 and 60 degrees. The primary factor influencing these results appeared to be the simultaneous contraction of the quadriceps and hamstrings.

Conclusion.—Exercise in the standing position with the knees flexed and the trunk anteriorly flexed can be performed in the early stages after reconstruction of the ACL. Such exercise should have favorable effects on muscle strength and prevent bone atrophy. The posture of standing with the knees flexed resembles that of an exercise method called "half squatting," used in rehabilitation of the cruciate ligament.

▶ Our rehabilitation programs for past ACL repair patients have moved rapidly into the "closed kinetic chain" type of exercises. There has not been a great deal of scientific experimentation done to support our move in that direction. This particular study does support the direction many of us in the clinics have chosen. More studies of this type should be done before an exercise can be deemed appropriate or safe to perform.—F.J. George, A.T.C., P.T.

9 Leg and Ankle, Miscellaneous

Achilles Tendon Rupture in Athletes: Histochemistry of the Triceps Surae Muscle
Maffulli N, Testa V, Capasso G (Newham Gen Hosp, London; Univ of Naples, Italy)
J Foot Surg 30:529–533, 1991   9–1

Background.—Spontaneous rupture of the Achilles tendon is a serious and increasingly common injury in athletes. Its pathologic causes are unclear. The biopsy findings in the triceps surae muscles in a group of 12 athletes operated on for ruptured Achilles tendon were examined.

Patients.—The 10 men and 2 women who underwent surgery for subcutaneous midsubstance rupture of the Achilles tendon had an average age of 34.1 years. All the injuries occurred during sports, most commonly tennis or soccer. Only 3 had previous Achilles tendon problems, and none had ever received any injections in the area. Bilateral percutaneous muscle biopsy specimens of the triceps surae muscle were taken and histochemical analyses were conducted.

Observations.—None of the specimens showed any necrosis, atrophy, or substantial fiber grouping or regeneration. On both sides the muscles consisted of about 70% type I fibers, with no significant differences in their histochemical characteristics. Area measurements of the fibers were within previously described limits and were similar on both sides. The contralateral side tended to have a greater average capillary density and average capillary-fiber ratio, but this was not significant.

Conclusions.—In athletes with spontaneous rupture of the Achilles tendon muscle abnormalities do not appear to be a significant factor. Although this study conflicts with previous reports, the timing and technique of biopsy were different. Gentle training and warm-up may lessen the risk of such injuries by enhancing the aerobic metabolism and mechanical characteristics of the triceps surae muscle.

Histopathological Changes Preceding Spontaneous Rupture of a Tendon: A Controlled Study of 891 Patients

Kannus P, Józsa L (Natl Inst of Traumatology, Budapest)
J Bone Joint Surg 73-A:1507-1525, 1991   9-2

Background.—The prevalence of spontaneous rupture of a tendon has increased in recent decades. The most common finding in tendons that have ruptured spontaneously is degenerative tendinopathy, but calcification and mucoid-like changes have also been seen. The histologic changes in spontaneously ruptured tendons from different locations in humans were compared with changes and their frequencies in age and sex-matched control tendons.

Methods.—Biopsy specimens removed at the time of repair of spontaneously ruptured tendons included 397 Achilles tendons, 302 biceps brachii tendons, 40 extensor pollicis longus tendons, 82 quadriceps tendons and patellar ligaments, and 70 other tendons. The age- and sex-matched control specimens were taken from cadavers. Light and polarized light microscopy and scanning and transmission electron microscopy were used to analyze histopathologic changes.

Findings.—Sixty-five percent of the control tendons were structurally healthy, but none of the spontaneously ruptured tendons showed any healthy structures. The pathologic changes associated with rupture in 97% of the cases were classified as degenerative and the most common lesion was hypoxic degenerative tendinopathy. The next most frequent lesion was mucoid degeneration followed by tendolipomatosis and calcifying tendinopathy. In the remaining 3% of ruptured tendons, pathologic changes included an intratendinous foreign body, rheumatoid tendinitis, a xanthoma, a tumor, or a tumor-like lesion such as an intratendinous ganglion. Degenerative changes were also observed in 34% of the control lesions. Only one third of the patients with a ruptured tendon had previous symptoms such as tenderness, stiffness, pain, or discomfort.

Conclusions.—Degenerative changes in tendons may be common in people older than 35 and may predispose to spontaneous rupture. The degenerative changes include hypoxic degenerative tendinopathy, mucoid degeneration, tendolipomatosis, calcifying tendinopathy, or a combination.

▶ Maffulli et al. (Abstract 9-1) clearly demonstrate that "muscle abnormalities do not appear to be a significant factor in determining Achilles tendon rupture in healthy athletes." However, Kannus and Józsa (Abstract 9-2) clearly demonstrate that spontaneous tendon rupture in general and that of the tendoachilles specifically are commonly associated with a preexisting degenerative tendonopathy. They further point out that in 66% of tendon ruptures, the predisposing degenerative process is asymptomatic. This observation questions the "popular theory that degeneration of a tendon goes through acute, concurrent, subacute, subchronic, and chronic phases of ten-dinitis before actual degeneration develops." Although these 2 articles iden-tify the location and pathologic process involved, they do not answer why degeneration occurs. Also, important from the clinical standpoint is whether or not a supple, well-conditioned triceps will protect an Achilles tendon un-dergoing a degenerative process from complete rupture.—J.S. Torg, M.D.

Repair of Achilles Tendon Ruptures With a Polylactic Acid Implant: Assessment With MR Imaging
Liem MD, Zegel HG, Balduini FC, Turner ML, Becker JM, Caballero-Saez A (Presbyterian Med Ctr, Philadelphia; South Jersey Sports Med Ctr, Cherry Hill, NJ; MRI Diagnostics, Philadelphia)
AJR 156:769–773, 1991   9–3

Background.—A device for the surgical repair of tendons and liga-ments is undergoing multicenter clinical trials. The device is composed of multiple filaments of a polymer of lactic acid (PLA) twisted together, with suture needles placed at both ends (Figs 9–1 and 9–2). The PLA is attractive for tendon repair because it has high tensile strength and in-duces rapid tissue healing, which may shorten the rehabilitation period. The appearance of this device on MRI was examined in 10 patients.

Findings.—Sixteen MR examinations were done in 10 patients 3 to 35 months after repair. Every T1-weighted sagittal image revealed a thick-

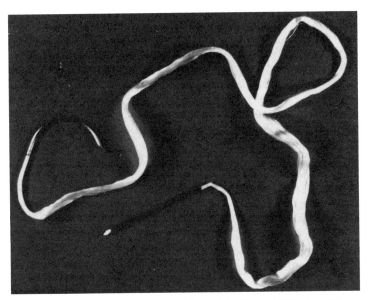

9–1.—The tendon repair device. (Courtesy of Liem MD, Zegel HG, Balduini FC, et al: *AJR* 156:769–773, 1991.)

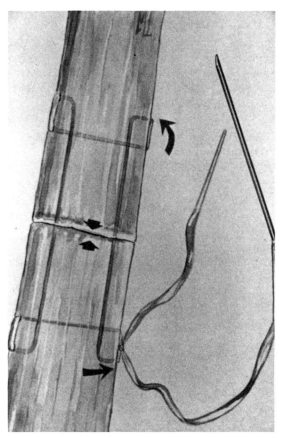

Fig 9–2.—Modified Kessler stitch used to repair Achilles tendon ruptures (*short arrows*) is a rectangular stitch with stabilizing corner loops (*long arrows*) oriented along longitudinal axis of tendon. (Courtesy of Liem MD, Zegel HG, Balduini FC, et al: *AJR* 156:769–773, 1991.)

ened fusiform tendon with streaks of moderate signal that corresponded to the PLA device and its surrounding collagenogenic response. On double-echo T2-weighted axial images, there were progressive changes in the signal pattern at the mid-tendon level, reflecting the maturation of the healing tendon. Mid-level spin-density axial images showed a group of punctate foci corresponding to strands of polylactic acid (Fig 9–3). Tendons repaired with PLA appeared hypertrophied because of the induced proliferative collagenogenic ingrowth.

Conclusion.—On MR examination, a tendon repaired with PLA is markedly thickened in a diffuse, fusiform manner and has diffuse thin streaks of intermediate signal throughout. A conventionally repaired tendon has less pronounced and more localized thickening and a thicker, localized zone of intratendinous signal. The diffuse hypertrophy of the

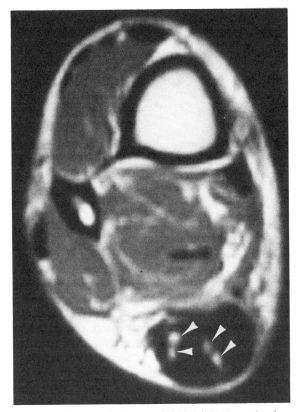

Fig 9–3.—Mid-level spin-density axial MR image (SE 2000/20) 12 months after repair showing a group of sharply defined punctate foci (*arrowheads*) corresponding to strands of polylactic acid against low-signal background of fully healed tendon. (Courtesy of Liem MD, Zegel HG, Balduini FC, et al: AJR 156:769–773, 1991.)

tendon repaired with PLA may contribute to the continued strength and integrity of this repair.

▶ As a participating investigator in the clinical trials of this device, I can attest to its efficacy. Presumably, one of the advantages of using polylactic acid as a suture for a rupture of the Achilles tendon is that it is biodegradable. However, this paper does not demonstrate the adequacy of this property. Requiring comment is the inappropriateness of an orthopedic investigational device being first reported in the radiographic literature.—J.S. Torg, M.D.

Achilles Tendon Ruptures Operated on Under Local Anesthesia: Retrospective Study of 81 Nonhospitalized Patients

Sejberg D, Hansen LB, Dalsgaard S (Koge Hosp, Denmark; Herlev Univ Hosp, Denmark)

Acta Orthop Scand 61:549–550, 1990   9–4

Background.—As an alternative to inpatient surgery under general anesthesia for a ruptured Achilles tendon, a surgical outpatient treatment was introduced. A total of 97 patients were treated surgically as outpatients over a 6-year period.

Methods.—The 76 men and 21 women were operated on under local anesthesia, within 6 hours of the subcutaneous rupture of the Achilles tendon. After surgery a below-the-knee plaster splint was applied. Sutures were removed after 1 week and a circular plaster cast was applied. After 6 weeks the cast was removed and the ankle joint was exercised for 2 weeks. Weight-bearing increased after 2 months to full weight-bearing at 3 months.

Results.—At follow-up 79 of 81 patients walked normally and 2 walked with a slight limp. Three reruptures occurred 2 months after operation. Plantar flexion was normal in 63 patients and dorsiflexion was normal in 62.

Conclusion.—This outpatient surgical procedure under local anesthesia yielded the same good results as surgical in-patient treatment of a ruptured Achilles tendon and avoided costly hospitalization.

▶ As a proponent of the numerous advantages of performing surgery with local anesthesia, this paper has great appeal. However, from a scientific standpoint, I find it to be somewhat lacking. Specifically, the authors report a 25% decrease in plantar flexion and a 25% decrease in dorsiflexion postoperatively. However, because of their failure to accurately describe who has what, the reader can't be sure if 25% or 50% of the patients have limited motion postoperatively or if the number falls somewhere in between. Because of the authors' failure to randomize the series, they cannot make the statement that "this outpatient surgical procedure under local anesthesia yields the same good results as surgical inpatient treatment."—J.S. Torg, M.D.

Chronic Rupture of the Achilles Tendon: A New Technique of Repair

Mann RA, Holmes GB, Seale KS, Collins DN (Thomas Jefferson Univ, Philadelphia)

J Bone Joint Surg 73A:214–219, 1991   9–5

Introduction.—Patients with untreated ruptures of the Achilles tendon often have large gaps between the proximal and distal portions of the ruptured tendon or between the tendon and the posterosuperior surface

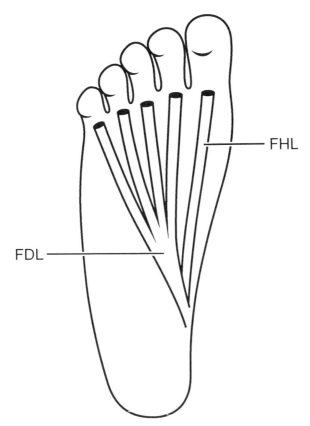

Fig 9–4.—Plantar view of the flexor digitorum longus (*FDL*) tendon and the adjacent flexor hallucis longus (*FHL*) tendon. (Courtesy of Mann RA, Holmes GB, Seale KS, et al: *J Bone Joint Surg* 73-A:214–219, 1991.)

of the calcaneus. A new technique, in which the flexor digitorum longus is used to repair chronically ruptured Achilles tendons, was used to treat 7 patients with symptoms of 3–36 months' duration. The patients were followed up for 2–6 years.

Technique.—A hockey-stick-shaped 8-10-cm incision was made beginning proximally, medial to the tendon, then curving laterally, distal to the insertion of the tendon. A second 7-cm incision was made on the medial aspect of the foot, extending along the upper border of the abductor hallucis toward the first metatarsophalangeal joint. Dissection permitted localization of the digital branches of the flexor digitorum (Fig 9-4), which was cut proximal to its division into digital branches. The proximal aspect of the distal stump of the flexor digitorum longus tendon was sutured to the flexor hallucis longus tendon (Fig 9-5). The proximal part of the flexor digitorum longus tendon was passed through a drill-hole placed in the calcaneus and sutured to itself (Fig 9-6).

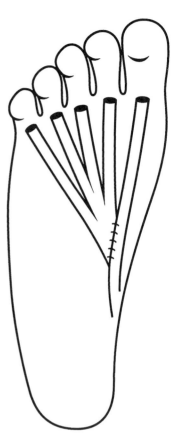

Fig 9–5.—Anastomosis of the distal stump of the flexor digitorum tendon to the flexor hallucis longus tendon. (Courtesy of Mann RA, Homes GB, Seale KS, et al: *J Bone Joint Surg* 73-A:214-219, 1991.)

Results.—Results were excellent in 4 patients. Results were good in 2 patients, requiring secondary soft-tissue procedures because of superficial necrosis of the wound. In 1 patient the result was fair, with a return to daily activities but with intermittent pain and a limp. All patients walked without walking aids and had return of function. No reruptures were observed during average follow-up of 39 months.

Conclusion.—Transfer of the tendon of the flexor digitorum longus seems to be an effective and durable operation for patients with chronic rupture of the Achilles tendon. This procedure might prove useful for treatment of acute rupture when the defect cannot be bridged by primary anastomosis alone.

▶ The authors report an innovative method of dealing with chronic rupture of the Achilles tendon that can aptly be described as good news and bad news. The good news is they have used autogenous tissue with satisfactory functional results. The bad news is that they also report a 30% (2/7) major complication rate. Specifically, these patients had wound necrosis requiring

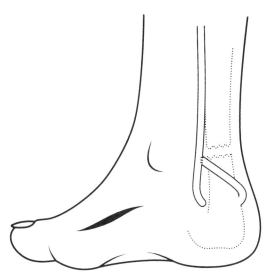

Fig 9–6.—The flexor digitorum longus is pulled through a transverse drill-hole in the calcaneus. (Courtesy of Mann RA, Homes GB, Seale KS, et al: *J Bone Joint Surg* 73-A:214-219, 1991.)

skin grafting procedures with associated functional decrease in strength and inability to return to preinjury activities. It is my opinion that attempting to repair either acute or chronic Achilles tendon rupture with the patient in the prone position places the surgeon at a disadvantage. We recommend that the surgery be performed with the patient supine, the knee flexed to 90 degrees with the hip externally rotated and the ankle and foot placed in maximum equines. In this position, with either an acute or chronic injury, end to end anastomosis should not be a problem.—J.S. Torg, M.D.

Stress Fractures of the Anterior Tibial Diaphysis
Beals RK, Cook RD (Oregon Health Sciences Univ, Portland)
Orthopedics 14:869–875, 1991   9–6

Introduction.—Stress fractures of the anterior tibial diaphysis, which occur mostly in leaping athletes, are rare. Data on patients reported in the literature and those on 35 patients with 36 anterior stress fractures of the mid-tibia were reviewed. An additional 15 such fractures in 11 patients were discussed, for a total of 51 fractures in 46 patients. The patients were 11–30 years old; most were male.

Results.—Many of the patients were professional athletes, and almost all were involved in high performance leaping sports activities. The sports included basketball, track and field, ballet, and football. When the various treatments were compared, there was a high risk of complete fracture if patients were allowed full activity. Treatment by rest alone

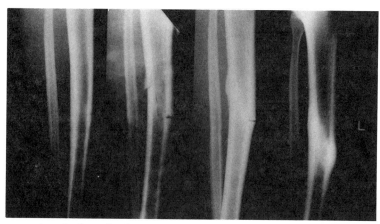

Fig 9–7.—Lateral radiographs of a college football player with an anterior tibial stress fracture (*left*). He became asymptomatic with rest, and on return to full activity, incurred a complete fracture on the first day of practice (*second from left*). The fracture healed posteriorly in 4 months with increased anterior bowing and with persistence of the anterior defect (*third from left*). He was unable to return to full activity for 2 years, when healing of the stress fracture had occurred (*right*). (Courtesy of Beals RK, Cook RD: *Orthopedics* 14:869–875, 1991.)

permitted only 40% to return to full activity, even after their symptoms improved (Fig 9–7).

Conclusion.—The optimal treatment for patients with stress fractures of the anterior tibial diaphysis is excision of the fissures, transverse drilling at the fissure site, and cancellous bone grafting of the defect. Open reduction and internal fixation is better than closed treatment in patients with a complete fracture.

Diagnosis and Treatment of Stress Fractures Located at the Mid-Tibial Shaft in Athletes

Orava S, Karpakka J, Hulkko A, Väänänen K, Takala T, Kallinen M, Alén M (Univ of Oulu; Keski-Pohjanmaa Central Hosp, Kokkola, Finland; Research Inst for Physical Activity and Health, Jyväskylä, Finland)
Int J Sports Med 12:419–422, 1991   9–7

Introduction.—The tibia is the most common site of stress fractures, which usually are located medioposteriorly at the upper or lower third of the bone. Conservative management may be prolonged, and delayed union is a considerable risk for athletes.

Patients.—Seventeen patients with stress fractures at the anterior cortex of the midtibia were seen in 1973–1989. Mean age of the 12 men and 5 women was 26 years. All the patients had trained intensively and 6 were international-level athletes. Runners, jumpers, and pole vaulters were included.

Clinical Findings.—Diffuse dull pain in the leg, made worse by activity, was the chief symptom. The anterior tibia was thickened and tender to palpation, especially after exercise. Late radiographs showed a small fissure line passing transversely at the midtibial level, which on CT passed halfway through the cortex. Bone scans showed increased uptake in this region.

Course.—Nine patients required surgery for delayed union or nonunion. Eight other patients avoided undue activity for an average of 6 months. One operated patient had a refracture after returning prematurely to full activity. All patients ultimately returned to athletic activity.

Recommendations.—Rest for up to 6 months is appropriate. If delayed union is suspected, the hypertrophied cortex should be drilled. Surgery is best if there is considerable diagnostic delay.

▶ Incomplete stress fractures involving the anterior midtibial shaft have been aptly described as the "dreaded black line" by Bergfeld. These 2 papers are in keeping with the observations of Green et al. (1) who reported 6 similar nonunion stress fractures of the tibia, 5 that went on to complete fractures. Rettig et al. (2) have reported 8 patients with similar fractures that were treated with rest and external electrical stimulation for minimum time of 3–6 months. Except for 1 patient who required bone grafting, all 8 showed complete healing and were able to return to full activity after an average of 8.9 months of treatment. Clearly, this lesion presents a major management problem. In view of the prolonged time required for healing, it appears that early aggressive surgical intervention is indicated.—J.S. Torg, M.D.

References

1. Green NE, et al: *Am J Sports Med* 13:171, 1985.
2. Rettig AC, et al: *Am J Sports Med* 16:250, 1988.

Stress Fractures: Identifiable Risk Factors
Giladi M, Milgrom C, Simkin A, Danon Y (Tel Aviv Med Ctr, Israel; Hadassah Univ Hosp, Jerusalem; Israel Defence Forces Med Corps)
Am J Sports Med 19:647–652, 1991   9–8

Background.—Increased participation in sports has led to an increase in overuse injuries such as stress fractures. Stress fractures are common in some populations and rare in others. There is a high incidence of stress fractures among Israeli military recruits. Risk factors were prospectively analyzed in 312 Israeli male military recruits by orthopedic examination; foot and tibial radiographs; measurements of tibial bone width, bone mineral content, and density; measurements of aerobic fitness and leg power; assessments of somatotype and smoking habits, and evaluation of psychological and sociological factors.

Results.—Multivariate analysis indicated narrower tibial and a high degree of external rotation of the hip were independently and cumulatively associated with stress fracture.

Conclusions.—Two risk factors that predispose to stress fracture were identified. These risk factors can be used to identify those at risk, so their regimen can be altered. Variation between populations for these risk factors may explain the reported variation in the incidence of stress fractures.

▶ The authors state that the purpose of this study is to "answer the question why such large differences in stress fracture morbidity rates exist in different countries." They point out that stress fractures occurring in military recruits range from a low of 2% in the United States Army to a high of 64% among Finnish soldiers. Although they never really answer the question, by inference we must assume that their conclusion would be that American soldiers have fat tibias as opposed to the Finnish soldiers having thin tibias. Actually, the answer to their question is that this wide range of occurrence of stress fractures is predicated on criteria used to make the diagnosis. Specifically, Israeli military physicians historically have taken the erroneous position that "cintigraphy was considered to be diagnostic of stress fracture when a focal area of increased uptake was found." Thus, they demonstrate a propensity to confuse stress reactions of bone with stress fractures. Obviously, their American counterparts diagnosed a lesion on the basis of positive roentgenograms demonstrating a stress fracture. So much for the skinny tibia concept.—J.S. Torg, M.D.

Iliotibial Band Friction Syndrome
Anderson GS (Univ College of Cape Breton, Sydney, Nova Scotia)
Aust J Sci Med Sport 23:81–83, 1991   9–9

Background.—Knee pain is cited in approximately 42% of all running injuries and the complaint is frequently lateral knee pain. Lateral knee pain is often associated with an inflammation of the iliotibial band resulting from friction between the band and the underlying lateral femoral epicondyle, called iliotibial band friction syndrome or "runner's knee."

Discussion.—Lateral knee pain associated with iliotibial band friction syndrome (ITBFS) is aggravated by continuous activities that involve a smooth steady pace and repetitive flexion and extension, like running. It is characterized by a sudden intense pain on one stride. Pain is reduced quickly with the cessation of activity and does not normally limit daily activities. The authors suggest that muscle fatigue is an important factor in the development and onset of ITBFS. Prior to muscle fatigue, the pelvis is stabilized by muscular contraction. Muscular fatigue allows the pelvis to drop toward the non-support leg, creating increased tension on the iliotibial band on the supporting leg side. The pelvic tilt and in-

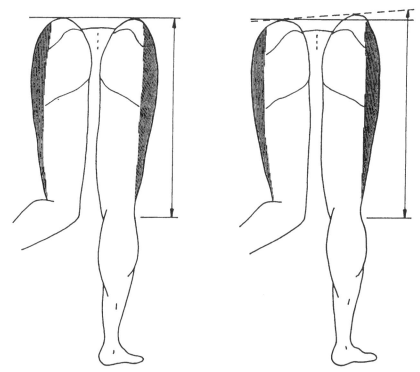

Fig 9–8.—During running, before muscle fatigue, the pelvis is stabilized by muscle contraction as in the diagram on the left. Muscular fatigue, however, allows the pelvis to drop toward the nonsupport leg as in the diagram on the right, increasing the length and tension of the iliotibial band. (Courtesy of Anderson GS: *Aust J Sci Med Sport* 23:81–83, 1991.)

creased tension in the iliotibial band create a greater friction between the lateral femoral epicondyle and the iliotibial band, which would set up an inflammation resulting in the sudden onset of pain. (Fig 9–8) This proposed mechanism of injury could explain why runners can run for extended durations asymptomatically and why certain sports such as cycling, which supports the pelvis, can be undertaken with no pain. Modification of training and the development of muscular strength and endurance in muscles involved in stabilizing the pelvis during running should be the goal of rehabilitation for ITBFS.

Conclusion.—As muscle fatigue develops, a pelvic tilt places increased tension on the iliotibial band. The increased tension increases the friction occurring between the lateral femoral epicondyle and the iliotibial band, explaining the sudden onset of pain. Rehabilitation for ITBFS should concentrate on modifying training and the development of muscular strength and endurance in the muscles stabilizing the pelvis.

▶ The authors have proposed that muscle fatigue of the pelvic stabilizers (gluteus medius, gluteus maximus, and tensor fascia lata) may be the underlying cause of ITBFS. "Fatigue in these muscles may lead to a pelvic tilt and increased tension will increase the friction between the lateral femoral condyle and iliotibial band." Rehabilitation of athletes with ITBFS should emphasize strengthening and endurance training of the pelvic stabilizers.—F.J. George, A.T.C., P.T.

Quadriceps Contusions: West Point Update
Ryan JB, Wheeler JH, Hopkinson WJ, Arciero RA, Kolakowski KR (United States Military Academy, West Point, NY)
Am J Sports Med 19:299–304, 1991   9–10

Background.—Based on previous study, a modified protocol for treatment of acute quadriceps injuries has been followed at the United States Military Academy, including rest with the injured leg in flexion and early passive pain-free motion emphasizing flexion, in the mobilization phase of therapy.

Methods.—One hundred seventeen contusions in 115 cadets were studied. All were followed up for at least 6 months. The average age was 19 years, and only 6 patients were female. Injuries were classified according to knee flexion range of motion at 12–24 hours: more than 90 degrees being mild, 45–90 degrees being moderate, and less than 45 degrees being severe. The final evaluation was based on subjective complaints, measurement of range of motion, and performance on a physical fitness test and obstacle course. The protocol followed was that of Jackson and Feagin, except the leg was rested in flexion rather than extension and early flexion instead of extension exercises were done.

Results.—There were 71 mild, 38 moderate, and 8 severe injuries. Most injuries occurred in football players, but a high percentage occurred in rugby and karate or judo. Disability times average 13 days for mild, 19 days for moderate, and 21 days for severe injuries. Twenty-eight patients were hospitalized for an average of 3 days. All patients returned to full activity, although 5 had residual symptoms. Nine percent of patients had myositis ossificans; risk factors for this condition included knee motion less than 120 degrees, football injury, previous quadriceps injury, delay in treatment more than 3 days, and ipsilateral knee effusion.

Conclusions.—A 3-year study of quadriceps contusions was evaluated. A three-phase program of rest, mobilization, and restrengthening, modified to include knee flexion to pain tolerance and early restoration of flexion, appears to be effective. Risk factors for myositis ossificans are identified.

▶ Prior to reading this study, we had used a treatment regimen for quadriceps contusions very similar to the one used at West Point. After reading this study, we have changed our protocol as they have changed theirs. In the first stage of treatment we use ice, compression, and now rest the hip and knee in a flexed position. A wide strap or elastic wrap around the lower leg and upper thigh may be used to maintain the knee in a flexed position. Early passive and active, pain free, knee flexion exercises are also used early in the treatment program. We also use a great deal of ice, ice, and more ice.—F.J. George, A.T.C., P.T.

Comparison of Vastus Medialis Obliquus: Vastus Lateralis Muscle Integrated Electromyographic Ratios Between Healthy Subjects and Patients With Patellofemoral Pain
Souza DR, Gross MT (Univ of North Carolina at Chapel Hill)
Phys Ther 71:310–320, 1991   9–11

Background.—One suggested mechanism for abnormal lateral tracking of the patella is imbalance in activity between the vastus medialis obliques (VMO) and the vastus lateralis (VL) muscles. The VMO:VL integrated electromyographic (IEMG) ratios of healthy subjects and of patients with patellofemoral pain (PFP) were compared during isotonic and isometric quadriceps femoris muscle contraction.

Methods.—The subjects were 10 women and 6 men, 18 to 35 years old. In group 1, which consisted of 7 healthy controls with no history of knee abnormality, both knees were tested. Group 2 consisted of 9 patients with unilateral PFP, in whom only the painful knee was tested, and in group 3, made up of the same patients, the nonpainful knee was tested. Both normalized and nonnormalized VMO:VL IEMG ratios were computed for ascending and descending stairs and for submaximal isometric contraction, and nonnormalized ratios were only computed for maximal isometric contraction.

Results.—According to 2-way analysis of variance for repeated measures, VMO:VL ratios for isotonic stair climbing were significantly greater than those for isometric contractions. Group 1 subjects had significantly greater nonnormalized VMO:VL ratios than either of the other groups.

Conclusions.—Abnormal VMO:VL activation patterns may be noted in patients with PFP; these patients may have more favorable responses to isotonic quadriceps femoris muscle exercise than to isometric exercise. However, further study is needed before these findings can be applied to treatment regimens for PFP.

▶ Scott D. Minor, Ph.D, P.T., has written a commentary to this study that questioned study design and interpretation of the EMG results. My reason for selecting this study was to comment on the use of isotonic exercises and some of the changes we have recently made in our rehabilitation program for these athletes. All of these patients are evaluated for patella "tilt" and "rotation." A McConnell type of taping procedure is used to correct any type of tilt or rotation that may be found. Our exercises are done with the patella "re-

aligned," and all exercises are done in a pain-free range of motion. The predominance of exercises are of the "closed kinetic chain" type. We continue
to use open chain isokinetic and isometric, pain free arc, exercises on a limited basis. Please read Abstract 9–12 and my comments.—F.J. George,
A.T.C., P.T.

**Effect of Contraction Type, Angular Velocity, and Arc of Motion on
VMO:VL EMG Ratio**
Sczepanski TL, Gross MT, Duncan PW, Chandler JM (Univ of North Carolina;
Duke Univ)
J Orthop Sports Phys Ther 14:256–262, 1991   9–12

Introduction.—The underlying cause of patellofemoral pain syndrome
(PFPS) is malalignment of the patellofemoral joint. The components of
the quadriceps muscle that influence patellar alignment are the vastus
medialis obliques (VMO) and the vastus lateralis (VL). An alteration in
the activation pattern or strength of the VMO and the VL may disrupt
the muscular balance between the 2 muscles. Effects of arc of motion,
angular velocity, and contraction type on the VMO:VL absolute averaged
EMG (AAEMG) ratio were investigated.

Methods.—Electromyography data from the VMO and VL was obtained as 30 individuals performed maximum concentric and eccentric
isokinetic quadriceps muscle contractions on a dynamometer at velocities of 60 and 120 degrees per second. A VMO:VL AAEMG ratio was
calculated for all combinations of the 3 independent variables.

Results.—The performance of isokinetic exercise through a 60–85—
degree arc of motion and at a faster angular velocity may be more effective than a more extended arc of motion or a slower angular velocity in
activating the VMO. An increase in patellofemoral contact force concomitant with an increase in patellofemoral contact area may function to
minimize changes in patellofemoral contact pressure as the knee is
flexed. Exercises prescribed to treat PFPS should avoid increased patellofemoral contact pressure and not necessarily increased patellofemoral
contact force. Concentric exercise performed at a faster angular velocity
may be beneficial on the basis of decreased patellofemoral contact force
and relatively greater VMO:VL EMG ratios elicited. Contingent on the
angular velocity of the contraction, concentric isokinetic contractions
may produce a significantly greater VMO:VL EMG ratio than an eccentric isokinetic contraction. Isokinetic exercise to activate and strengthen
the VMO must be specific for angular velocity and type of muscle contraction.

Conclusion.—Isokinetic exercise through a 60–85 degree arc of motion may be more effective than isokinetic exercise through a more extended arc of motion in producing a greater VMO:VL EMG ratio. Concentric isokinetic exercise at 120 degrees per second may be more
effective than concentric isokinetic exercise at 60 degrees per second or

eccentric isokinetic exercise at 120 degrees per second in producing a greater VMO:VL EMG ratio. Producing a greater VMO:VL EMG ratio may be effective in altering a muscular imbalance between the VMO and VL in patients with PFPS. Further clinical studies should investigate if specific isokinetic exercise parameters identified in this study influence the VMO:VL EMG ratio and symptoms of patients with PFPS.

▶ Please read Abstract 9–11 and my comments regarding taping and exercise for patients with patellofemoral pain. The authors of Abstract 9–12 reinforce the importance of VMO:VL ratio for patients with PF pain. They recommend exercising isometrically through an arc of motion of 60–85 degrees, concentrating at 120 degrees per second to increase the VMO:VL ratio. Clinically, our goal is to reduce the pain of patients with PFPS. This is done by increasing VMO strength and improving tracking of the patella.—F.J. George, A.T.C., P.T.

Magnetic Resonance Imaging of the Foot and Ankle: Correlation of Normal Anatomy With Pathologic Conditions

Ferkel RD, Flannigan BD, Elkins BS (Valley Presbyterian Hosp, Van Nuys, Calif; Univ of California, San Francisco)
Foot Ankle 11:289–305, 1991   9–13

Introduction.—Magnetic resonance imaging offers a possible alternative to conventional radiography in diagnosing abnormalities of the foot and ankle. To define the normal MR anatomy 110 normal feet and ankles were examined, and 150 scans were obtained to characterize various abnormalities. Slices 3 mm thick were acquired with a 1-mm interslice gap.

The Ankle.—Medially, a retracted tendon can be identified in patients with rupture. Tenosynovitis is recognized as fluid within a tendon or sheath. A range of Achilles tendon abnormalities is seen on MRI. Insertional tendinitis presents as focal high-signal intensity at the site of insertion of the distal Achilles tendon. Laterally, ligament disruption can be recognized, as well as accumulation of debris or a meniscoid type lesion in the anterolateral gutter producing anterolateral impingement syndrome. Centrally, the most common pathology includes osteochondral lesions of the talus, loose bodies, and avascular necrosis of the talus.

The Foot.—Magnetic resonance imaging of the foot has demonstrated angiosarcoma, ganglion cysts, plantar fibromatosis, and osteomyelitis.

Technical.—Oblique-angle imaging often allows a structure to be seen entirely on a single slice rather than having to piece it together. It is necessary in examining this region to use thin slices with small gaps. Current head and knee coils provide good spatial resolution, but dedicated foot and ankle coils are expected to provide even better images.

▶ This is an excellent anatomical study.—J.S. Torg, M.D.

Fracture of the Medial Sesamoid Bone of the Great Toe: Controversies in Therapy
Weiss JS (Univ of Massachusetts Med Ctr)
Orthopedics 14:1003–1007, 1991   9–14

Introduction.—A fractured sesamoid is difficult to diagnose. Individuals with high arches and long first metatarsals, who engage in activities that result in chronic repeated stress to the forefoot, have a greater risk of fracturing their sesamoid.

Case Report.—Woman, 32, experienced sudden pain in the ball of her right foot while jumping during a high impact aerobics class. She continued with her normal activities after anteroposterior and lateral radiographs of the foot were normal. An orthopedist diagnosed a ligamentous injury and told the woman that pain would be prolonged during healing. When severe pain recurred 2 months later, she returned to the orthopedist. A radiograph at this time showed a nondisplaced fracture of the right medial sesamoid. No healing had occurred after 6 weeks of using a controlled ankle motion walker. A second orthopedist recommended a nonweight-bearing short leg cast and crutches for 6 weeks. No healing was seen when the cast was removed 18 weeks after the initial injury. A bivalve cast was used for an additional 12 weeks, with naproxen prescribed for pain. The patient was able to walk with marked reduction in pain 6 months after the injury.

Conclusion.—Pain may arise suddenly or insidiously with a fractured sesamoid. Tenderness on physical examination may fall short of the patient's subjective symptoms, and diagnosis cannot be based on physical findings alone. Initial foot films may not show fractures of the sesamoid; thus, additional films or a bone scan are often necessary. Improper treatment may result in prolonged and debilitating pain, yet the optimal treatment for this injury is controversial.

▶ To determine the proper therapeutic modalities for problems involving the sesamoids of the great toe, an accurate diagnosis is a prerequisite. Specifically, it must determine if one is dealing with symptomatic bipartite sesamoid, acute fracture of the sesamoid, or stress fracture of the sesamoid. With regard to symptomatic bipartite sesamoids, we believe that these can be treated conservatively with a relief "donut" pad. Acute fractures on the other hand, should heal with non–weight-bearing immobilization from 4 to 6 weeks. It is generally accepted that stress fractures of the sesamoid that fail to respond to conservative treatment may necessitate surgical extirpation.—J.S. Torg, M.D.

Chronic Compartment Syndrome of Both Feet
Lokiec F, Siev-Ner I, Pritsch M (Sheba Med Ctr, Tel Hashomer, Israel; Israel Dance Medicine Ctr, Tel Aviv, Israel)
J Bone Joint Surg 73-B:178–179, 1991   9–15

Introduction.—Compartment syndromes of the foot have been reported, but only related to acute injury. Chronic compartment syndrome of both feet was found in a professional ballet dancer.

Case Report.—Man, 18 years, complained of pain in both feet. The pain began after 10 min of warm-up exercise and eased after 10 min rest. It had gradually worsened over its 6-month' duration, and had interrupted the patient's dancing. Examination showed swelling of the medial aspects of both midfeet. Swelling became tender, tense, and cyanosed after strenuous exercise, but all symptoms subsided after rest. Magnetic resonance imaging showed hypertrophy of all muscles of the medial and central compartments of both feet; bone scans and radiographs were normal. Using a 20-in indwelling catheter, pressure measurements of 80 mmHg in the central compartments and 35 mmHg in the medial compartments were recorded, after vigorous exercise, much higher than the

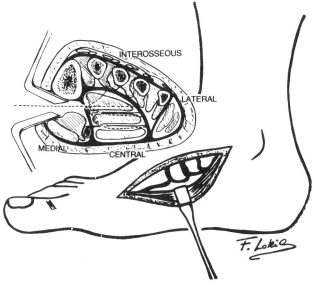

Fig 9–9.—A 5-cm incision along the medial aspect of the midfoot allowed good exposure of the medial and central compartments. Bilateral decompressive fasciotomy was performed by incision of the medial extension of the plantar fascia and the intermuscular septum laterally, relieving pressure in both compartments. (Courtesy of Lokiec F, Siev-Ner I, Pritsch M: *J Bone Joint Surg* 73-B:178-179, 1991.)

10 mmHg recorded in all compartments at rest. After exercise, the pressures gradually returned to resting levels.

A bilateral decompression fasciotomy was performed through a 5 cm incision along the medial aspect of the midfoot just under the proximal half of the first metatarsal (Fig 9–9). This approach permitted easy access to the medial and central compartments. Incision of the medial extension of the plantar fascia and the intermuscular septum laterally relieved both compartments. Recovery was complete, including return to full ballet activity.

Discussion.—Although no other cases of chronic compartment syndrome of the foot have apparently been reported, this condition may be commonly undiagnosed rather than rare. As with all reported cases of compartment syndromes of the foot related to acute injury, treatment of this patient with decompressive fasciotomy relieved symptoms. Chronic compartment syndrome should be considered in the differential diagnosis of foot complaints in athletes and dancers.

▶ The authors have presented what is certainly an interesting and unusual condition. Although, not at the top of the list of differential diagnoses in dancers and other athletes with foot pain, certainly chronic compartment syndrome of the foot should be a consideration.—J.S. Torg, M.D.

Stress Avulsion Fracture of the Tarsal Navicular: An Uncommon Sports-related Overuse Injury
Orava S, Karpakka J, Hulkko A, Takala T (Deaconess Inst of Oulu; Univ of Oulu, Oulu; Keski-Pohjanmaa Central Hosp, Kokkola, Finland)
Am J Sports Med 19:392–395, 1991   9–16

Introduction.—Overuse injuries to the foot are common exertional injuries. Stress fractures of the tarsal navicular, usually seen in athletes engaged in sports involving sprinting and jumping, are rare. Data on 9 patients treated for stress-related avulsion fractures of the superior corner of the tarsal navicular in 1980–1989 were reviewed.

Methods.—The patients sought medical attention because of long-lasting midfoot pain. Radiologic assessments using anteroposterior and oblique nonweight-bearing and lateral weightbearing radiographs helped establish the diagnosis (Fig 9–10). Isotope scan and/or tomography findings confirmed the diagnoses.

Results.—In 4 patients, treatment was conservative, and 5 were treated surgically. Those treated conservatively had the shortest delay of diagnosis from symptom onset. Conservative treatment consisted of rest from athletic activities and orthoses or thick-soled athletic shoes. Local corticosteroid injections were given in 3 patients with painful injuries. In those treated surgically, all loose fragments were excised. In 2 patients, the involved area was drilled. Ankle and foot exercises were started 3 weeks after surgery, and return to sports was allowed 5–6 weeks later.

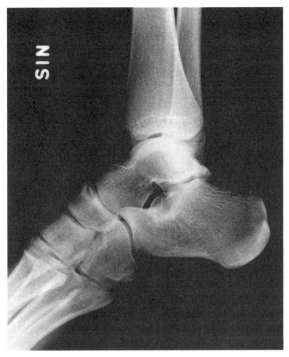

Fig 9–10.—Stress fracture of the proximal superior corner of the navicular bone. The lesion simulates osteochondritis dissecans (preoperative radiograph). (Courtesy of Orava S, Karpakka J, Hulkko A, et al: *Am J Sports Med* 19:392–395, 1991.)

Both conservatively and surgically treated groups had good results, defined as full return to preinjury levels of sports activity. There were no complications.

Conclusion.—This uncommon injury is believed to result from repetitive cyclic compressive loading secondary to an impingement of the tarsal navicular. The small dorsal triangular fragment is visualized best on weightbearing lateral view radiographs. Isotope scan and/or tomography help confirm the diagnosis. Surgery appears to be the method of choice in highly symptomatic patients and for top athletes because the recovery time is shorter.

▶ The most characteristic stress fracture of the tarsal navicular, located in the central one third of the bone and oriented in the sagittal plane, has been described as being either partial or complete (1). This fracture uniformly responds to conservative non–weight-bearing treatment and rarely, if ever, requires surgery. The less common dorsal transverse fragment, described as a "stress avulsion fracture" by Orava et al. requires surgical extirpation in the symptomatic patient. The dorsal transverse fragment may be associated with a sagittal fracture and persistent symptoms following healing of the former are due to the presence of this dorsal transverse fragment.—J.S. Torg, M.D.

Reference

1. Torg JS, et al: *J Bone Joint Surg* 63-A:700, 1982.

Tarsal Tunnel Syndrome in Athletes: Case Reports and Literature Review
Jackson DA, Haglund B (Univ of Kentucky)
Am J Sports Med 19:61–65, 1991   9–17

Introduction.—Tarsal tunnel syndrome is associated with foot pain and paresthesias and has only recently been reported in the literature and identified. Two patients with the syndrome were studied.

Case 1.—Woman, 39, experienced foot pain, numbness, and weakness while on a ski trip. Examination revealed a positive Tinel's sign over the tarsal tunnel at the level of the medial malleolus on the affected foot, and abnormal nerve conduction of the medial and lateral plantar nerves was also detected on the affected side. After treatment with NSAIDs, steroid injection into the tarsal tunnel, and physical therapy with ultrasound and a strengthening program, the patient had a good recovery and no further complaints.

Case 2.—Woman, 42, was a runner with foot pain and numbness. Tinel's sign at the medial malleolus was positive, bilateral plano-valgus deformities were noted, and decreased sensation to sharp/dull and light touch was found along the plantar aspect of the affected foot. Lateral plantar nerve distal latency was not obtainable on the affected side. After a 6-week course of therapy consisting of NSAIDs, steroid injection into the tarsal tunnel, and custom-made orthotics, the patient returned to running without complaint.

Discussion.—Abnormal foot mechanics appear to cause the tarsal tunnel syndrome in runners. Electrodiagnostic studies, electromyographic studies, and complete roentgenographic work-up should be completed in any patient with foot pain, numbness, and weakness. Treatment with NSAIDs, steroid injections, flexibility exercises, and custom-made orthotics will usually be helpful.

▶ This paper presents an excellent description of the tarsal tunnel syndrome and is strongly recommended to those caring for athletes. Symptoms include pain at the medial malleolus radiating to the sole of the foot, the heel, and sometimes the calf. There are associated paresthesias, diasthesias, and hypasthesias with worsening of symptoms at night, with walking, and with dorsiflexion of the foot. Also noted are weakness of toe flexion, increased fatigue of the foot, and trophic changes of the foot and nails. Numbness and burning paresthesias in the plantar aspect of the foot and toes, which radiate up into the leg, may occur. Although the actual incidence of this syndrome is unknown, it should be considered of all athletes complaining of foot pain. The authors point out that it must be differentiated from plantar fasciitis, which tends to cause more heel pain at the origin of the plantar fascia, whereas tarsal tunnel syndrome tends to produce more medial heel and arch pain. Also, pain caused by plantar fasciitis may improve with stretching and gradual running, whereas tarsal tunnel symptoms worsen with running.—J.S. Torg, M.D.

Os Trigonum Syndrome: A Clinical Entity in Ballet Dancers
Wredmark T, Carlstedt CA, Bauer H, Saartok T (Karolinska Inst, Huddinge Univ Hosp, Huddinge; Karolinska Inst, Stockholm, Sweden)
Foot Ankle 11:404–406, 1991   9–18

Introduction.—Ballet dancers often stand on the tips of their toes after forceful plantar flexion of the foot. Posterior impingement pain in the ankle can reflect a posterior bony block by an os trigonum, an accessory bone present in about 1 of 10 ankles, which ordinarily does not produce symptoms.

Methods.—In 9 female and 4 male dancers aged 14–31 years, there was progressive pain and soreness behind the medial malleolus of the ankle while dancing. None had a history of acute trauma to the involved ankle. The symptoms developed gradually and were treated conservatively.

Surgery.—The os trigonum was removed after incising the tendon sheath of the flexor hallucis longus longitudinally. If a prominent lateral posterior process of the talus was noted, an ostectomy was performed. If the tendon or sheath was thickened, the sheath incision was extended in both directions.

Results.—Symptoms resolved in all but 1 of the patients who were able to return to performance dancing after a mean of 7 weeks. At a mean of 22 months after surgery, 12 dancers were performing at the same level.

Conclusion.—A symptomatic os trigonum in a ballet dancer can be effectively treated operatively. Removal of an os trigonum or the lateral posterior process of the talus does not impede classical ballet dancing.

▶ The authors' conclusion that "progressive symptoms of pain in the posterior area of the ankle in ballet dancers can be due to an os trigonum syndrome, and that this can be successfully treated with surgery" is in keeping with my own clinical experience.—J.S. Torg, M.D.

Posterior Tibial Tendon Rupture in Athletic People
Woods L, Leach RE (Boston Univ)
Am J Sports Med 19:495–498, 1991   9–19

Introduction.—Tendon inflammation is becoming more frequent as more athletes train for extended periods. Peroneus muscles are involved less often than the Achilles tendon.

Patients.—Surgery was necessary for 6 athletes of varying age with chronic posterior tibial tendon problems. In 3 patients there was a total rupture of the posterior tibial tendon. In 3 others there was a partially intact but dysfunctional tendon that was partially ruptured and chronically inflamed (Fig 9-11). In 5 patients, diagnosis was made at a late stage, compromising their ability to return to athletic activity. In the remaining patient, the condition was diagnosed before the longitudinal arch became flattened, with an excellent outcome. The partial ruptures required only removal of damaged tissue and side-to-side repair.

Recommendations.—Early diagnosis is the key to successfully treating these injuries. A patient with chronic posterior tibial tendinitis who fails to respond to conservative treatment may do well after débridement of the tendon and opening of the tendon sheath. Tendon advancement or transfer may relieve pain from total tendon rupture, but flatfoot deformity will remain and may impede a return to athletic activity at the former level.

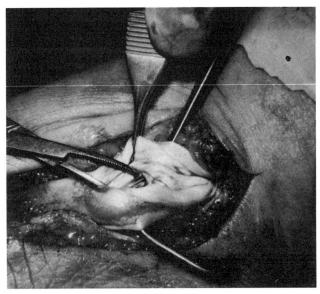

Fig 9–11.—Degenerative tear of posterior tibial tendon. (Courtesy of Woods L, Leach RE: *Am J Sports Med* 19:495–498, 1991.)

▶ The point that "loss of function of the posterior tibial tendon may be devastating to the athlete and nonathlete alike" is well taken. It has been my own experience that partial and complete ruptures of the posterior tibial tendon occur infrequently and when they do, they present a diagnostic challenge. A recent paper by Rosenberg et al, has established the role of MRI in dealing with this problem (1). They concluded that MRI is the method of choice for detecting posterior tibial tendon ruptures having a sensitivity of 95% and a specificity of 100%.—J.S. Torg, M.D.

Reference

1. Rosenberg ZS, et al: *Radiology* 169:229, 1988.

Arthroscopic Treatment of Anterolateral Impingement of the Ankle
Ferkel RD, Karzel RP, Del Pizzo W, Friedman MJ, Fischer SP (Southern California Orthopedic Inst, Van Nuys, Calif)
Am J Sports Med 19:440–446, 1991   9–20

Introduction.—The cause of chronic lateral ankle pain after inversion injury is often difficult to establish, especially when the ankle is stable. This condition has been labelled "anterolateral impingement of the ankle."

Clinical Features.—A group of 31 patients with this diagnosis was studied. None of the patients had fractures; the average age was 34 years. All patients had sustained a "sprain" injury, and 6 patients had multiple sprains before the most recent major event. A sprain was fol-

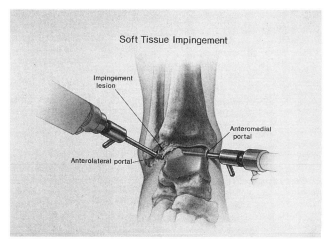

Fig 9–12.—Arthroscopic visualization of hypertrophic soft tissue in lateral gutter. (From Ferkel RD: Ankle arthroscopy, in *An Illustrated Guide to Small Joint Arthroscopy*. Andover, Mass, Dyonics Inc, 1989. Courtesy of Ferkel RD, Karzel RP, Del Pizzo W, et al: *Am J Sports Med* 19:440–446, 1991.)

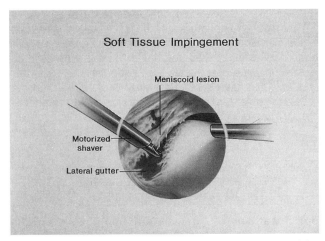

Fig 9–13.—Débridement of soft tissue is performed arthroscopically. (From Ferkel RD: Ankle arthroscopy, in *An Illustrated Guide to Small Joint Arthroscopy.* Andover, Mass, Dyonics Inc, 1989. Courtesy of Ferkel RD, Karzel RP, Del Pizzo W, et al: *Am J Sports Med* 19:440-446, 1991.)

lowed most often by persistent ankle pain on walking, weakness, and a sensation of giving way. Localized tenderness was present at the antero-lateral gutter of the ankle.

Management.—All of the patients received conservative treatment for a prolonged period. Arthroscopic surgery was done an average of 2 years after injury; a distractor was used only when necessary. The abnormalities were confined primarily to the lateral side and included synovitis and scar tissue (Fig 9–12). Hypertrophic soft tissue was débrided (Fig 9–13) and, when necessary, chondroplasty of the talus was performed.

Outcome.—Synovial hyperplasia and subsynovial capillary proliferation were constant findings; many patients also had hyaline cartilage degeneration and fibrosis. Follow-up at an average of 33 months postoperatively revealed excellent results in 15 patients, good results in 11, and fair results in 4; only 1 patient had a poor outcome.

Conclusion.—Arthroscopic surgery relieves pain and disability caused by anterolateral impingement of the ankle in a high proportion of patients who fail to respond to conservative treatment.

▶ There can be no question that chronic pain following injury and/or surgery to the ankle occurs with great frequency. In addition to what the authors describe as anterolateral impingement, they also attribute chronic ankle pain to result from chronic instability, osteochondral lesions of the talus, calcific ossicles beneath the malleoli, peroneal sublaxation, dislocation or tear, tarsal coalition, subtalor joint dysfunction, and degenerative joint disease. Also included in the differential are sinus tarsus syndrome, anterior capsular impingement, anterior lateral corner compression syndrome, and meniscoid lesion. To put things in perspective, the authors point out in a 6-year period they treated approximately 2,000 patients for ankle sprains, of which 43, or 2%, were diagnosed as having anterolateral impingement. They emphasize that the diagnosis is predicated on the absence of ligamentous laxity or instability and the presence of "moderate synovial hyperplasia." Also of note, 50% of the patients were observed to have lateral talor dome chondromalacia. It appears to this observer what they are actually describing is what we term the incompletely rehabilitated ankle, an entity that responds to an intraarticular steroid injection and appropriate active dorsiflexion exercises. The failure to delineate their preoperative physical therapy program leaves in question the necessity for surgical intervention.—J.S. Torg, M.D.

Syndesmotic Ankle Sprains
Boytim MJ, Fischer DA, Neumann L (Braemar Sports Medicine Ctr, Minneapolis)
Am J Sports Med 19:294–298, 1991   9–21

Introduction.—Ankle sprains require accurate diagnosis for proper treatment and recovery period. The syndesmotic sprain is less common than the lateral ankle sprain and requires more treatment and prolonged recovery time. It is important for the sports physician or trainer to recognize the difference between these 2 types of ankle sprains.

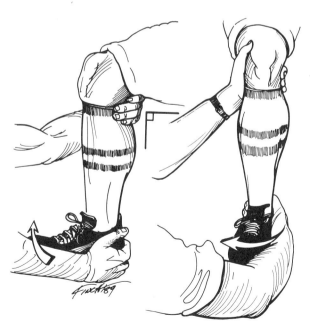

Fig 9–14.—External rotation stress test is applied to ankle in neutral position with knee flexed 90 degrees. (Courtesy of Boytim MJ, Fischer DA, Neumann L: *Am J Sports Med* 19:294–298, 1991.)

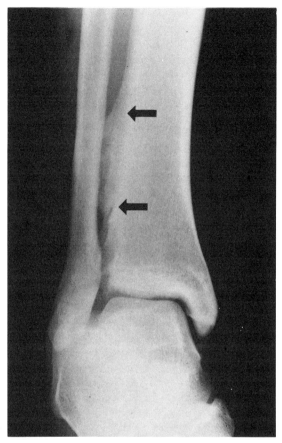

Fig 9–15.—Interosseous calcification (*arrows*) seen 4 months after injury. None was present in original postinjury radiograph. (Courtesy of Boytim MJ, Fischer DA, Neumann L: *Am J Sports Med* 19:294-298, 1991.)

Data Analysis.—Fifteen professional football players (Minnesota Vikings) who sustained syndesmotic ankle sprains during a 6-year period were studied and compared to 28 players with significant lateral ankle sprains. Syndesmotic ankle sprains were distinguished from inversion sprains by a history of external rotation injury, tenderness over the syndesmosis or posterior tibiofibular ligament, and also tenderness over the anterior tibiofibular ligament proximal to the anterior talofibular ligament. The external rotation stress test allowed a more specific diagnosis of syndesmotic ankle sprains. The knee was held at 90 degrees of flexion and the ankle was in a neutral position while external rotation stress was applied to the involved foot and ankle (Fig 9–14). Pain over the anterior or posterior tibiofibular ligaments and over the interosseous membrane was a positive indication.

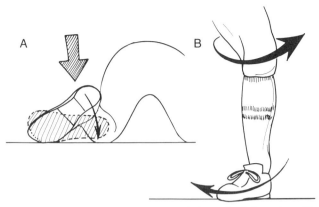

Fig 9–16.—Mechanisms of external rotation sustained during football. **A,** direct blow to leg of downed player whose foot was held in external rotation. **B,** force applied to lateral aspect of knee while player's foot was planted in external rotation. (Courtesy of Boytim MJ, Fischer DA, Neumann L: *Am J Sports Med* 19:294–298, 1991.)

Results.—Roentgenograms taken at least 1 month after injury in 6 of 8 players demonstrated calcification of the interosseous membrane (Fig 9–15), which was not visible on immediate postinjury roentgenograms. Players with syndesmotic sprains missed significantly more games and practices and received significantly more treatment than players with lateral sprains. Treatment modalities included cryotherapy, exercise, contrast bath, massage, ultrasound, injection, whirlpool, electric stimulation, and transcutaneous electric nerve stimulation.

Discussion.—A significant force is most likely necessary to produce syndesmotic sprains (Fig 9–16), which are not often seen in basketball or running but in collision sports such as football, hockey, and, sometimes, soccer. The external rotation stress test that creates pain in the anterolateral aspect of the leg well proximal to the ankle joint is a good indication of severe ankle injury. Physicians and trainers should recognize the long recuperation period for syndesmotic sprains.

▶ This is an excellent paper that describes the pathomechanics and salient clinical features of syndesmotic ankle sprains. I fully agree with the authors that physical examination is the key to diagnosis. They point out that "an external rotation stress test causes pain in the anterior lateral aspect of the leg, well proximal to the ankle and is indicative of a severe injury." Also pointed out is that prolonged recovery can be anticipated. The authors make it quite clear that the purpose of the report deals with diagnosis rather than treatment of syndesmotic sprains. Hopefully, their next endeavor with this problem will be to deal with treatment parameters.—J.S. Torg, M.D.

Long-Term Results of the Evans Procedure for Lateral Instability of the Ankle

Korkala O, Tanskanen P, Mäkijärvi J, Sorvali T, Ylikoski M, Haapala J (Lahti City Hosp, Lahti, Finland)
J Bone Joint Surg 73-B:96–99, 1991   9–22

Introduction.—Severe ankle sprains left untreated or treated inadequately are often complicated by persistent lateral instability. The long-term results of the Evans procedure for lateral instability of the ankle were reviewed.

Methods.—A modified Evans procedure was used to treat 42 consecutive ankles. A static tenodesis was fashioned using the peroneus brevis tendon. The patients were followed up for 9–12 years; 40 ankles were available for review.

Results.—Results were excellent or good in 33 (82.5%) ankles, fair in 3, and poor in 4. These clinical findings were matched by the radiographic findings, which showed significant talar tilt or anterior talar translation in 3 ankles only. Functional results were not correlated with the stress-radiographic analysis (Fig 9–17).

Conclusion.—The modified Evans procedure appears to be simple and safe. It can be performed through 2 small incisions. There is no

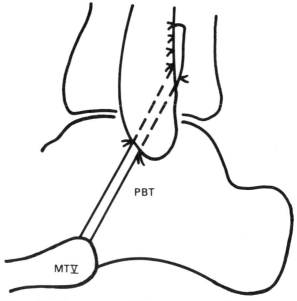

Fig 9–17.—The modified Evans operation. *PBT* indicates peroneus brevis tendon; *MTV*, fifth metatarsal. (Courtesy of Korkala O, Tanskanen P, Mäkajärvi J, et al: *J Bone Joint Surg* 73-B:96–99, 1991.)

damage to the talus. The tendon is not vulnerable to rupture at the sharp edges of the bony tunnel, as it is not acutely angulated.

Reconstruction of Lateral Ligaments of the Ankle With Allogeneic Tendon Grafts
Horibe S, Shino K, Taga I, Inoue M, Ono K (Osaka Univ, Japan)
J Bone Joint Surg 73-B:802–805, 1991   9–23

Introduction.—The lateral ankle ligaments are commonly injured in sports. Many ligamentous reconstruction procedures have been proposed, all of which sacrifice normal tissue and result in nonanatomical ligaments. In 17 patients, allogeneic tendon grafts were used to reconstruct the ligaments in an anatomical fashion.

Technique.—Fresh frozen allogeneic toe flexor or extensor tendon, or both, from amputation specimens are used as the graft material. The anterior talofibular (ATFL) and calcaneofibular (CFL) ligaments are exposed. If the ATFL alone is to be reconstructed, 2 holes 4.5 mm in diameter are drilled, 7 from the fibular attachment to the posterior aspect of the distal fibula and the other from the talar attachment to the medial aspect of the talus. If the CFL is also to be reconstructed, the fibular hole is drilled to half-depth from the fibular attachment of the ATFL and likewise from the fibular attachment of the CFL. Another hole is made from the calcaneal attachment of the CFL to the medial aspect of the calcaneus. The tendon grafts are thawed and prepared with 3 polyester sutures (1-0) at each end, which are passed through the drill holes and tied over buttons under tension. The ankle is immobilized in a below-knee cast, full weight-bearing is allowed at 6 weeks, and sports are allowed at 5 months.

Patients.—A total of 17 patients with a mean age of 23 years underwent this operation. Thirteen returned for follow-up examination. Ten had ATFL repair only, and 3 had CFL repair as well. There we no infections or rejections. Nine patients had excellent and 4 had good results, with only mild pain during sports or strenuous work. Talar tilt and anterior drawer both decreased significantly after surgery. One patient had the button used for fixation removed at 6 months; the new tendon appeared taut and thick and showed a crimp pattern similar to that of a normal ligament.

Conclusions.—Allograft reconstruction of the lateral ligaments of the ankle is a new method of treatment which restores stability without sacrificing tendons. The procedure restores normal kinematics, and results are good to excellent. Immunologic rejection and, with sterile technique and cryopreservation, cross infection have not been problems.

▶ On the basis of my own clinical experience, I agree with Korkala et al. (Abstract 9–22) that in patients with symptomatic, 2-plane, ankle instability, reconstruction of the anterior-lateral supporting structures using the peroneus brevis tendon yields consistently satisfactory results. Because of possible HIV transmission, I would question the approach of Horibe et al. (Abstract 9–23) using allogenic tendon grafts.—J.S. Torg, M.D.

The Effects of Intermittent Compression on Edema in Postacute Ankle Sprains

Rucinski TJ, Hooker DN, Prentice WE Jr, Shields EW Jr, Cote-Murray DJ (Milwaukee County Med Complex-Sports Medicine Ctr; Univ of North Carolina at Chapel Hill)
J Orthop Sports Phys Ther 14:65–69, 1991   9–24

Background.—Ice, compression, and elevation are widely recognized as the standard treatment protocol to control edema in postacute ankle sprains. The effects of 3 treatment protocols on pitting edema in patients with first- and second-degree sprained ankles were compared.

Treatment.—Thirty subjects with postacute ankle sprains and pitting edema, which did not require cast immobilization or surgery, were treated. In all subjects, the ankles were elevated by raising the foot section of an adjustable table to a 45 degree angle during treatment. In 10 subjects, an elastic wrap was applied from the heads of the metatarsals to 12.7 cm above the malleoli. Another 10 subjects had intermittent compression, that was set at 40–50 mm Hg with a 60-second on time

Compression Effects on Ankle Volume

TREATMENT	VOLUME MEASUREMENT (mL) PRETREATMENT	POSTTREATMENT	CHANGE (mL) MEASUREMENT
Pump (n = 10)			
Mean	1222.0	1229.4	7.4
Standard Deviation	166.7	166.5	5.9
Standard Error	52.7	52.6	1.9
Wrap (n = 10)			
Mean	1340.2	1343.9	3.7
Standard Deviation	128.0	127.4	14.6
Standard Error	40.5	40.3	4.6
Control (n = 10)			
Mean	1350.4	1335.5	-14.9
Standard Deviation	201.6	203.2	13.7
Standard Error	63.8	64.3	4.3

Means, standard deviations, and standard errors of pretreatment and posttreatment ankle volume measurements and volume changes (N = 30).
(Courtesy of Rucinski TJ, Hooker DN, Prentice WE Jr, et al: *J Orthop Sports Phys Ther* 14:65–69, 1991.)

and a 15-second off time. The other 10 subjects received the elevation treatment only. Using the water-displacement method, volumetric measurement of the subjects' ankles were obtained before and after treatment.

Outcome.—Only the subjects who received elevation treatment alone had significant reduction in edema (table). Both elastic wrap and intermittent compression device increased the amount of edema in the subjects' sprained ankles after treatment.

Conclusion.—Elevation remains the most appropriate method to reduce edema in the postacute phase of rehabilitation of ankle sprains.

▶ Surprise! Surprise! Surprise! I have been a proponent of using compression in acute ankle sprains for many years. I have alternated frequently between compression and ice as to which of these I thought was most important to prevent or reduce edema. The authors of Abstract 9–24 have concluded that elevation is the most important factor in reducing edema. I won't give up the ice, but I will be sure to include the elevation and continue to use adhesive tape and a rigid ankle brace for compression and support. Please read Abstract 9–25 for related information.—F.J. George, A.T.C., P.T.

Treatment of the Inversion Ankle Sprain Through Synchronous Application of Focal Compression and Cold
Wilkerson GB (Trover Clinic, Madisonville, KY)
Athlet Train, JNATA 26:220–239, 1991   9–25

Background.—Edema may contribute to prolonged functional impairment after an inversion ankle sprain. When damaged ligaments are sufficiently protected from excessive tensile stress, early use of the ankle may greatly enhance the recovery rate. The treatment of inversion ankle sprains through synchronous application of focal compression and cold was evaluated.

Cryotherapy.—Contrary to popular belief, there is no scientific evidence supporting the theory that cryotherapy decreases edema immediately after injury. Cold may actually increase edema just after injury. However, immediate application of cold therapy may provide long-term benefits. Chilling may reduce secondary hypoxic injury to cells by decreasing their metabolism and oxygen needs. By this mechanism, early cryotherapy may reduce total tissue damage and, in turn, delay edema. Another hypothesis is that cold decreases the synthesis of prostaglandins.

Compression.—Clearly the most effective deterrent to edema is the early application and continuous use of external compression. Compression increases interstitial fluid pressure, which reduces outflow from capillaries and increases lymphatic drainage. Elevation complements the effects of compression. Focal compression consists of pressure on the

A

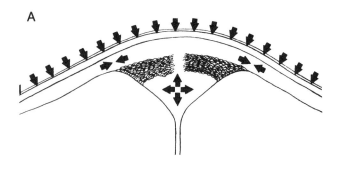

B

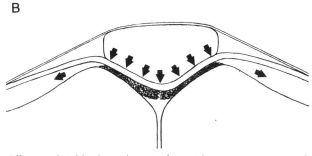

Fig 9–18.—Effects produced by the application of external compression over an edematous area that normally has a concave surface contour: (**A**) uniform compression; (**B**) focal compression. (Courtesy of Wilkerson GB: *Athlet Train, JNATA* 26:220–239, 1991.)

surface concavities. Adjacent proximal convex bony prominences are not compressed. This procedure greatly enhances the centripetal effect of collateral compression (Fig 9–18).

Conclusions.—Although many practitioners treat inversion ankle sprains with the combination of elastic wrap, periodic cold application, and avoidance of early weight-bearing, there is little scientific evidence to support this approach. Two interrelated factors appear to determine the rate of restoration of function: the exact mode of compression application, and the degree of protected use of the injured ankle in the early stages of recovery. Uniform circumferential compression and complete avoidance of early weight-bearing may adversely affect long-term outcomes. As long as injured ligaments are protected from excessive inversion stress, the combination of focal collateral compression, cold, and early functional weight-bearing may enhance long-term outcomes (Fig 9–19).

▶ "Clearly the most effective deterrent to edema is the early application and continuous use of external compression." That is the conclusion of the author of Abstract 9–25 and certainly an assumption I have been working un-

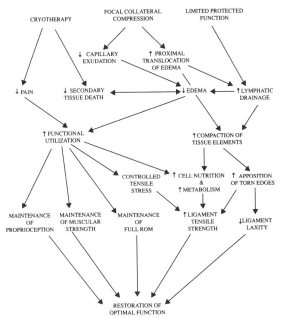

Fig 9–19.—Theoretical interrelationships among factors that may facilitate a rapid return to full ankle function and minimize susceptibility to reinjury. (Courtesy of Wilkerson GB: *Athlet Train, JNATA* 26:220–239, 1991.)

der for many years. However please read the conclusions of the authors of Abstract 9–24, who state, "elevation alone is superior to elastic wrapping and intermittent compression." As stated previously, I'll continue using ice, elevation, and adhesive tape for compression and support with a rigid ankle brace.—F.J. George, A.T.C., P.T.

Comparative Biomechanical Effects of the Standard Method of Ankle Taping and a Taping Method Designed to Enhance Subtalar Stability
Wilkerson GB (Trover Clinic, Madisonville, Ky)
Am J Sports Med 19:588–594, 1991   9–26

Objective.—Ankle taping, although never proven effective, is the most commonly used method for preventing ankle sprains and protecting previously injured ankle ligaments. The restriction of forced passive ankle motion by the standard method of taping was compared with that of a taping method incorporating a subtalar sling.

Subjects and Methods.—Thirty college football players had 1 ankle taped using the standard method and the other using the modified method. Measurements of 4 ankle motions were obtained for each foot

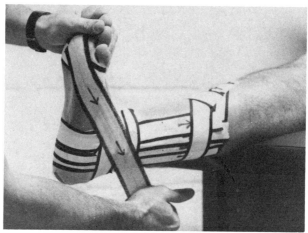

Fig 9–20.—Origin of the subtalar sling over the head of the second metatarsal (modified method). (Courtesy of Wilkerson GB: *Am J Sports Med* 19:588-594, 1991.)

before and immediately after taping, and after a 2–3 hour football practice.

Taping Technique.—The modified taping method differed from the standard method only by the addition of an extra component after application of the standard stirrup and horseshoe strips. This subtalar sling consisted of 2 strips with a course approximately perpendicular to the functional axis of the subtalar joint complex. The first strip was adhered to the plantar aspect of the forefoot over the head of the second metatarsal (Fig 9–20), passed over the central portion of the fibular malleolus,

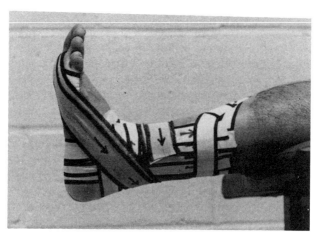

Fig 9–21.—Completed application of the subtalar sling component (modified method). (Courtesy of Wilkerson GB: *Am J Sports Med* 19:588-594, 1991.)

wrapped around the posterior aspect of the leg, and terminated on its anterolateral aspect. The second strip overlapped the first by about 75% of its width, following a course generally the same but slightly more posterior and inferior than the first (Fig 9–21). Short distal forestrips were used to pull the subtalar sling against the surface of the foot, and application of a continuous heel lock and circumferential strips completed the modified method.

Results.—Multiple statistical procedures showed that addition of the subtalar sling significantly enhanced protection against an inversion sprain. This benefit occurred at the expense of slightly increased restriction of plantar flexion. Tape applied in the standard method loosened during exercise more than the modified method and provided less restriction to both supination and inversion.

Conclusions.—The less restrictive standard method is probably the best choice for prophylactic use, due to performance considerations. However, for the protection or stabilization of ankles with injured ligaments or chronic instabilities, the disadvantages of the restrictive abilities of the subtalar sling may be outweighed by its advantages.

▶ We are always looking for a better way to tape injured ankles and add stability to lax ankles. I will certainly try the authors' subtalar sling (see Figs 9–20 and 9–21). In recent years I also added a lace-up ankle brace, which is made specifically for unstable ankles, over the completed tape application for even a more rigid vinyl support.—F.J. George, A.T.C., P.T.

Achilles Tendinitis: Don't Let It Be an Athlete's Downfall
Leach RE, Schepsis AA, Takai H (Boston Univ; Tokushima Univ, Tokushima, Japan)
Physician Sportsmed 19:87–92, 1991   9–27

Introduction.—The clinical manifestations, diagnosis, and treatment of Achilles tendinitis are examined.

Setting.—Achilles tendinitis is frequently associated with the chronic repetitive stresses of running and jumping sports. Fusiform swelling of the tendon may be the only physical finding in many patients. Another common finding is loss of passive dorsiflexion of the foot (Fig 9–22). Diagnostic imaging procedures may show calcification and inflammation.

Treatment.—There is no quick cure for Achilles tendinitis. Conservative treatment remains effective, and it includes rest or significant reduction in activity, moderate stretching to increase passive dorsiflexion of the foot, light progressive-resistance exercises for the calf muscles, and nonsteroidal anti-inflammatory drugs. Maximum benefit from slow, controlled stretching can be achieved in 5 or 6 stretches. Activity should be reduced during nonsteroidal anti-inflammatory drug therapy. Providing

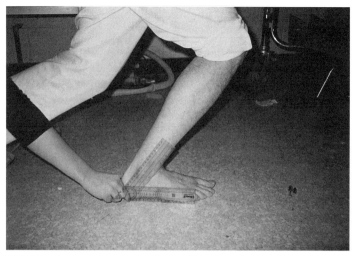

Fig 9–22.—How to measure passive dorsiflexion: Have the patient step forward, keeping the toes pointed straight ahead. Instruct the patient to keep the heel flat on the floor and flex the knee and ankle as much as possible. Subtract the resulting angle between the tibia and the foot from 90 degrees to determine the degree of passive dorsiflexion. (Courtesy of Leach RE, Schepsis AA, Takai H: *Physician Sportsmed* 19:87–92, 1991.)

orthoses or changing shoes does not produce a quick cure for Achilles tendinitis. Surgical treatment remains an option among patients who are still limited by pain after 6 months of conservative management. Surgery can be performed for patients with localized fusiform swelling, those with generalized involvement of the tendon sheath and tendon, and those with retrocalcaneal bursitis and associated tendinitis.

▶ The authors have described an innovative method of measuring ankle dorsiflexion (see Fig 9–22). They also state that "rest from running and jumping benefits virtually all Achilles tendinitis patients. The patient who has short-term but acute symptoms is much more likely to benefit from rest for 3 to 6 weeks." They also recommend slow, controlled stretching, which decreases stress on the Achilles tendon. Maximum benefit is attained in 5 or 6 stretches when done below the limits of pain. We also advise all our Achilles tendinitis patients to never walk in their bare feet and to always use a shoe with a heel lift.—F.J. George, A.T.C., P.T.

Sensations of Cold Reexamined: A Study Using the McGill Pain Questionnaire

Ingersoll CD, Mangus BC (Sports Injury Research Ctr, Univ of Nevada, Las Vegas)

Athletic Training 26:240–245, 1991   9–28

Introduction.—When an athlete is to receive cold applications, it is customary to describe what he can expect to feel. A wide range of sensations are described in cryokinetics, including a recognition of cooling, burning, aching, and relative cutaneous analgesia or anesthesia.

Methods.—A modified version of the McGill Pain Questionnaire was used to elicit descriptions of cold-induced sensation from 28 normal persons of both sexes with an average age of 21 years. A 21-minute foot-angle immersion in a 2°C ice bath was followed by a 21-minute recovery period.

Results.—The 23 persons who completed the study most often mentioned freezing, a penetrating feeling, sharpness, stinging, cold, numbness, tingling, and coolness.

Conclusion.—Burning and aching, descriptors typically used to describe cold-induced pain, were infrequently chosen in this study. The period typically associated with numbness, 7 to 20 minutes, was dominated by reports of stinging, freezing, and cold. It may, in fact, not be possible to provide athletes with a concise and accurate list of descriptors to define cold-related pain. It is, however, appropriate to confirm that pain will become less intense over time.

▶ What do you tell an athlete when you are about to immerse an injury in a cold water whirlpool or place an ice pack on them? What type of sensation are they about to experience? Tell them that it will hurt, but the pain will diminish as the treatment time progresses. Usually the first cryokinetic treatment produces the most pain. After 1 treatment the athlete usually tolerates subsequent treatments with considerably less discomfort.—F.J. George, A.T.C., P.T.

The CO_2 Laser in Arthroscopy: Potential Problems and Solutions
Garrick JG, Kadel N (Saint Francis Mem Hosp, San Francisco)
Arthroscopy 7:129–137, 1991   9–29

Introduction.—The use of lasers in both general and specialized surgery has increased over the past 2 decades. Since 1988, when the Food and Drug Administration approved the laser for arthroscopy, at least 5,000 procedures have involved the CO_2 laser. Some of the potential problems encountered with use of the CO_2 laser in arthroscopy were reviewed.

Problems.—Lasers are known for their considerable destructive capabilities, but medical lasers are chosen for their precision. Damage to unintended targets is usually superficial and clinical consequences appear to be minor. The major potential complication in arthroscopy involves the gas medium. Because CO_2 laser energy is invisible, an additional red, helium-neon laser is coupled coaxially with the CO_2 laser. Escape of gas from the confines of the joint is the only documented significant complication associated with the CO_2 laser in arthroscopy. The vaporization of tissue results in carbonization (charring). The charred material obscures visualization of the target and reduces the effectiveness of the laser. Charring can be minimized by pulsing the laser. Tissue vaporization also results in a plume of smoke, most easily cleared by using active suction throughout the procedure. A potentially dangerous problem is the inadvertent activation of the laser. The CO_2 lasers used in arthroscopy are turned on and off with a foot pedal. Because the surgeon cannot easily tell when the laser has been activated, an audible tone accompanying laser activation is recommended to solve this problem. Safety concerns require that a thoroughly trained, experienced nurse be present during laser surgery.

Conclusion.—Lasers are used with increasing frequency during arthroscopic surgery, despite a lack of compelling clinical or biomedical advantages associated with the procedure. The CO_2 laser appears to offer increased visibility and precision, improved hemostasis, and enhanced access of difficult-to-reach structures.

▶ The authors' failure to explicity delineate indications, criteria for use, and results of laser arthroscopic surgery indicates that perhaps the role of the laser in arthroscopic surgery remains a treatment looking for a disease.—J.S. Torg, M.D.

Septic Bursitis: Experience in a Community Practice
Pien FD, Ching D, Kim E (Univ of Hawaii-John A Burns School of Medicine; Straub Clinic and Hosp, Honolulu)
Orthopedics 14:981–984, 1991   9–30

Introduction.—Septic bursitis is an uncommon and usually benign condition, but can require prolonged treatment and hospitalization. Data were reviewed on 47 episodes of septic bursitis in 42 patients treated in 1979–1988. Approximately half of the patients were treated on an outpatient basis with antibiotics alone.

Patients.—Most (72%) infections occurred in the olecranon bursa. Prepatellar bursitis accounted for only 28% of the cases, but these patients were more likely to be hospitalized. About half of the patients had previous trauma of the infected bursa or an occupation involving frequent pressure to the bursa. Surrounding cellulitis was present in 18 patients.

Results.—*Staphylococcus aureus* was aspirated from 70% of bursal fluid aspirations. Other etiologic organisms included gram negative bacteria and *Mycobacterium marinum*. Bursal cell counts and crystal analysis were important in differentiating non-infectious causes of inflammatory bursitis. Those requiring hospitalization were primarily febrile with severe prepatellar bursitis in need of bursal drainage. Aggressive oral antibiotic therapy was given to outpatients for at least 4 weeks. Incision and drainage were done only when bursitis did not respond to at least 1 aspiration. The need for therapeutic drainage was variable and appeared to depend on the severity and site of infection.

Conclusion.—Septic bursitis can be refractory to therapy in immunocompromised patients. In others, however, the condition is often successfully treated with antibiotics on an outpatient basis. All of these patients were eventually cured without serious complications.

▶ It is my belief that a septic bursitis, whether involving olecranon or prepatella bursa, should be treated aggressively with open drainage and intravenous antibiotic therapy.—J.S. Torg, M.D.

Acute Compartment Syndrome From Anterior Thigh Muscle Contusion: A Report of Eight Cases
Rööser B, Bengtson S, Hägglund G (Varbergs Hosp; Univ Hosp, Lund, Sweden)
J Orthop Trauma 5:57–59, 1991   9–31

Introduction.—Data were reviewed on 8 patients with contusion or muscle rupture in the anterior compartment of the thigh in whom an acute anterior compartment syndrome developed. All patients had severe pain at rest, which usually did not respond to narcotic analgesia. Tenderness was maximal where a hematoma was found at exploration.

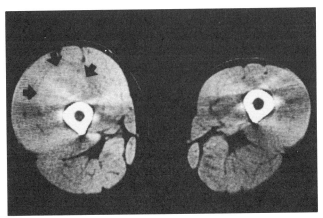

Fig 9–23.—Patient 7. Man, aged 34 years, was kneed on his right thigh while playing handball. He continued to play but was admitted 18 hours later with progressive pain at rest and a tense and tender anterior thigh compartment. There was no distal neurologic or circulatory deficit. The pressure in the anterior compartment was 76 mm Hg. This CT scan shows hematoma (*arrows*) and edema of the quadriceps muscle. (Reproduced with permission from Rööser B: *Acta Orthop Scand* 58:170–172, 1987. Courtesy of Rööser B, Bengtson S, Hägglund G: *J Orthop Trauma* 5:57–59, 1991.)

Methods.—Surgery was performed within 6 hours of admission. All the patients had increased quadriceps muscle pressures of 41–80 mm Hg. A hematoma was found in the rectus femoris muscle in 3 patients and in the vastus intermedius in 4. Only 1 patient had edema of the anterior compartment, but edema was a constant finding (Fig 9–23). Active knee joint exercises began within 2 days after surgery; patients were mobilized on crutches for 5–7 days. Continuous passive motion exercises were used by several patients.

Results.—Pain was immediately relieved in all patients, and all had normal function after about 4 weeks, walking independently without a limp. The patient with the highest recorded pressure had moderately restricted knee flexion at follow-up.

Conclusion.—Broad indications for fasciotomy and evacuation of hematoma are appropriate in patients with thigh muscle contusion or rupture. The operation is safe and the consequences of untreated compartment syndrome are serious.

▶ This paper makes several interesting points. The authors note that because major nerves in the thigh were not confined to the involved compartments, a disturbance in sensation was not characteristic of this problem. In each case it is reported that the problem developed from what is described as "a very moderate trauma" and all patients involved in an athletic activity continued to play after the injury. Also, it is pointed out that "it cannot be excluded that symptoms may have resolved with nonoperative measures." They further point out that "since no morbidity could be demonstrated from fasciotomy in this series and considering the serious consequences of an unrelieved compartment syndrome, we believe that the indications for fasciotomy and evacuation of a hematoma should be broadened in blunt thigh muscle injures."—J.S. Torg, M.D.

Traumatic Subluxation of the Hip Resulting in Aseptic Necrosis and Chondrolysis in a Professional Football Player
Cooper DE, Warren RF, Barnes R (Hosp for Special Surgery, New York)
Am J Sports Med 19:322–324, 1991   9–32

Introduction.—Aseptic necrosis and posttraumatic arthrosis are usually not associated with only subluxation of the hip. A professional football player was seen with posterior hip subluxation and subsequent aseptic necrosis and posttraumatic arthrosis.

Case Report.—Man, 23, a professional football player, was injured and a fracture fragment at the posterior aspect of the hip was demonstrated and confirmed by CT. Rest and activity modification were prescribed, and pain persisted at 6 weeks. A MRI showed a wedge-shaped focal region of aseptic necrosis in the superior aspect of the femoral head. The patient was treated with nonsteroidal anti-inflammatory medication and stayed on crutches for 4 months. Roentgenograms at 4 months revealed marked loss of the joint space. With the potential for collapse of the femoral head and continued joint space narrowing, the patient was advised of possible progressive arthrosis. He subsequently returned to full participation in professional football, and at 8 months postinjury he was pain free and had a full range of motion.

Discussion.—Interruption of the blood supply to the femoral head is a common cause of posttraumatic aseptic necrosis. In this case of sublaxation of the hip, hip congruity was only instantaneously disrupted. Therefore, aseptic necrosis may be less extensive.

▶ This carefully documented case report is interesting from 2 aspects. First, as the authors have pointed out, with aseptic necrosis as a complication of a dislocation of the hip, the time between injury and reduction is usually considered a critical prognostic factor. In this case, hip congruity was only instanteously disrupted. Yet evidence of a focal pattern of necrosis was demonstrated on magnetic resonance imaging at 4 months. And second, at 3-year follow-up, although radiographs demonstrated moderate arthritis, the patient had full range of motion, no hip pain, and continued to play football at the professional level.—J.S. Torg, M.D.

Skier's Hip: A New Clinical Entity? Proximal Femur Fractures Sustained in Cross-Country Skiing
Frost A, Bauer M (Östersund Hosp, Östersund, Sweden)
J Orthop Trauma 5:47–50, 1991   9–33

Introduction.—Cross-country skiing always has been considered to be safe and an excellent path to fitness, but injuries do occur and there may be a trend toward more serious ones.

Patients.—In 10 patients, a proximal femoral fracture was incurred while engaged in Nordic skiing. An example is shown in Fig 9–24. In 5 patients, there was a trochanteric fracture; in 4, a collum femoris fracture; and in 1, a combined trochanteric-subtrochanteric injury. Most patients underwent repair with a plate and sliding screw or with pins.

Conclusion.—Release bindings, as are used in downhill skiing, have been proposed as a mean of preventing these injuries. It appears, however, that significant force is applied to the injured extremity and that direct impact is a likely mechanism. Probably some form of protective padding would be helpful. Participants should recognize that even cross-country skiing can be dangerous, especially today with fast tracks and sophisticated equipment.

▶ The authors recognize that coining the term "skier's hip" to describe proximal femoral fractures is "somewhat presumptuous." However, the paper certainly does "point out that significant injuries occur not only in downhill skiing, but also in cross country skiing." To be noted, the average age of

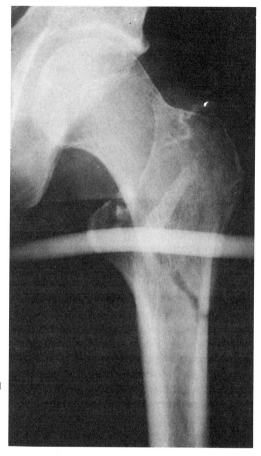

Fig 9–24.—Left hip, anteroposterior view, proximal femoral fracture. (Courtesy of Frost A, Bauer M: *J Orthop Trauma* 5:47–50, 1991.)

these 10 patients is 49 years. This, of course, raises a question of age-related susceptibility.—J.S. Torg, M.D.

Acute Lumbar Paraspinal Compartment Syndrome: A Case Report
DiFazio FA, Barth RA, Frymoyer JW (McClure Musculoskeletal Research Ctr, Burlington, Vt)
J Bone Joint Surg 73-A:1101–1103, 1991   9–34

Introduction.—A compartment syndrome in the lumbar region may cause low back pain. A case of acute lumbar paraspinal compartment syndrome was documented by intracompartmental pressure measurements and MRI.

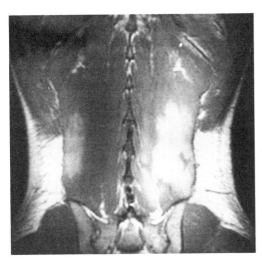

Fig 9–25.—Three days after the onset of symptoms, this coronal T1-weighted MRI shows a generalized increase in the signal in the paraspinal muscles. The increase is greater on the left side than on the right. (Courtesy of DiFazio FA, Barth RA, Frymoyer JW: *J Bone Joint Surg* 73-A:1101–1103, 1991.)

Case Report.—Male, 27 years, complained of low back pain that began after 3 days of downhill skiing. The findings on physical examination were generally normal except for hypoactive bowel sounds, mild abdominal tenderness, and bilateral rigidity of the paraspinal muscles with tenderness from the 12th thoracic to the 5th lumbar level. Straight-leg raises exacerbated the back pain. Sensation was diminished only in the lumbrosacral area. Laboratory results showed marked elevations of creatine phosphokinase and serum glutamic-oxaloacetic transaminase, and a slight elevation of serum amylase. The only radiographic abnormality found was an abnormal pattern of bowel gas. The initial diagnosis was acute rhabdomyolysis secondary to exertion, and the treatment consisted of intravenous fluids, bed rest, and analgesics.

Two days later the patient was transferred and further evaluated. The physical and laboratory findings were essentially unchanged at this time, except that serum amylase level had normalized. An MRI showed increased signal in the paraspinal muscles (Fig 9–25). These findings were consistent with a diagnosis of intramuscular hemorrhagic necrosis. Lumbar paraspinal compartment pressures were 80 mm Hg on the left side and 70 mm Hg on the right, much higher than the normal range of 5–30 mm Hg. Over the next few days, the patient improved, and his serum enzyme levels and compartment pressure fell. A decrease in abnormal signal densities of the paravertebral muscles was seen on MRI done 8 days after the onset of symptoms.

The patient was discharged, able to walk while wearing a lumbosacral corset. He continued to have mild intermittent low-back pain with increased activity 6 weeks after discharge, but by 4 months after discharge he had resumed normal activities, including some skiing, with only slight discomfort. Abnormalities on MRI had generally resolved.

Interpretation.—Documented acute lumbar paraspinal compartment syndrome did not seem caused by mechanical trauma, infection, or idiopathic rhabdomyolysis. Operative decompression was not necessary for successful clinical recovery.

▶ The authors report a rare and unusual form of compartment syndrome originally described by Styfm and Lysell, who reduced the intramuscular pressure by fasciotomy (1). Of note is that the 2 cases reported by DiFazio et al. achieved a successful clinical recovery with nonoperative management.—J.S. Torg, M.D.

Reference

1. Styf J, Lysell E: *Spine* 12:680, 1987.

Spin-Echo and STIR MR Imaging of Sports-Related Muscle Injuries at 1.5 T
Greco A, McNamara MT, Escher MB, Trifilio G, Parienti J (Ctr Hosp Princesse Grace, Principality of Monaco; Assn Sportive Monaco; Olympic Gymnaste Club de Nice, France)
J Comput Assist Tomogr 15:994–999, 1991   9–35

Introduction.—Athletes with suspected muscle trauma were studied with MRI to compare the performances of SE T-weighted with the short TI inversion recovery (STIR) technique for the detection and characterization of the injury.

Methods.—All of the 70 males aged 16–40 years, had pain involving the lower extremities following either a specific injury or athletic overuse. All patients underwent MRI at 1.5 T$_j$; 20 patients underwent follow-up MRI. The SE T1-weighted and double-echo T2-weighted pulse sequences were supplemented by the STIR sequence in 36 patients. The MRIs were examined for the presence of muscle strains, muscle tears, and organized hematomas.

Results.—Strains, detected in 28 patients by both techniques, were more readily visible on STIR images (Fig 9–26). The STIR technique allowed the greatest lesion/muscle contrast in both the initial assessment and follow-up of tears. Organized hematomas in 11 patients were viewed in anatomical detail with short TR, short TE SE images. Follow-up MRI revealed regression of the tear in 11 patients, recurrence in 4, and fibrous scar formation in 5. In 3 patients, evolution of hematomas into scar or cyst was apparent.

Conclusion.—Because of the additive effect of T1 and T2 mechanisms, the STIR sequence improves lesion detection and is well suited for both initial screening and follow-up of muscle injuries. A T1-weighted SE sequence is recommended for anatomical detail and hematoma characterization.

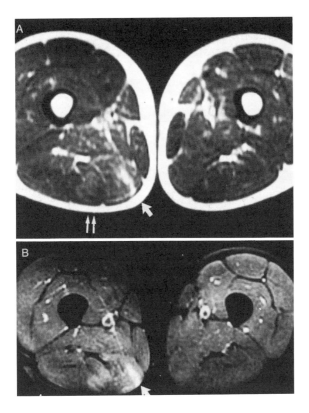

Fig 9–26.—Soccer player with acute onset of posterior right thigh pain. Axial SE 2,000/80 **(A)** and STIR 1,8000/170/27 **(B)** images at 48 hours show partial tear of the right semimembranosus muscle *(single arrows)*. Strained semitendinosus muscle shows increased signal intensity *(double arrows)*. Note the greater conspicuity of the lesions on the STIR image. (Courtesy of Greco A, McNamara MT, Escher MB, et al: *J Comput Assist Tomogr* 15:994–999, 1991.)

▶ STIR techniques alone can obscure bony pathology. However, once an osseous lesion is excluded, this is an excellent method for detection and follow-up of muscle pathology. The authors' protocol to shorten the time required for the examination by using a smaller matrix and a single excitation is helpful. Communication of the clinical suspicion of a muscle injury should be provided to the MRI personnel before the MR examination so the appropriate study can be obtained.—J.S. Torg, M.D.

Patient Activity, Sports Participation, and Impact Loading on the Durability of Cemented Total Hip Replacements

Kilgus DJ, Dorey FJ, Finerman GAM, Amstutz HC (VA Med Ctr-West Los Angeles; Ctr for the Health Sciences, Los Angeles)

Clin Orthop 269:25-31, 1991

9-36

Background.—Several authors have associated high patient activity levels and high-impact activities with deleterious effects on hip implant durability. Others have suggested that regular exercising does not increase the risk of implant loosening and that nonimpact exercise may actually have a stimulating effect on the bone. The effect of sports participation and heavy labor on the durability of cemented hip replacements and the effect of participation in high-impact vs. low-impact activities on the hip were assessed using a large university center data base.

Methods.—Patients were divided into groups by the type of prosthesis, 1 conventional total hip arthroplasty (THA) or resurfacing THA; the characteristic of less active or active, and by preoperative diagnosis of osteoarthritis or nonosteoarthritis. Although the most accurate method of stress measurement on the hip would be the use of pressure transducers to measure force transmission, that approach was not possible.

Findings.—The active patients with either the conventional or resurfacing prosthesis types had more than twice the risk of aseptic loosening in comparison with the less active group. In patients with conventional THA, the greatest adverse effects of exercise were with a preoperative diagnosis other than osteoarthritis. The effects were seen about 6 years after surgery in patients with THA and 10 years after surgery for patients with conventional stemmed prostheses. In resurfacing THA for osteoarthritis, the long-term loosening is primarily in patients who participate in high-impact activities.

Conclusions.—A low-impact activity level in patients with resurfacing has a more adverse effect in those with an etiologic factor other than osteoarthritis. High activity levels are associated with increased hip-replacement failure rates for both conventional and resurfacing THA.

▶ No Comment.—J.S. Torg, M.D.

Subject Index

Author Index